THRIVAL IN THE

CHEMTRAIL HOLOCAUST

Youthifying From Within

Jana Dixon

Published by Amazon Kindle Direct Publishing

First Edition February 2019
ISBN-13: 978-1-7336664-0-4

Cover Painting by Jana Dixon
Make of it what you will.

http://biologyofkundalini.com
http://jana-sovereignstate.blogspot.com
https://biologyofkundalini.academia.edu/JanaDixon

DISCLAIMER: I offer lists of potential remedies, while I advise the reader to be self-aware of their counter indications and sensitivities. As sovereign individuals we aspire to be self-intelligent and dismiss false authority—becoming solely responsible for all factors related to our own health and that of our community. Truth is the ultimate elixir—the path to love, radical openness and unbroken connection. This book is a compilation of investigative research, by which the reader can address dis-ease and imbalance through restoring the elements of nature's perfect design. This book is an anti-aging manual and if it upsets you, consider it a work of science fiction. It goes without saying that we are the ones we have been waiting for. Loving ourselves enough to care for our own thrival is the ultimate place to start in caring for the whole.

The complex, interrelated nature of this book makes a linear document less than ideal, so please dear reader mark in the margins page numbers and notes to interconnect the book for your own personal needs. There is empty pages at the end of the book to write your own index.

FORWARD

It is obvious that the current environmental, economic, and cultural breakdown results from an outdated mental framework and a lack of genuine spirituality, or higher human consciousness. We need to redefine our cultural values and beliefs regarding our collective karmic relationship with nature and the planet in order to establish a meaningful, culturally responsible humanity. The worse off "the world" gets, the more we have to believe in a transcendent future, while dealing with our present reality and planning for collective thrival. We are at the turning point where all of us are being called to a deeper and more profound experience of being human.

Thus I have written a self-help manual to help reduce the insidious anthropomorphic damage to our body, mind and soul, so that we may meet the upcoming challenges with physical and spiritual strength and thrive! To the extent that we can come alive and heal ourselves we can go on to heal the planet. There are places on the globe where we might run to for the rest of our lives, but for those who cannot leave the spray zones or the polluted urban centers, this chemtrail thrival manual is particularly useful. For we are under constant attack by a deadly enemy—namely Stupidity! See the last page of this book on the dangers of increasing the conductivity of the atmosphere.

Thrival in the Chemtrail Holocaust: Youthifying from Within is a basic manual for thrival under soft-kill extermination conditions. As outrageous as that sounds—this is the reality we must face, for we have a responsibility to thrive, not just the continuum of life on earth—not just human life, but all living creatures. It is the duty of all good citizens of the world to rise up in their sovereignty, freedom and creativity and be enthusiastically motivated to set about bringing on Civilization Next. Together we may become whole. Together we Thrive!

This book is dedicated to the Sovereign warrior of the New World
With the Force in their Heart
And the Fire of Life in their Mind
Freedom is a right which is only expressed when it is explored
Together let us free the earth from the madness of the
Death Machine

"There is only one reason why you would build a weather control device - to take over the world." ~ Jean-Claude Van Johnson

I

PREFACE

While living in Boulder, Colorado I noticed that all trees in the area began dying beginning in 2013, whereas 17 miles upwind in the mountains at Nederland the trees were still fine. The only significant difference between the two locations was that in Nederland there was no chemtrail spraying. Thus it was that I realized that 100% of the trees in Boulder and the Front Range were dead and dying due to oxidation and poisoning from heavy metal toxicity from the chemtrail nanometals; and to a lesser degree the increased UVC solar radiation, loss of ozone layer and radiation from Fukushima. What is happening on the Front Range of the Rockies is happening everywhere that chemtrailing is undertaken. By extrapolation—knowing the interconnectivity of nature—what is happening to the vegetation is also happening to all living things including human beings.

Chemtrails and geoengineering are destroying people's health, killing pets, and shortening the lifespan of our children via accelerated aging and disease, including Alzheimer's, cancer, infections, influenza and pneumonia. It is also apparent that people are generally becoming brain damaged from the heavy metal and aluminum poisoning, they are losing their minds, their hearing and other senses. If this environmental collapse continues it is inevitable that humans, and practically all other life will go the same way as the trees. I came to realize we are under a chemocidal assault by a deadly enemy at the very top of global governance.

They spray for a while, get the population sick—they let up so people go get antibiotics and heal up and then they whomp'em with another disease dump several weeks later. With the chemtrail program and the pneumonia epidemics—now the doctors are being told not to keep administering antibiotics after the initial crisis. They appear to be saving critical patients, but are withholding extended care, and failing to educate patients on boosting the immune system. Since the immune system declines 2-3% each year after our 20's this leaves older people more vulnerable to the monkey business of chemtrails and the skull-druggery of pharmica mania.

Chemtrails are likely causing Parkinson's' disease, autism, Alzheimer's disease, headaches, respiratory ailments, liver failure, neurological failure, and hormonal imbalances, reproductive failure, cancer and a host of other diseases. Doctor warns world about "chemtrail lung," a new health epidemic causing brain and lung problems across society. We all live in our own little prison of enculturation—it is time to break out. Living within a culture of institutionalized out-of-control-greed we are facing extinction pressures from all sides, "the vaccine, GMO, radiation, chemtrail and EMF holocaust." What is occurring is nothing less than slow, premeditated genocide. We must fortify ourselves against the degenerate world, which is clearly insane—being dense and offensive—a diversion from an ascendant future. Thus we must learn how to survive and avoid the multiple affronts to the lifeforce and the living planet.

Remaining sane and thriving on a planet under attack by the techno-kraken is one of the greatest challenges humans have faced throughout of species existence. It is my hope that *"Thrival in the Chemtrail Holocaust"* will help many of us "be the best we can be" under nefarious, calamitous conditions. These are the best of times and the worst of times—the apocalypse can be turned around if each of us wakes up to the reality of what is really going on and hacks the full spectrum dominance mainframe that would hold humanity and the planet hostage for eternity.

WHO WOULD HAVE THUNK? Some stupid scientist in the 1940's ago must have thought about shading the earth with aerosols, so they came up with the idea of global warming, and the carbon-pirates thought they could cover their asses by pumping the sky full of shit, the manufacturers and the miners jumped on board and gave the project their industrial waste to conveniently get rid of. Then the pharmaceutical companies made a wicked stew of deadly infectious agents to throw into the mix so that they could sell drugs to the sickening population. The banksters bankroll the whole thing because they end up with the property and houses when the people get sick, default on their mortgages and die. The flyboys coming back from the illegal wars in the oil rich nations get an extended call of duty killing their own families and countrymen.

Wars are games on a chessboard, played by international disaster capitalists for the spoils of war. Sounds like a great plan concocted by a machiavellian psychopaths high on drugs."

The extent of global warming from CO2 emissions is minuscule compared to the primary climate driving influence of the sun. However the chemtrailer's airplane exhaust and aerosol spraying does warm the earth by holding in reflective radiant heat. The aerosol spraying program costs trillions while doing nothing good, only bad—at a time when civilization is going to face its most extreme survival challenge yet, of going into the Grand Solar Minimum. Human emissions and poisons are changing climate, not the least of which is by promoting deforestation. However it is the solar cycles that are the dominant force, and we are already 5 or more years into a Grand Solar Minimum. Anthropomorphic influence tends to drive extremes in climate and earth changes by eliminating "buffers and self-regulators."

Edward Snowden says the CIA first orchestrated the spread of the "Global Warming scare" in the 1950s. *"I have documents showing that the CIA invented the whole thing. Global Warming was invented to both scare people, and divert their attention from other human-made dangers like nuclear weapons. The CIA gave millions of dollars to any scientist who would confirm the theory, so many unscrupulous scientists did what they were told in order to get the money. Now, there is so much fake data to confirm that Global Warming "exists," that they actually convinced everyone that it was real."* Edward Snowden.

In the Symposium on Science and Spirituality in Germany in 2013, Claudia Von Werlhof pointed out that the officially propagated thesis of CO2 as the reason behind the growing climate chaos in the world is not true. This cover story is instead hiding the consequences of 70 years of development of a new military geo/climate warfare, applied internationally. www.pbme-online.org/

The Solar Radiation Management program will go down as one of the greatest catastrophic blunders in history—killing the biosphere at a time when it is already under massive stress from the Grand Solar Minimum. Profit and industrial expediency—a method of eliminating industrial waste via aerial dispersal, could cause the death of millions or billions of citizens around the world. This as a matter of fact appears to be the principle intention of the debacle.

CONTENTS

I

INTRODUCTION

THE HEINOUS CRIME OF WEATHER WARFARE

"Man is never smarter than nature, and a greedy mindless man immersed in dogma as science, a disconnected man is a plague." ~ Mia Efrem

Geoengineering is forcing increasingly erratic climate processes resulting from rapid anthropomorphic atmospheric disruption into a cascade of unpredictable, self-reinforcing, chaotic, catastrophic events. Solar Radiation Management (SRM) is aggravating climate extremes by killing the forests and ocean plankton and creating a desert planet. The ultimate result of weather wars and global climate interference is greatly reduced food harvests, leading to the potential collapse of civilization. Solar Radiation Management is part of the full spectrum dominance of the planet, which is motivated by a fascistic mental illness. Besides the desire to kill off the majority of humans on earth — the metallic ionization and microwave frying of earth's atmosphere is precipitating the 6th Great Extinction.

A perfect storm is brewing, of abject piracy and greed, meeting criminal lawlessness and homicidal mania. The storm is gathering on all fronts, from climate disruption, to the global economy, to blind industrial hegemony and political extortion via geo-warfare. War for profit is the #1 is the number one business on earth right now, and it is the number one crime. But there is a different war afoot, and the war victims both are people and planet. Biochemical-warfare is the ideal soft kill solution. The slow war of aerial chemical spraying is a clandestine/in-your-face war against the earth and her people.

The plausible deniability of slow genocide, makes chemtrailing the perfect method of global eugenics. The question is — how are the perpetrators preventing their own health from declining due to the slow poisoning of the planet? Stratospheric Aerosol Geoengineering via chemtrails and microwaving the atmosphere represent a grave danger to the biological heritage of the planet — ultimately nothing survives.

Chemtrails are ostensibly to increase the conductivity of the atmosphere so the weather can be more easily manipulated by HAARP to create weather disasters in the form of drought, floods, tornadoes, hurricanes, earthquakes, tsunamis etc…to force small farmers off the land and to open up areas for corpro-military occupation and Agenda 21 "sustainable" redevelopment. Corporate science is being used to forward the globalist agenda which includes population reduction and the loss of personal liberties and rights, variously referred to by the would-be perpetrators as "The Depopulation Agenda, The Culling of Useless Eaters, Agenda 21, or The UN Charter of Global Democracy."

1

It is not just living things that the chemtrails are destroying, it is the very foundational infrastructure of civilization. The chemtrails and other aspects of Stratospheric Aerosol Geoengineering are "eating" the material infrastructure of civilization and are killing people daily, while setting up generations for early onset dementia and worse. The chemtrails and the EMF frequency smog is weakening the power poles, eating the wires, aging plastic and rubber, dissolving the concrete, corroding the bridges, roads, houses, buildings, rusting cars and other metal, weakening planes etc....

The infrastructure of civilization is being consumed by nano technology, radiation and frequencies. Chemtrailing with corrosive chemicals is depreciating the value of houses, cars and all man-made and biological structures. Chemtrail nanometals eat away at concrete, roads, steel, paint, wood and all man made structures—thus all the infrastructural components of civilization are under grave threat of rapid deterioration—greatly accelerating depreciation costs.

Chemtrailing breaks down the thermodynamic environment conducive for Life in the universe, and for what? The enormity and unprecedented nature of this man-made disaster will require unprecedented approaches to survival, comprehensive remediation and thrival. If the population becomes enlightened there won't be any interest in the competition games that lead to personality politics, sports, fake boobs and bombs.

All our efforts now must be spent on going in the upward direction towards emergence of the soul-life of the individual and the evolution of culture. Or at least creating ecovillages that serve as Arks of Advancement to preserve genetic integrity, higher consciousness and spiritual development. We cannot let capitalist corporations dictate reality for the good people of the planet. We must start a collective storm of critical thinking, open communication and joint courage to right these ethical and scientific errors, before they destroy the possibility for higher life on earth.

Thus our most urgent imperative as a species is to stop the cultural processes leading to dehumanization, biocide and omnicide, in order to grow up cognitively, morally and spiritually and undo the corpro-military stranglehold that is suffocating human society. Only those who are free of Western Deculturation, or who are able to protect and detoxify themselves from the evil forces of anti-life technology will have strong enough genetic integrity to carry viable genes into the future. Wholebrain culture is focused on understanding Nature, preventative-proactive lifestyle and evolutionary medicine.

Hindbrain culture is focused on manifesting disease in humanity and the planet, and then capitalizing on pretending to heal it. Predatory medicine, predatory government, predatory business, predatory military, predatory religion and predatory education—these are obsolete in the 21st Century, and completely outdated for the level of consciousness that we SHOULD embody at this late stage of civilization. This intolerably sad lack of social/cultural development is symptomatic of the retardation of spiritual evolution due to the reptilian brain hijacking the limbic and prefrontal regions of the brain. Humanity has a power addiction because it is spiritually disempowered. Such a Thanatos focused civilization can only end one way—in an unholy mess of murder-suicide.

The predators at the top of the food chain that have set up the game so they can freely exploit the people and the planet. We can no longer simply call the Hindbrain Borg culture a patriarchy, for it is more rather a Piratearchy!

Retardation of human evolution through addiction to power keeps the species in compartmentalized Hindbrain mode. The prison planet has been created not by one gender, "namely male," but by a class of competent, organized criminals who have willed it so, and worked tirelessly for thousands of years to manifest the hive. Peterson points out that "the hierarchy" is not due to male dominance over the tribe, but due to merit and competency. However, merit and competency is carefully controlled within a class system of "access" to opportunity, resources, capital and connections. Thus we have a certain band of pirates who have gained great power, wealth, influence and freedom to act. They are possessed with the will and responsibility to act not in the planet or the people's behalf, but in their own self-interest with the aim of ever greater power, wealth, influence and freedom to enact their will.

CONNECTING THE DOTS

Chemtrails spread incendiary chemicals comprised of pyrotechnic metal nano powders — Aluminum/Barium are conductive — Ionizing the atmosphere increasing lightning number and intensity — Chemtrails reduce the ozone layer by reducing the Oxygen from reaching the upper the stratosphere (12 to 19 miles) — The atmospheric dome of Chemtrail aerosols cause solar lensing like a magnifying glass causing intense heat and desiccation of vast regions — Reflective aerosols refract/reflect sunlight changing its frequency and increasing its burning quality — Chemtrail overseeding of clouds creates droughts — Chemtrail aerosols conduct wireless signals better so drones or satellites can pick up on communications or smart meters — Smart meters can be GPS'ed from the air and houses can be targeted with Directed Energy Weapons — By using HAARP technology from ground or satellite on aerosol ionized air, jet streams can be moved around for weather-attacks and geo-warfare on states or countries. Raytheon's SBX radar platform - is a mobile HAARP/Tesla Unit that can sailed to any ocean on earth and used as a 'tectonic weapon.'

The chemtrailing is a money making scheme by industralists that want to get rid of their poisonous industrial waste, by spreading it all over the globe. Any sane person would know that dilution is obviously no solution. If the chemtrails are protecting us from something, then that something must be worse than the loss of ozone, the death of the forests, the poisoning of agricultural land, poisoning of the water, the collapse of food production, rapid depreciation of infrastructure and man-made structures, collapse of the economy, cancer, dementia, destruction of the genetics of all life, collapse of the electromagneticosphere necessary for life. As the land loses its vegetative cover, it loses its protection from the rain eroding the soil away to dust. America is heading for another dust bowl, and **famine.** Trees dying is also due to increased cosmic rays due to lowered magnetic field due to reduced solar wind.

Geoengineering is amplifying climate variations we are experiencing by increasing atmospheric conductivity through man-made dispersal of nano-particulate matter from various sources and creating a heat blanket effect with their fake cirrus clouds. With regular chemtrailing the whole atmosphere becomes ionized, therefore even regular clouds are streaming out of consolidation and coalescence into strange fake cirrus clouds. Persistent contrails (Cirrus homogenitus) are human generated cirrus clouds. The chemtrail cirrus clouds have been classified as Homomutatus...ie: Human mutating clouds!

3

Meanwhile we are going into a Grand Solar Minimum mini ice age, and the Ice Age Proper after that. The Grand solar minimum, loss of magnetosphere, diminished ozone layer, increased galactic cosmic rays, increased UVC, changes in the solar spectrum especially from the coronal holes, toxic frequencies from the Nemesis system, toxic alkalizing metals from chemtrail aerosols, toxic acidifying sulfur, Wifi, HAARP, 5G technology, pulsed-radio/radar frequency, loss of soil organic material and demineralization of the soil—and all these forces acting to kill soil microbial life—are killing the trees and all flora and fauna. If the current trend continues then humanity will quickly follow this death cycle.

Besides illegal resource wars, CIA drug running, false flags, stealing gold from the treasury and bank bailout scams, they now are dipping into the people's Social Security, Medicare and Medicaid benefits. This is why 5G is coming, so citizens will have an early expiration date. The roll out of 5G at extremely high (millimetre wave) frequencies is planned to begin at the end of 2018, despite the evidence that radio frequency (RF) radiation is harmful to life is already overwhelming. No life on Earth will be able to avoid exposure, 24 hours a day, 365 days a year, to levels of RF radiation that are tens to hundreds of times greater than what exists today, without any possibility of escape anywhere on the planet.

Ionizing the atmosphere with chemtrail particulates makes 5G radiation all the more pernicious by increasing EMF wave conductivity. The 5th Generation Microwave communications in general use will sicken the population, turn them into zombies and remove all descent and fight. It is so toxic the people won't be able to grow their own food and it can also be can be used as a weapon. Microwave radiation is invisible and not trackable forensically! This is why it is such an excellent stealth "weapon."

One of the principle reasons they spray aerosols is to "overseed" and prevent rain over the fracking fields. Global Warming was an ogre concocted by the ELite to scam more taxes off the people so they could drill and frack more and melt the poles with their microwaves. The oil dinosaurs have been suppressing advanced non-fossil energy generation systems at least since Tesla. Thus they are imperiling the survival of civilization and our compliance with the hydrocarbon cabal will be the death of us all unless we can break free from their death grip.

We are in a war against corruption, evil, greed and ignorance in high places. The governments work for the oil cartels, thus they have been suppressing and stealing New Energy technology for a hundred years. The energy cartels are so powerful that they control the governments that control them. There is no city or governmental response to what is occurring, because they are either ignorant of or complicit in the geoengineering fiasco. We need a global push towards energy alternatives to free ourselves from the banker/oil cabal. Protesting just feeds into the NWO's agenda. There are dozens of energy alternatives already established and thousands of patents locked away in the US patent office.

At present the Global Eugenic Deep State technology seems focused mostly on geo-climate warfare and depopulation and total dominance/total surveillance. Misguided manics who would play God have weaponized the sky to the detriment of all life on earth. Chemtrails and geoengineering are a travesty against the earth and the evolution of life. The biosphere should always be put above militarization and power grabs. The climate meddling geoengineers are making extreme weather worse, with unprecedented climate and ecosystem destabilizing effects—combine that with Grand Solar Minimum, pollution, very bad Hindbrain/Flatland land management, the uncompromising greed of industrialists, Fukushima radiation and the strange visitation of our binary twin solar system—and we are definitely in the middle of the 6th great extinction. The loss of genetic heritage will take millions of years to recover.

The chemtrail holocaust amounts to a global anthropogenic pandemic of epic proportions!

THE FALL

The great permaculturalist Andrew Faust said: *"No civilization that pollutes the air, water, soil and genetic integrity of its people, is truly advanced."* Nothing could be more primitive than contemporary culture as it can only lead to the breakdown and death of all life on earth. We can barely even conceive of life beyond the Death Culture, and yet all of us are called back toward LIFE should we care enough to listen. The human race is splitting into the degenerators, and the regenerators. The eternal war between Thanatos and Eros. Those who have profited the most from industrial capitalism, now seek to impose socialists austerity measures on the serfs with Agenda 21 "sustainability." It is ill advised for the lamb to ask the wolf how best to survive.

We are living in an increasing era of insane technological experimentation that is cutting us off from the Sun and the stars as a milky haze of metal oxides creates layers of toxic pollution which can be used by the military and the corporatocracy that is profiting. There are at least 15 companies worldwide participating in metalizing and weaponing our planet's atmosphere. We have been under attack for more than fifty years of geoengineering our planet, the 'metalizing' and weaponizing of our atmosphere with toxic materials, the poisoning with radiation and chemicals of our oceans, water sources, foods that are synthetic & toxic with preservatives, GMO seeds, the polluted air we breathe, and our bodies — all of which takes place with the cooperation of the secret governments, the Global Eugenic Deep State, the CIA, NSA, and the banks that fund them. These effects will eventually render the human body obsolete for incarnation by Human Angelic Souls.

Rather than admitting that chemtrails and Fukushima radiation is killing all the trees and bushes along the Colorado Front Range—.the city and forestry people make up stories about beetles and get the home owners to pay for the cutting down of the urban forestry. Beetles, viruses, bacteria and fungi etc... attack trees that have already been compromised, their immunity destroyed and are in fact already dying from radiation, heavy metal and aluminum poisoning, loss of soil microbiome, and oxidation of all the tissues. A substance is oxidized when electrons are removed, forming highly damaging oxygen-based free radicals (ROS). The bark of the trees, the rocks, the soil surface, along with the human structures including cars, houses and concrete have all been highly oxidized by the chemtrails, Fukushima radiation, solar UVC and galactic Galactic cosmic rays from the reduced magnetosphere.

Alzheimer's is caused by aluminum and other heavy metals in the brain in conjunction with Candida and other parasites. A condition derived from leaky gut and leaky BBB, resulting from the cooked food civilization. Autism is derived from massive brain inflammation and GI tract bacteria microbiome collapse due to vaccination (with aluminum adjuvant) of the child or the mother.

Both conditions foreshorten life and end in dementia. Both conditions require a similar lifelong protocol of increasing ATP, oxygen, zeta potential, antioxidants, anti-inflammatories, remineralization, Omega-3, phytonutrients, anti-pathogenic herbs, healing tight junctions in GI tract and BBB and detoxification in order to reverse the symptoms.

The principle cause of Alzheimer's and Autism is vaccination in combination with the increase in the inflammatory nature of our human bodies in this denaturing, anti-biological culture, which makes us prone to infection, inflammation, oxidation, hypoxia and aging. With industrial farming and the shift to eating cereals and the modern degenerative diet—we don't have the energy for higher (spiritual) consciousness, detox, repair and sanity.

One of the principle causes of humanity's Fall was the decline in ATP production due to the ratio of Omega 3 to Omega 6 going from 50:50 to 1:20 after leaving the paleolithic age. We are not producing enough ATP to detox our cells and body because our Omega 3 to Omega 6 ratio is off since cereal agriculture began—hence we have been in a 12,000 year degenerative decline. Dr Jack Kruse recommends a Paleo Diet based around seafood for Omega-3 and reestablishing Mitochondrial/ATP function. The raw vegan diet with focus on Omega-3 is the most refined, eliminating excess weight, and raising energy and consciousness. Thus we have to grow or find excellent quality produce, vary our diet, sprout and make seed cheeses, etc....

Basically all evidence points to the decline in Homo sapiens since the beginning of agriculture and cereal cultivation, which ultimately led to the loss of physical, mental and spiritual integrity from Metabolic X syndrome and the spectrum of degenerative diseases. The metabolic stresses have increased massively in the last 100 years, while the soils and food have deteriorated greatly and now we are exposed to a toxic onslaught of life-harming EMFs, chemicals, chemtrails and pathogens. It is only an accelerated downhill trip from here unless we rectify our ways. The body and the earth is forgiving if we give it all that it needs.

The morphology of plants are changing rapidly—all the trees and other plants are dying, and so they are dropping the genetic expression of "parts" that cost energy to produce that aren't absolutely essential to immediate survival. For example certain flowering plants are losing their petals and reverting to a more primitive genotype. What was a flowering bedding plant, now becomes a mere weed. There are reports on global insect and bird populations being critically reduced by 3 quarters from previous numbers. The world's Bee populations have been decimated due to sensitivity to neonicotinoid insecticide poisons and other chemicals produced by Monsanto-Bayer and DuPont.

Strange how there is talk of terraforming Mars, when THEY are systematically killing this planet. Lichen is proposed as one of the first organisms introduced into Mars to aid in establishing an Earth-like planet. I have notice an up-tick in lichen growth on the rocks in the Front Range of the Rockies since the Chemtrails and the changes in the sun's output has decimated the ecosystem. Environmental conditions are approaching their zenith for the continuum of life. Geoengineering and anthropomorphic environmental changes are reverting the biosphere back to the BEGINNINGS OF LIFE—billions of years ago.

The chemtrails, UVC and galactic cosmic rays have oxidized all surfaces including the rocks, freeing up fresh minerals for the lichens to flourish. Lichen is a composite organism composed of algae or cyanobacteria living symbiotically in association with fungi filaments. The constitute partners gain water and mineral nutrients mainly from the atmosphere, through rain and dust. The fungi protects the algae by retaining water, serving as a larger capture area for minerals and providing minerals obtained from the substrate. If a cyanobacteria are also present they can fix atmospheric nitrogen, complementing the activities of the green algae.

MAGNETO-APOCALYPSE

The magnetic shield is our first line of defense against harmful UV rays, and any thinning of the atmosphere could increase the risk from skin cancer. The atmosphere, the ionosphere, and the magnetosphere is all that stands between us and oblivion! The earth's magnetic field is vital to life and has weakened by 15 % over the last 200 years. This protective field acts as a shield against harmful solar radiation and extends thousands of miles into space and its magnetism affects everything from global communication to power grids.

Our magnetosphere has been dwindling since the Cretaceous (from the end of the Jurassic Period 145 million years ago to the beginning of the Paleogene Period 66 million years ago). According to the stratified fossil record, earth's magnetic field has gone from 300 Gauss down to our present day (.5 to .3 Gauss). The earth's magnetosphere shields us against outbursts of highly-charged solar emissions caused by **coronal mass ejections** (CME) & solar flares. Due to the decline in solar wind pressure the earth's magnetosphere is at its thinnest point in recorded history, and even has holes in it at times.

The greatest fear for industrialized nations, is that of an Earth-facing CME or solar storm, hitting a hole or thin spot in the magnetosphere. The earth's poles and magnetic field are shifting fast, and the solar wind from the coronal holes is buffeting the magnetosphere, plus the magnetosphere itself is weakening. The chemtrail aerosols, UVC and Cosmic rays and radiation is oxidizing the birds feathers, therefore probably reducing the birds ability to fly long distances, and lowering their lifespan. Geoengineering is killing the birds along with everything else.

The magnetosphere shifts and drops to almost nothing during the polar reversal, which is presently under way. This polar flip could take thousands of years, so are they going to keep up the chemtrailing for many thousands of years, when the planet is ALREADY dying from the toxic aerial assault? If they want to protect their electrical grid, they should change over to implosion physics and cold electricity which is not affected by EMPs and CMEs.

That is—bring technology up to date, rather than kill the planet in an attempt to support arcane technology, the primitive oil industry and criminal dominion over the energy industry. We are already living under weaponized skies! THEY are using the oceans, Earth's magnetic field and earthquakes, tsunamis, fires and hurricanes for political extortion. In fact the climate meddlers are increasing the levels of ultraviolet radiation, increasing methane release from the melting of the polar regions, also radiation from Fukushima and many other sources, spraying toxic-to-all-life metal oxides into the atmosphere, poisoning our oceans and killing the plankton, leading to the collapse of the food chain and thus starvation for millions. All of these factors and more will bring the inevitable collapse of the biosphere, the destruction of civilization as we have known it, and the end of the Rule of Law sooner than we may imagine.

The development of nano-technology has made this aerosol dispersion more difficult for the untrained eye to detect, but everyone can be aware of the milky haze that lays over the land, and the fact that our Sun has become impossibly piercing as its rays pass through these layers of refractive metal particles in the air that are being used to ionically charge the atmosphere. Any particulates in the atmosphere negatively impact the ozone layer, and just as the trees are suffering extreme UV damage, so too humans and other creatures will experience an increase in cancers.

Solar dimming effect resulting from chemtrailing is only temporary for the nanoparticles (called aerosols) will wash out of the atmosphere within a year or so and would have to be constantly replenished. Thus the shading and albedo effect created by chemtrailing fake clouds is undone by the massive burning of fossil fuels necessary to get all those trails into the atmosphere via plane, drone and ship. Their solar dimming efforts do not cool the earth one bit—THEY are undeniably collapsing the life support system of the planet with their toxins and destroying the electromagnetic basis of life. Those who are establishing a prison camp planet are burning the forests to reduce the O2 supply, and removing places where people may escape and retreat to and live. As the atmosphere loses oxygen due to the killing of the biosphere the ozone layer is no longer adequately replenished—precipitating an even steeper decline in the survival of life on earth. Thus all the heating and cooling climatic processes have been amplified.

GRAND SOLAR MINIMUM & THE ICE AGE

We are experiencing the beginning of the Grand Solar Minimum, with a lot of preliminary weather disruption all over the world and then the Ice Age Proper.

Besides the chemtrails, EMF poisoning, city ozone production, and radiation, the tree's are also dying due to the fact that the earth is experiencing the effects of the Grand Solar Minimum, which precipitates the following effects: The ozone layer bleeds off into space as the Magnetosphere is reduced, this is one of the reasons why there is increased UVC reaching the surface of the earth along with increased galactic cosmic rays. The Grand Solar Minimum sun's large coronal holes have a higher cosmic ray % which strips the ozone also. The loss of magnetic shields means the galactic cosmic rays heat the earth's core speeding magma movement, increasing sulfur acid rain from increased volcanicity, increased cloud cover and flooding, wild temperature swings and weather chaos due to disrupted jet streams, accelerated leaching and erosion, plus soil demineralization at end of interglacial.

The sun's circulation patterns go through cycles including periods of solar quiet. We can track these cycles through written history and by reading tree rings and ice cores. We are said to go into a Maunder Minimum or grand solar cooling cycle by 2020. The sun is presently going into a Grand Solar Minimum which could last 200 years and then possibly into the ice age cycle which lasts around 90K years. The Black Sea drains into the Mediterranean Sea, via the Aegean Sea and various straits, and is navigable to the Atlantic Ocean. Which is why Putin took back Crimea to ensure Russia had a warm water port for during the Grand Solar Minimum and ice age.

The Earth always warms prior to the onset of The Grand Solar Minimum because the reduction in our magnetosphere allows ozone and atmosphere to escape into space—and the residual heating of the earth and ocean keeps things toasty even as the solar output decreases. The initial stages of the Grand Solar Minimum are already occurring, meanwhile the Solar Radiation Management folks are presently destroying the earth's immune system, along with our capacity to grow food and to prepare for an ice age. Solar shading at a time of increased cloud cover due to heightened galactic cosmic rays is a surefire way to prevent populations from getting the necessary Vitamin D needed for their immune systems. And the toxic aerosols directly impact immunity by causing heavy metal poisoning and chronic inflammation.

The earth is undergoing increased heating AND cooling. Circulation patterns more extreme and cosmic rays pouring out of the sun's coronal holes and the oceans are rapidly heating from the activated magma. The galactic and solar cosmic rays heat the earth's core expanding the earth, generating earthquakes and increasing volcanic activity. The lowered solar wind of the Grand Solar Quiet increases the amount of galactic cosmic rays that get through earth's magnetic shields, which in turn increases cloud cover and precipitation, which generates deluges and mega storms—hence the extraordinary flooding. The great worldwide flooding has already begun and will continue until the ice age proper sets in. Consequently the farmers have to be warned that we have to prepare for biblical flooding and cities need to upgrade their drainage systems. There will be around 50 more years of this mega-disruption prior to settling down into 150 years of Grand Solar Minimum freeze.

There is an enormous increase in cloud cover over the globe compared to the 1970s and 1980s, which is readily observable comparing old satellite pictures with NASA Worldview. Back then the clouds looked normal, sensible, logical and artistic, but now we only get diabolical plasmafied clouds, which make no sense at all and are painful to observe. Over millions of years the human eye has evolved to appreciate the perfection of nature, whereas the spastic geoengineered clouds fill the heart with fear and loathing, and the belly with disgust. Clouds cannot conform to Nature's design in man-made ionized skies. I have nostalgia for the real clouds that thrilled me in New Zealand and the Pacific 25 years ago, and I wonder if I will ever see natural clouds again.

The last polar reversal event happened 780,000 years ago during the stone age. The next reversal is underway but could take 1,000 years to occur, at which point the Earth's magnetic field which prevents the Sun's dangerous radiation getting through, would be neutralized for around 200 years, during which time we would lose part of our atmospheric oxygen and ozone layer to space. Because the sun is operating at half power already you can expect the sun 'dying' towards the next ice age when the full solar minimum hits in 2024. From 100% in 1998 the solar wind has reduced down to 40% in 2018. By 2038 the temperature of the sun drops and the primer fields collapse at which point the ice age proper begins.

See Rolf Witzsche's YouTube video *"The Sun is 'dying' - build a New World."*

Planetary upheaval could simply be a sign of visitation by the Nemesis solar system. The north pole is being pulled towards the Nemesis solar system which was coming in from the south. The dark star fed on Sol changing the sun's spectrum so that it was no longer yellow in color around 2005 or earlier, but it took us a while to notice. The visitation of the Nemesis system is ripping holes in the sun and siphoning off the suns corona. From 2015 for last two years the

9

sun was marred by extreme coronal holes from pole to pole. The cosmic ray solar wind from these coronal holes was very harsh on the plant life and vulnerable species like frogs. The coronal holes have subsequently reduced somewhat as Sol moves into a more stable EMF arrangement associated with the Grand Solar Minimum. We also have to include electromagnetic and gravitational effects from the Nemesis system. The Tidal anomalies we have been experiences in the last few years are no doubt related to the close proximity of the red dwarf star Nemesis and its planets and moons.

If you look on NASA worldview you will see the planet is covered with extensive cloud as the magnetosphere falls during Grand Solar Minimum permitting more cosmic rays. The jet-steams are wandering as they are liberated from their usual tracks due to the lowered magnetosphere and the changes in solar radiation intensity and frequency. This is drawing more water up from the poles towards the equator creating massive deluges around the planet—thus providing the potential to green the deserts. The reduced solar wind pressure causes the breakup of the standing waves of the Jet Streams causing them to break and go all over the place, even crossing the equator.

The wandering jet streams are what is causing many current anomalies and extreme weather events and persistent heat domes and drought due to jet streams getting stuck. Reduced solar wind pressure destabilizes the jet streams. Sand was streaming out of the Sahara in 2017, and even more so in 2018 with the disruption to the jet streams, due to reduced solar wind pressure of the Grand Solar Minimum. This disruption of regular weather due to broken jet streams is causing drought in some regions and deluge in others. I imagine this jet stream destabilization will occur for the majority of the Milankovitch solar quiet—for as long as the solar wind pressure is reduced.

Increased galactic cosmic rays from the lowered heliosphere/magnetosphere, raising of ocean temperature, combined with extensive disruption of the jet-streams, sulfur from volcanoes and the general "heating" of the solar system are contributing to massive deluges around the globe. Geoengineered overseeding to prevent rain allows for the atmospheric rivers to build up over time, and also leads to the accretion of massive sized hail. Polar Storms out of Antarctica and the Arctic are probably going to be the regular thing now as the hot and cold drivers of weather increase with increased galactic cosmic rays due to the lowered magnetosphere, and reduced solar wind—as we go into the grand solar quiet.

The earth's crust is already in destabilization mode due to reduced magfields and increased cosmic rays. There is also a massive increase in volcanism around the globe. Bad men are doing bad things like setting off fake volcanic eruptions, because they are too stupid to do good things like plant trees, permaculturalize the landscape and grow food for the upcoming global famine. The human continuum is in the hands of mad men.

The rise in volcanic activity will occur for hundreds of years due to the solar system moving through a cosmic ion cloud (The Local Fluff), along with increased galactic cosmic rays which heat the earth's core. Astronomers reportedly call the cloud the Local Interstellar Cloud. It's about 30 light years wide and contains a mixture of hydrogen and helium atoms at a temperature of 6000 degrees Celsius. But the true mystery of the cloud has to do with its surroundings—the "Fluff" (as it's called) is surrounded by high-pressure supernova exhaust that should be either crushed or dispersed by it.

As we go into the Grand Solar Minimum, the mag-field is weakening, the plates are shifting and the magma is on the move and so volcano activity is increasing worldwide. Large eruptions can have a global cooling effect for several years, because volcanic sulfur dioxide gas forms microscopic particles high in the atmosphere that reflect some sunlight back into space before it can warm the earth's surface. One of the triggers for earthquakes is the "shifting" of rotation speed due to changing in the solar wind intensity/speed that creates crustal shift. Now, however volcanism is up due to the reduction in earth's mag-shields and increased galactic cosmic rays heating the core. The earth grows when the mag-shields go down due to reduction in solar wind as the grand solar minimum comes on, and possibly due to the Nemesis binary twin star system in close proximity also. Simple reduction in solar output seems insufficient to account for the massive increase in magma movement, earthquakes, fault cracking and volcanic activity.

Of course humanity had not prepared for this and so most of this water will simply cause great flooding, erode the land and runoff into the oceans. The world's landscapes should have been permaculturalized with swales, ground covers, forests, river clearing and bank reinforcement. The focus should have been to get the water into the acquifers to recharge the underground stores and thus prevent a scorched earth-desert planet. However humanity is infected with a criminal ĒLite who think only of personal acquisition from arcane-destructive technologies, murderous wars, trickery, deceit and destruction. Governments are captive to these arch pirates and so humanity as a whole is running blind into a brick wall of systemic systems failure.

Why Shade The Sun During The Grand Solar Minimum?

Efforts toward humane mastery of survival will promote human evolution during the Grand Solar Minimum and the major Ice Age. The question is does this "mastery" involve active euthanizing of the majority of the human population, or the effort to keep as many people alive as possible? Whether by mismanagement or by design the vaccine, GMO, radiation, chemtrail and EMF holocaust appears to be intentional to ensure maximum cull rate during the upcoming ice age. Since we are going into an ice age, chemtrailing must come to an end when the cooling effect of the Grand Solar Minimum is plainly obvious to all, and the rise in the galactic cosmic rays increases the cloud cover (and consequent precipitation and flooding) to such an extent that Solar Radiation Management MUST be outlawed by the UN and WHO, or some global legal enforcement capable of restraining the war against planet earth.

The toxic fallout from chemtrailing is destroying our capacity to produce the food we need to survive the cooling and extreme weather. Fact is, the fake cloud creation of chemtrailing solar radiation management could cool the earth more and so the solar quiet global cooling will kill off a lot more people than it otherwise would. Either the Solar Radiation Meddlers are misinformed or they are trying to induce sickness and famine so the maximum number of people die off during the 200-400 year Grand Solar Minimum. However a contradictory viewpoint is that both airplane fuel emissions and chemtrailing with coal fly ash creates an atmospheric heat blanket that aggravates global warming by holding in the radiant infrared heat at night. As well as the coal fly ash in the aerial spraying program, there is carbon black dust, which is the residue from jet diesel fuel. Jim Lee says there is a program to use high sulfur fuel in the

11

upper atmosphere to block sunlight. Using sulfur compounds could have the negative side effect of reacting with atmospheric ozone that would slow the recovery of the "holes" in the ozone layer. Sulfur also creates acid rain when it washes down to earth.

During solar minimums, the sun's magnetic field weakens and there is a decrease in the outward pressure of the solar wind, which allows more galactic cosmic rays from deep space to penetrate earth's atmosphere. Also the coronal holes that form on the sun during Grand Solar Minimum creates allows more solar cosmic rays down to the earth to heat the core and seed the clouds. Plus the current weakening of earth's magnetic field and polar excursion/reversal is further amplifying the Galactic Cosmic Ray situation. The upshot of these changes – will be a cooling of the planet, climate chaos and massive flooding.

Keep up on facebook and youtube with the exciting changes related to the onset of the Grand Solar Minimum with the electric universe folks Wallace Thornhill and David Talbott. www.electricuniverse.info/ and https://electroverse.net/

Join YouTube:: The Grand Solar Minimum, Adapt 2030 , the Oppenheimer Ranch Project and Ice Age Farmer for more on the upcoming earth changes.

HOMO EXPLOITUS & CLIMATE DISRUPTUS

"He who controls the weather, will control the world." Lyndon Johnson, 1962.

Homo exploitus is doing a thorough job of destroying the life support system of the planet, so he won't be around much longer. Just as the trees and bees are dying from chemtrails, radiation, electro-smog, pesticides and other chemicals—so too is *Homo exploitus*. The uptick in drought, fire, floods, tornadoes, hail, earthquakes and volcanism is partly due to man-made influence, but also because the Grand Solar Minimum has started.

We may like to contemplate why the poles are still melting? Is this the volcanic and magma heating from the magnetosphere changes, coupled with less cosmic protection due to reduced mag-shields? Or is it the residual heat from solar max and increased UVC from the loss of ozone layer? Or perhaps the ionization of the atmosphere via chemtrails is acting to heat the poles along with microwave HAARP technology. Since there are so many HAARP arrays scattered around Antarctica at various nations bases, we can only assume that the melting of the poles is intentional for mining and exploitation purposes.

Although there is no hope for *Homo exploitus* there is still hope for *Homo beautious*—he who has redeemed himself and undertaken the change process to correct the state of dis-ease/disease, whereby their journey is aligned with the natural order things. This is "Walking in Beauty," or following the natural order—*"Hozho Naasha."* "Hozho" – means "natural order," in Dineh/Navajo. Our job as conscious global citizens is to salvage and repair ourselves from the waning death culture, and to set about creating the regenerative culture before it is too late. Generally anything Hindbrain humanity tries as a fix does the opposite of what is intended, because false power uses force to work against nature and not with her. The Borg hive-mind doesn't Grok complexity, synergy, consequence, lateral thought, astrotheology, holarchy, nor geometric progression. Plus the complexity and wholism necessary for understanding the sacred science of nature (Tao) is unavailable to fractured minds.

The regenerative Tao of Life is a gnostic science that is given to those who are ripe for Apotheosis, via their capacity for connection/communion/communication. Apotheosis means "making divine," the beatification, or glorification of a subject to divine level. We have no alternative but to unleash or evolve higher human consciousness. To this end we each do what we are called to do. We have no control over what others do, nor are we responsible for their awakening. We offer what we can and we must, and hope for the best. Hope turns on the medial prefrontal lobe—affording us foresight, insight, clearsight, and futuresight to Civilization Next!

If we fail to heed the approaching **Black Swan Event** and act responsibly towards the reality of the upcoming changes much unnecessary suffering will ensue. We are up against the wall with the grand solar minimum. However it is hard to organize for the good, when the organizational bodies are corrupt. Due to Grand Solar Minimum this could go on for at least another 50 to 200 years, and will increase in intensity. Civil engineering and architecture will have to get with the meta-program and up their game immensely. We must plan to accommodate massive flooding, mudslides, hail, crop loss, freezing, raging heat, fierce winds, firestorms, and all manner of disasters. To weather the Grand Solar Minimum economic collapse people need to be build hot beds, sunken glass houses, shade houses, composts and start saving seeds now.

Building the soil microbiome counteracts some of the harmful effects of the chemtrail holocaust, and for this you need to apply lots of compost, mushroom compost and soil amendments and cover with a layer of mulch, because the UVC sterilizes the soil surface. Natural soil amendments such as bat guano, leonardite, green sand, kelp, ground egg shells, shungite, and micronized azomite etc... All the trees are dying, but we can still produce food by shading and ensuring soil-organic matter and microbiome is high. Octagonal (Tesla frequency) water, deuterium depleted water, deep spring (high H-) water can be sprayed on the leaves to counter the oxidative and ion-disrupting effects of chemtrail nanometals in the air and water.

GLOBAL FAMINE - IMMUNODEFICIENCY

The immune-system apocalypse is well underway with the ensuing soil-gut-planet senescence. All physical and mental disease arise from the diet and the digestive system, which relies on the health and vitality of the soil. Chemical agriculture has all but killed the soil, and the chemtrails are doing a fine job of finishing it off. If the present trajectory of deteriorating soils continues, this means human populations will experience ever greater degeneration and disease, cognitive decline, mental illness and burden on the sustainability of "higher" culture. Cut, burn and poison merely creates more destabilization, and doesn't address the underlying ecosystem and food chain imbalance. To work with nature and not against her is the way of all medicine, ecology, agriculture and land/ocean management.

Crop choice and growing systems will have to be geared up for this, and the increased flooding situation managed and "taken advantage of." The jet streams meander when the solar wind reduces which changes weather patterns and makes weather unreliable—creating snow in summer, along with the floods and burning UVC this worsens conditions for agriculture. With the associated bee die off, and upcoming Grand Solar Minimum, global famine and mass starvation is a given. It is apparent that the systematic poisoning of water by fracking and radiation etc… is destroying the potential for the continuum of higher life, and certainly higher human civilization.

They are setting up the famine now, making sure there are few food stores, wild foods and stable food growing areas. Poisoning the soils with their toxic aerosols. Chemtrails and geoengineering is undermining the immune system of the biosphere, both due to the fungal based nano-particles and the atmospheric microwaving destroys the electrical properties and bonding angles of water needed to sustain life. Along with the accumulative poisoning by aluminum, barium, strontium, fluoride and other chemicals in the chemtrails.

The global food supply is under eminent risk of collapse, even pasture grass is dying in tropical Queensland, Australia. Unexplained patches of dead pasture are occurring on a grand scale, rendering paddocks useless and whole farms wiped out. While so far the condition has been largely coastal, there is evidence the dieback is moving south and west, but researchers are still unsure what is causing the condition. Radiation from Fukushima, evaporating from the ocean and spreading out over the land from the sea in the rainfall would impact Northern Queensland first. Some remediation could be achieved with industrial scale compost tea, and rockdust spread by planes. The humate organic matter and microbes could mediate some of the heavy metal and radiation, giving plants natural resistance.

Presently we are experiencing the forests burning off, as they do at the end of interglacial periods as the earth becomes demineralized, and the nuclear winter effect from large volcanic eruptions also contributes to the cooling of the planet. The trees die off and burn off prior to ice ages possibly because the reduced magnetosphere associated with a Grand Solar Quiet means the earth's shields go down and the galactic cosmic rays go up. Trees are dying worldwide from chemtrails and increased UVC from the sun. The tree die off started in earnest in 2013, so that it can likely be attributed to Fukushima destruction of the northern ozone layer, chemtrail aluminum poisoning, along with the increased UVC and galactic cosmic rays which are going up each year. The symptoms of the tree die off are those of radical aluminum poisoning, UV damage and intense oxidation.

The northern hemisphere is in for major disruption in the next 200 years due to lowering of Earth's magnetic field, Grand Solar Minimum "Global Cooling," the disruption of the jet streams and war-capitalization. The northern hemisphere will be plunged into a cold era that could last between 35 to 200 years, which will reduce food production and cause mass famine and unprecedented deaths. The weather will be rather extreme, anomalous and disrupted going into the solar minimum. If say the Grand Solar Minimum is going to be 200 years—before the mini ice age starts you need to move to a survival village where it won't get too cold, and away from fracking and chemtrailing, 5G and smart meters, that is you need to escape from Western Culture. By the luck of the draw of geography some places will be safe from extreme weather events, floods, earthquakes, volcanoes and the like.

Ocean Heating increases evaporation creating global cloud cover that adds to the deluge! The oceans are presently heating up with the millions of underwater volcanoes, now brought to life with the cosmic ray heating of the earth's core, and the consequent cycle of "The Growing Earth." To really study why the oceans are heating, you have to read Viktor Schauberger's books to understand that Borg human water treatment, engineering, conveyance, storage, damming, along with industrial farming, forestry, fracking, chemtrails and pollution is destroying the life-giving potential of water on this planet. As we kill the water, we destroy all life on the planet. It requires education and awakening to the spiritual awareness of Nature but this mistreatment of water can be fixed.

There is probably deeper aquifers to deal with the fact that cities like Delhi, India are running out of water. However with the increased cloud cover from heating oceans, cosmic ray increase and increased cloud seeding from volcanic sulfur dioxide, all countries need is a massive engineering project to create catchment systems. The deluge can be harvested in the hills and settled in holding dams, swales, and forests then diverted back down into the water table and aquifers. As long as the point of use was quite some distance from the point of catchment, this system could be feasible—however aquifer water normally takes 100,000 years to create, so the recharged aquifer water will never be quite the same.

We are entering a period of civil engineering challenge greater than any previous civilization—farming, cities, housing, bridges, dams and drainage systems will need to change to adapt to extreme conditions throughout many areas of the world. The present human infrastructure is built for stable interglacial conditions and is not going to last long in its present form due to increased extreme weather so it might be good to get a portable solar generator, that you can move indoors during the storms. Chemtrails are the last nail in the coffin of a viable industrial civilization!

CHEMTRAIL COCKTAIL CONTENTS

Aluminum Oxide Particles, Methyl Aluminum, Arsenic, Barium Salts, Barium Titanates, Strontium, Cadmium, Calcium, Chromium, Nickel, Radioactive, Cesium, Radioactive Thorium, Uranium, Selenium, Lead, Mercury, Sharp Titanium Shards, Silver, Nano-Aluminum-Coated Fiberglass, Carbon Nanotubes, Nitrogen Trifluoride Known as CHAFF), Polymer Fibers, Ethylene dibromide, Acetone, Dibromide, Desiccated Human Red Blood Cells, Human white Blood Cells, Restriction Enzymes used in laboratories to cut DNA into smaller fragments, Enterobacter cloacae, Enterobacteriaceae, Bacilli, Mold Spores, Mycoplasma, Streptomyces, Pseudomonas Aeruginosa, Pseudomonas Fluorescens, Serratia Marcescens, Sub-Micron Particles (Containing Live Biological Matter), Unidentified Bacteria, Yellow Fungal Mycotoxins.
~ *List provided by StopSprayingCalifornia.com*

Stratospheric Aerosol Injection involves the spraying of millions of tons of nanoparticulates of aluminum, 26 heavy metals including barium, strontium, arsenic, lead, mercury and uranium, and other ingredients such as anthrax and pneumonia, acetylcholine chloride, molds and fungi, viruses, carcinogens and sedatives. The annual cost of delivering 5 million tons of an albedo enhancing aerosol to an altitude of 20 to 30 km is estimated at \$2 to \$8 billion USD. From the 1980's biochemists at Tinker Airbase, located in Oklahoma City, have been employed to research and create nano pharmaceutical, psychoactive chemtrail cocktails designed to create general malaise, ineffective sleep cycles, blood instability, mood swings, short term memory loss, chronic fatigue syndrome, antidepressant, riot control, and other symptoms for social control.

"Polymer chemist Dr. R. Michael Castle has studied atmospheric polymers for years. He found that some of them contain bioactive materials, which can cause "serious skin lesions and diseases when absorbed into the skin." He has identified microscopic polymers comprised of genetically-engineered fungal forms mutated with viruses. He says that trillions of fusarium (fungus)/virus mutated spores), which secrete a powerful myco-toxin, are part of the air we breathe."Furthermore the chemtrail cocktail also is said to contain DNA, and GNA. GNA is a Man-Made Synthetic Version of DNA. This GNA is reportedly entering the bodies of Humans and Animals, using Nano Technology and changing the DNA .This synthetic DNA, is ferroelectric, which means that it responds to external frequencies. So our bodies are much more sensitive to the microwave, WiFi, etc. See *Chemtrails to Pseudo-Life: The Dark Agenda of Synthetic Biology* by Sophia Smallstorm.

People all over the world are coming down with Chemtrail Syndrome: frequent headaches, sinus congestion, pneumonia, asthma and ear infections. Nano-particles of aluminum, barium, strontium, arsenic and other toxic particulates have a detrimental effect on the brain and spinal cord. A growing list of neurological diseases, respiratory illnesses, and autoimmune diseases including Alzheimer's, dementia, Parkinson's disease, and Lou Gehrig's disease (ALS) are all strongly linked to exposure to environmental aluminum and the effect of these nano-particles. The chemtrail aerosols drift down to the lower atmosphere and contaminate vegetation, crops, along with animal and human lungs. Micro-sized mechanized "dust" is inhaled and mechanically bores into lung tissue producing various pathologies. One version of this "dust" is said to be composed of phytalate (used to create PVC plastic) particles coated in aluminum, titanium and barium.

When aluminum is in nano-particulate form it is infinitely more inflammatory, and also more easily penetrates the brain by a number of routes, including the blood and olfactory nerves in the nose. Scientists have found that there is long-term aluminum adjuvant bio-persistence within phagocytic macrophage cells which causes a build up of aluminum in the brain via the Trojan horse translocation method. Thus the nano-aluminum in vaccines and chemtrails represent a major health concern by promoting chronic neurotoxic damage. Aluminum, according to Wilhelm Reich, neutralizes positrons (the antiparticle of a negative electron) in the atmosphere.

The consequences of coal ash dispersal on public health are profound, including exposure to a variety of toxic heavy metals, radioactive elements, and neurologically implicated chemically mobile aluminum released by body moisture after inhalation or through transdermal (skin) induction. Besides aluminum, barium and strontium, fly ash contains arsenic, beryllium, boron, cadmium, chromium, chromium VI, cobalt, lead, manganese, mercury, molybdenum, selenium, strontium, thallium, and vanadium, along with dioxins and PAH compounds and uranium. See the YouTube video: *"Chemtrails are Coal Ash,"* by nicholson1968.com

I believe the chemtrails are responsible for a chemical intoxication of the public, which would then cause a general immunosuppression, low grade to high grade, depending on exposure. The immune dysfunction allows people to become susceptible to opportunistic infections, such as this mycoplasma and other opportunistic infections." Dr. Horowitz.

SMELLING CHEMTRAILS

As we become increasingly poisoned with mercury from chemtrails, we are able to smell and taste chemtrails as our inhibitory neurotransmitter GABA levels drop. Some of the strange smells people are reporting from the different types of chemtrails include: Burnt Rubber, Dryer Sheets, naphthalene, sulfur rotten egg, phosgene gas, toluene, nail polish remover (butyl acetate or ethyl acetate), fresh cut grass, or a METALLIC smell in the air.

The burnt rubber smelling chemtrails are attributed to Bromine which is added to jet fuels under a Japanese patent, for both commercial and military planes. Feverfew is known to reduce the migraines that occur due to the burnt rubber and other types of chemtrails. Out-compete the bromine by keeping your iodine levels strong with kelp and Lugol's. When there is a spraying of the "Swamp Water" type chemtrail type chemtrail that continues for more than a few days, you will notice a "flu" going around town. These biologic chemtrails are often sprayed in association with immune suppressing chemtrails that smell like chrome. Chemtrails suppress our immune systems and lower disease resistance in the biosphere in general.

The volatile chemical that smells like a herbicide may be Ethylene dibromide, Acetone, Benzene or Dibromide. I need hardly add that ethylene dibromide is a highly toxic agricultural pesticide. When snow falls it efficiently scrubs these volatile compounds out of the air, so that they collect at ground level. When you first step outside early morning you may notice the smell of these volatile chemicals as the sun evaporates the snow and these vapors fill the air. "Normally" the smell of high alpine snow evaporating is a divine perfume. But after chem-spraying these volatile chemicals in the air can irritate your eyes, making us blink many times more than normal and our lungs feel irritated and damaged like one does when using paint spray cans. I have heard the this type of snow burns your hands and skin.

Ethylene dibromide (EDB) was used extensively as a soil and post-harvest fumigant for crops, and as a quarantine fumigant for produce. Ethylene dibromide in the jet fuel is a known human chemical carcinogen that was removed from unleaded gasoline because of its cancer-causing effects. Now suddenly it has appeared in the jet fuel that high-altitude military aircraft are emitting! Ethylene dibromide emitted from the jet fuels is causing immune suppression and weakening people's immune system. Then with the biologic chemtrails you've got a mycoplasma, bacteria or a fungus that causes an upper respiratory illness, and suddenly you develop a secondary bacterial infection.

It just so happens that these chemicals destroy the soil microbiome, and also amplify the infection rate from the high-atmosphere pathogens that coast down on the chemtrails and snow. When the lungs are already inflamed from volatile chemicals this raises infection rates for chemtrail flu and pneumonia. Ethylene dibromide is a mucous membrane irritant and exposures to high concentrations can cause eye, skin, and respiratory tract irritation, as well as pulmonary edema ie: chemtrail lung. Thus bumps, rashes, hives and itchy spots occur as your liver accumulates toxins that exit out through your skin and you get allergic reactions associated with the other chemicals.

The Eight Major Chemtrail Types: For a list of the different types of chemtrails see: https://bit.ly/2rwvXns

2

CHEMTRAIL SYNDROME AND CHEMTRAIL FLU

Industrial Agriculture, Cooked Food and the social stress of the power-over Borg hive-mind culture are the principle causes of madness, rapid aging and disease. Now however chemtrails may now be the principal agent of oxidation, inflammation, aging and disease. Chemtrail nano-particles accelerate aging, depreciate structures such as houses, cars, concrete and bridges, and constitute slow death to the environment and all life. Nano-sized aluminum and other nanometals greatly increases inflammation and oxidation, ie: rusting of the body! Oxygen unites with many metals, and in doing so, steals their outer orbit electrons. If an element steals electrons from another element in the process of forming a molecule, it is said to oxidize the element and to be itself reduced. Its valence drops (becomes more negative due to increased electrons).

You need more electrons from the earth (lying, walking on the grass and at the beach, and sunbathing). The key to overcoming inflammation and avoiding infectious diseases is to keep a good supply of electrons in the body through antioxidant foods, supplements and grounding. Plus adequate methylation via MSM, the cabbage family, Folic Acid, Vitamin B12, Vitamin B6, Choline & Green Tea. The body makes N-Acetyl-L-Cysteine (NAC) into cysteine and then into glutathione, a powerful antioxidant.

Cancer and other degenerative diseases occurs due to a mineral deficient, low enzyme, low oxygen state. Lack of enzymes (from generations of cooked diet) is one of the main reasons why people get cancer — it is the Dr. Beard theory. Dan McDonald the Liferegenerator on youtube will set you straight. CANCER EATS RIGHT SPIN MOLECULES: Dr. Antonio Jimenez mentioned in the Gaia series: *The Truth About Cancer: The Quest for the Cures"* with Ty Bollinger said that cancer can only absorb RIGHT spin molecules such as synthetic sugars and processed carbohydrates. Organic non-GMO, remineralized and unprocessed fruit is still OK to eat in moderation because it is LEFT spin. hope4cancer.com

Brain inflammation and cellular inflammation caused by the chemtrails leads to depression and torpor — making populations more easily manipulated, and less like to rise up in defense of their lives to challenge pathological authority. Inflammation (or free radical decay) is one of the major sources of inefficiency, "noise," or incoherence in the body-mind, thus a significant cause of our unenlightenment. Depression will be on the rise not only with the psychological torture of the chemtrail holocaust, but also the nanometals will directly create depression through an inflammatory cascade. We breathe these highly inflammatory agents directly into our brains through the nasal and sinus blood supply.

It so happens that people suffering from depression are loaded with inflammatory cytokines. Since inflammation creates depression this reduces our capacity to fight against the chemtrail holocaust and thrive. Depression and cognitive decline make us paralyzed and ineffective in dealing with the chemtrail assault that is causing us grievous bodily harm and threatening our survival, bringing the inevitable collapse of civilization itself. Vitamin C provides the electrons to quench cellular inflammation thereby removing the static on the central nervous system, so that it is easier to focus our energy. This way we can get the clear energy necessary to change our world. It is a full lifestyle shift that is required to Thrive in the chemtrail holocaust.

SYMPTOMS OF CHEMTRAIL SYNDROME

The Chemtrail Flu progresses from nostril lesions and cold symptoms, to a prefrontal lobotomy as the pathogens and nano-particulates enter directly into the brain through the nasal passages, then the infection progresses to a full body immune response that creates inflammation, fever and leaky cells. There is lasting effects with ongoing painful joints and reduced brain function due to inflammation, along with itchy lesions on the back and arms that can last for years. The overworked immune system, in permanent defensive state prevents the energy and resources needed for recovery, repair and regeneration. The symptoms show up differently in people according to their genetics, lifestyle and exposure. Chemtrail Flu exhibits a range of symptoms and normally hits us where we are most vulnerable. Many autoimmune diseases have been seen in the wake of the chemtrail spraying such as chronic fatigue, multiple sclerosis, lupus, and meningitis. Barium poisoning displays symptoms that are similar to flu. Acute exposure to very high levels of barium may induce gastrointestinal effects, cardiac dys-rhythmias, abnormal blood pressure, muscle weakness, and paralysis.

CHEMTRAIL SYNDROME SYMPTOMS INCLUDE:

Respiratory Problems, Coughing, Sneezing, Shortness of breath, and Acute Respiratory Distress, Abraded or infected nostrils, Sinusitis, Scratchy throat, Allergy symptoms, Hay fever out of season, Flu-like symptoms, Susceptibility to colds, Asthma, Bronchitis, Chronic Obstructive Pulmonary Disease, Skin discomfort, Skin itching/irritation, Morgellon's disease, Small sores on the ears, back and arms, Fibromyalgia and Chronic Pain, Joint inflammation pain, Muscle pain, Sore bones, Dizziness, Nausea, Vertigo, Lightheadedness, Tinnitus (distant ringing in ears or high pitched sound after spraying), Eye irritation, Red Eyes, Eye problems (blurred or fuzzy vision), Liver problems, Gallbladder dysfunction, General weakness, Neck pain, the rapid deterioration of Oral health, Teeth aching, Compromised immunity. Sense of Lack of Grounding, Disorientation and Difficulty paying attention and concentrating, Memory loss, Headache, Anxiety, Depression, Disturbed sleep, Inability to mentally focus, Loss of emotional affect, Prefrontal Lobe dullness, Complacency and Dissociation, Ennui, Low energy, Chronic Fatigue, Brain fog and Mental and Emotional Problems, Irritable, Anger/ Rage/Frustration and Social Reticence, Isolationism, Lack of Bonding, Social Indifference, Projection, Hate. **Social symptoms** relate directly to biochemical shifts The physical and metabolic symptoms of the Chemtrail Syndrome spectrum of illnesses lead directly to socioemotional symptoms in society, which ultimately degrade the inheritance of culture itself — breaking down human potential across the board, and our enjoyment of existence.

CHEMTRAIL SURVIVAL PROTOCOL

INTRODUCTION

I developed a protocol for surviving the chemtrail holocaust so we can be strong enough to stop the undeclared emergency of Global Genocide that is currently underway. The war against life is a perfect storm of heavy metals, radiation, trans-species infectious agents, EMFs and Microwaves weakening the Blood Brain Barrier, combined with compromised immune systems, plus nature-energy deprivation and malnutrition from depleted farm land. Virtually all aspects of immune system functions are compromised by the inhalation of heavy metal particulates.

In addition, toxic metals can increase allergic reactions, cause genetic mutation, compete with "good" trace metals for biochemical bonding sites and act as antibiotics killing both harmful and beneficial bacteria. Most chronic disease is not the failure of the immune system, but a conscious adaptation of the immune system to an otherwise lethal heavy metal environment. In response to the preposterous circumstances we find ourselves in we must "meta-adapt" in order to thrive beyond the slings and arrows of outrageous fortune that befall our communities daily, bought to us by crazy goons playing god.

Thus our personal chemtrail survival protocol must incorporate many angles to be effective. We need to support the detox organs, clean the liver and colon, then do chelators, binders, fibers, clays, zeolite, org-minerals, juicing, lots of silicon water, colloidal silver, sauna/infrared sauna, rebounding, lymph massage, anti-candida, anti-biofilm, enzymes, anti-parasite, antiseptic herbs, anti-inflammatories, probiotics. Researching and finding our way out of this inconceivable predicament is my principle goal in writing this book. I am using standard knowledge and suggesting some new recipes that work to detox and relieve the symptoms from the radiation, toxic chemicals and the "altered" biotech pathogens with pandemic potential.

We can take the passive route and tolerate slavitude and incremental extermination (soft kill) by further numbing the pain and killing ourselves with bad habits. Slaves have been doing this for thousands of years. Or we can take the active path to wake up more and free ourselves from wage dependency and the wily ways of our inner saboteur. Our soporific slave aids (alcohol, cigarettes, bread, sugar etc…) reduce our capacity to feel sensation or pain, thus deadened and anesthetizing us so that we are emotionally unresponsive, indifferent and disengaged. People use food, alcohol and drugs as an anesthetic to numb out a reality that is getting increasingly more scary by the day. This only serves to lock us into that morbid reality and to keep suffering from what has been foisted upon us. Having lost the positive incentive and investment in our own existence within a dying regime, we drift, unsure of the best course of action out of the collective nightmare. The perilous nature of the times we are in means that we must get out of our own way in order to be of service to the greater good and a beneficent future.

Pain has a tendency to confine character by limiting the free expression of Soul and shutting down our mind and body. To be free requires an innovating creative, free thinking brain—not the brain of an order follower. That is, the ability to think for ourselves rather than a follower of prior significance. In order to be our own person and think for ourselves we must "get on top of" the inbuilt orienting and defensive responses, including fight/flight/freeze, submission, collapse, dissociation, self-destruction and numbing. As Einstein said — "Blind belief in authority is the greatest enemy of truth." We slip even further from truth when authority is deliberately obscuring the truth and telling a pack of lies.

We live in a mad mirrored hall of lies — literally both insane and corrupt beyond belief. If the society doing the assessment is mad, then you would be declared insane if you were sane. We could have been supernatural creatures walking this earth. But the majority of humans are psychic virgins, so we cannot expect much from them. And the other point is that humanity is MAD, crazy mad, as we have been built on the wrong stuff for 200,000 years. It is a wonder that any of us have any psychic or visionary abilities, whereas we ALL should have multi-spectrum awareness, not simply sensory and mono.

To understand why *Homo sapiens* is insane view Tony Wright's YouTubes on our fall from grace after our species left the tropical forests thousands of years ago. In his books *"Return to the Brain of Eden: Restoring the Connection between Neurochemistry and Consciousness,"* and *"Left in the Dark."* In these books and his YouTube videos he explains how since moving away from a phytochemically rich fruitarian diet our brain development has been stunted and regressed to the more truncated left-brain mechanical, adaptive functioning. With limited cognitive and sensory capacity we then focus on the material, surface world for we have lost our higher psychic-spiritual capacities, and the "depth" potential of consciousness.

Proof of the chemtrail holocaust is plainly seen in the rapid dying of the environment and in the progressive symptoms of disease in ourselves and others. Peer review, scientific assay and research data are simply closing the gate after the horse has bolted. There is something terribly wrong with our scientific and political bodies that they let the global geoengineering carnage go on for more than 2 decades. The only logical reason could be that they are all in on the global cull, and are likely getting kickbacks along with their job security. We start to see that the civilization building process itself is broken as the wrong people are at the top. Even more bizarre than criminal compliance with corrupt orthodoxy is the "going along to get along" of the masses whom have not yet awoken to the fact that they are being farmed, and that the farmer is presently undertaking a harvest.

In a mutagenic society, it is apparent that cancerous cells have fallen out of sync with the body's own electromagnetic field, because the morphic field has become too weak to maintain its influence, due to lack of ATP, minerals and enzymes. Hence these maverick cells take up a "life" of their own and attempt to colonize the weakened life-form. This "overpowering by an invasive anti-life" force is occurring on all levels in cooked Borg humanity, as is plainly evident in the political, military, financial, medical, industrial and agricultural arenas. Intelligent, beneficent and enlightened humans use a spiritual understanding of "Nature's Force," not radiological, mechanical, chemical or military force. This is our last stand, and we need ALL the help we can get both natural and supernatural to survive and thrive under chemtrail, radiation and microwave assault.

Mastery of our body's own defense system allows us to live relatively free of the toxic impact of collective psychosis and the emotional plague.

21

THE CHEMTRAIL PROTOCOL CHECKLIST

Upgrade glutathione and other antioxidant levels
Remove Mercury Amalgams
Alkalizing (raw) diet, reduce acid pH
Rehydrate with silicon rich water to remove aluminum
Flood body with Antagonistic Organic Minerals
Chelate Heavy Metals
Remove Black Tar and other mucoid deposits
Dissolve Biofilms and Eliminate Candida
Enzymes, Antiseptics and Antivirals
Protect with Antioxidants and Anti-inflammatories
Colon cleanse and Colonics, assist elimination organs
Establish complex Microbiome
Binders and Brooms
Clean and support detoxifying organs
Prevent Reticulation
Maintain a detox lifestyle
Fast for regeneration and neurogenesis
Personal and Household protection against EMF pollution
Protect against inhalation and intake of chemtrail biohazards
Raise energy and establish flow to avoid self-destructive habits
Daily exercise/grounding/sunshine
Conform to circadian rhythms and avoid man-made EMFs
Teach others Chemtrail Thrival and create Thrival communities

CHEMTRAIL FLU PROTOCOL

Let us make ourselves immune to globalist chemtrail flu.

According to Dr. Len Horowitz, chemtrails and their subsequent immune suppression is causing a reported "mystery" flu for which flu vaccines are ineffective. The current state of the war against humanity is that wherever they spray, all of us harbor the biological warfare agents to one degree of another. How we express the infection depends on our genetic strengths and weaknesses, our immune strength and our lifestyle habits.

Chemtrails contain super-toxic chemicals and heavy metals, plus other 'mysterious ingredients like mycotoxins, mold spores, mycoplasma, human white and red blood cells, thus can express as flu/bronchitis/pneumonia type symptoms and mimic Multiple Chemical Sensitivity syndrome. The biological agents along with the aluminum and heavy metals represent a potent ongoing challenge to health and well-being.

For fast detox you have to open up the channels first. **Danjun Breathing** is a type of full body breathing exercise that greatly improves the immune system, digestion and metabolism, strengthening the body's internal energy and focuses in the **Danjun** (Dantien). So deep breathing, saunas, natural hot springs, vege juice, water and vitamin C, Enzymes, the beach, rebounding, yoga, body brushing, body tapping, clay inside and out, enemas/colonics, belly massage, local cleansing herbs, detox tea, put flaxseed into your teas. The Russians found that sunlight on the skin increases detoxification of the body by 20X. Sun gazing dawn and dusk while grounding is an ideal practice. Grounding on the earth and maintaining a super relaxed, stress free period in which you abstain from worry and mental anguish.

REMOVING AMALGAMS: Both chelation and antibacterials are used to get rid of nano-bacterial, viral and mycoplasmal plaques, but before an intensive chelation regime you have to remove your silver amalgams first! Mercury is the most toxic of the heavy metals because of mercury's interaction with sulfur-containing proteins that are critical to your brain function. Removing amalgams will help reduce the heavy metal load of the body, allowing stronger resources against the chemtrails. Mercury is a "biochemical train wreck in your body," causing your cell membranes to leak, and inhibit key enzymes your body needs for energy production and removal of toxins.

Mercury in your body can result in a variety of serious neurological, immunological, and endocrine problems. Mercury not only fuels the flames of inflammation, it also hampers your body's ability to detoxify itself. Mercury toxicity can lead to major inflammation and chronic illnesses such as Alzheimer's disease and Parkinson's disease. Oxidation-inflammation, including inflammation of the lining of your blood vessels is why people with mercury toxicity have damaged blood vessels, and elevated cholesterol and LDL levels. SEE documentary film, Mercury Undercover, exposes the dangers of mercury contamination to human health and to the environment.

See Dr. Christopher Shade YouTubes. Professional protocol for mercury removal read: *Amalgam Illness: Diagnosis and Treatment,* by Andrew Hall Cutler PhD.

ALKALIZING DIET, REDUCE ACID pH: The 0 to 14 pH scale measures the degree of acidity or alkalinity. Acidic solutions have pH values of less than 7, alkaline solutions more than 7. The pH (degree of acidity or alkalinity) of a liquid is determined by its concentration of hydrogen ions. Alkaline water contains positive ions of various metals such as sodium, calcium or magnesium. All water and all aqueous solutions contain both H+ and OH– ions. If there are more OH– ions than H+, the water is alkaline. An acidic pH water occurs when quantity of H+ exceeds that of the OH–. Pure water, which contains equal numbers of both ions and a pH of 7, is said to be neutral.

Negative thoughts and emotions are blockages in the free flow of life energy and ultimately manifest in the body as illness. For full health one must develop a positive attitude, seek balance and the feeling of being at peace with oneself, with others and nature. The stressed or angry person has an acid system with an abundance of positively charged H⁺ ions. This eventually leads to digestive problems, ulcers, arthritis and heart disease. If the blood is too acidic this produces feelings of fear, anger and depression and conversely these emotions produce and acid pH in the body.

Acidic people crave the very things that worsen their condition: coffee, sweets, starchy and fatty foods, alcohol, electronic distractions, aggravation and tension. Pollution, smoking, stress and the increased positive ions of urban areas further raise acidity. Since much of the average diet and lifestyle tends towards acidifying our bodies we must make an effort to ensure that we get adequate sunshine, grounding, exercise, hydration and raw food to alkalize and soothe our system.

RESISTING CHEMTRAIL FLU (C-FLU)

INFECTION RUNS: They seem to do disease saturation sprays in January and February to produce Chemtrail Flu for the medical industry after the Christmas commercial harvest, and the overindulgence in holiday food and alcohol. The disease process is influenced by the body's electromagnetic polarities and circuitry and that the different strengths of the immune system and health of the tissues will determine where and how the chemtrail disease process expresses itself.

The eugenics folks love to poison and infect people from the skies, and consequently the rapacious pharmaceutical-medical industry rakes in more money. It is a sick world we live in. It is hard watching people get C-Flu, bronchitis and pneumonia and not be able to tell them directly because they are your boss or manager, and you would be fired for being a "conspiracy theorist." How to encourage greater observation and dot-connecting skills in those in our community?

Some people only handle surface appearances and feel safety in the social programming . The pressure of Borg indoctrination is unrelenting, with wool is being pulled over the sheep's eyes again and again—just different colored wool! It is quite clear how we are all being mentally and physically affected by this outrageous chemical scourge that has overtaken our planet! Just look up the behavioral symptoms of aluminum toxicity for starters.

Chemtrail flu with its symptoms that include nostril lesions, ear infection, sinus infection, throat and lung infection often leading to bronchitis and pneumonia. The infection generally lingers in the body and manifests as chronic fatigue, brain fog, inflammation, arthritic joints, itchy sores, skin rash epidemic, immune suppression, candida and dysbiosis. Thus from the original Chem-Flu infection we end up with symptoms similar to the Lyme/Morgellons symptom complex. Thus as soon as you see an unusual up-tick in the chemtrailing you need to first protect yourself from "exposure" and to focus on a disciplined anti chemtrail flu regime. When defending against the Chemtrail flu you need to eradicate the infection before it establishes itself and builds protective biofilms… which lead to more permanent disease conditions as the disease agents get "inside" the cells, leaving one with a permanent infection. Successive bouts of chemflu and chemical pneumonia progressively weaken the immune system.

CHEM-FLU AND PNEUMONIA

Raising ATP production and strengthening immunity through diet, lifestyle, exercise, avoiding electro-smog and adhering to circadian (light) rhythms is essential to resist infection. But if you do catch it attack the Flu with a full-on protocol when it first expresses and you are less likely to end up with brain inflammation, permanent disabilities and chronic degenerative diseases. Mega dose Vitamin C, Alpha Lipoic, Vitamin D3, K2, Zinc, Selenium, Lugol's iodine, Colloidal Silver, Cayenne, and Garlic. Whenever a chemtrail day is underway overhead hit the natural flu and immunity measures such as: ginger tea, garlic, clove, cayenne, chaparral, echinacea, elderberry, 1-3 g of lysine, and vitamin B6 etc... Before you notice cold or flu symptoms, start taking 1000 mg of Vitamin C six to eight times a day and up your Vitamin D.

With something as simple as 100mg Zinc per day there is a 3-fold increase in the recovery rate from common cold. Zinc is essential for proper functioning of the immune system. Without zinc your Natural Killer cells won't work and you'll be susceptible to infection, thereby increasing inflammation. Make sure you soak, sprout or ferment your whole grains, legumes, lentils and nuts to remove the phytic acid which would otherwise interfere with zinc and iron use in the body.

Astaxanthin, Organic Lemons and fresh Ginger root tea, Japanese Knotweed, Red Sage, Cat's claw, Stephania Root and Andrographis (King of Bitters). Andrographis paniculata (kalmegh) is a popular Asian/Indian treatment for the common cold and as an anti-bacterial, anti-parasitic, anti-viral and prevents radical damage to your cells. This herb may be the most effective pre-treatment to take on heavy chemtrail days as a preventative to infection. Andrographis paniculata is available in pills or capsules, which is the best way to take this herb as it is very bitter. Andrographis paniculata is available in pills or capsules, which is the best way to take this herb as it is very bitter.

The fungi, viruses and bacteria cannot overgrow if the cell-voltage is normal, and bicarbonate works as an electron donor to raise the voltage. The alkaline effect of Baking Soda helps stop C-Flu transmission. Alkalinity helps put 10 times the oxygen in tissues and the flu virus cannot survive alkaline nor oxygen rich tissues. Thus a fizzy drink of buffered Vitamin C and ½ tsp of Baking Soda or Potassium Bicarbonate is an ideal quick fix for flu or metabolic distress. People are getting results drinking a warm version of the master cleanse (lemon, cayenne, raw honey) and taking 50 mg zinc twice a day.

Iodine and Selenium supplementation may also be advised when making an attack on your pathogen load and resisting a biological warfare attack from the skies. The small bumps on the thighs and the back of the upper arms are likely candida and sluggish lymph. Small bumps on the skin are often a sign of candida, while the tiny itchy red spots on arms and back are a sign of a mycoplasma or spirochete bacteria from chemtrails. Both are symptoms of a compromised immune system. Iodine has been used to cure syphilis, skin lesions, and chronic lung disease.

The body needs iodine to make thyroid hormones which are essential to a strong immune system and is anti-inflammation. High levels of iodine are necessary for optimal function of a number of body systems, including lactating breast, gastric mucosa, salivary glands, oral mucosa, arterial walls, thymus, epidermis, and the choroid plexus that produces the cerebrospinal fluid in the ventricles of the brain. Iodine is anticancer by causing apoptosis in cancer cells, whereas chlorine, fluoride, and bromide are carcinogenic.

Lugol's solution helps eliminate Candida and possibly viruses and other microbes from the bloodstream; this may be one of the methods by which iodine helps prevent cancer. Take 3 drops of Lugol's in a shot glass of water twice daily, but not together with antioxidants as Iodine is an oxidant and it is best to reduce the intake of antioxidants while using it. The Philosopher's silicon water strengthens collagen, removes toxins and plaques and can "push" toxins and pathogens towards the skin to "exit" the body.

Try saunas, kelp baths, green coffee enemas, dry brushing and clay-activated charcoal skin packs to stimulate skin detoxing. Drinking activated charcoal last thing at night is important during active infection and during detoxing. It is best to not heavy metal cleanse when you are experiencing Herx detox symptoms or during a bout of C-Flu. Best to focus on cleansing/supporting the eliminative organs and juice fasting till the body is clean and strong enough to start dealing with the Heavy Metals, mycoplasma, candida etc...

The corrosion of the eyes with chemtrail particulates cannot be good for the health of the corneas. I think that fresh coconut water mixed with distilled water might be a good eye wash to use after you have been outdoors under chem-assault. I suggest everyone get an eye washing glass. Nostrils, eyes and skin will need to be cleaned after being in out in a thick chemtrail stew! Wash you nose out with colloidal silver water during high chemtrail days, and when the ship-trailed air mass comes onto the land.

ANTIBACTERIAL HERBS

Aloe, Astragalus, Barberry, Bilberry extract, Black Cumin Seed, Black Walnut hull, Birch bracket mushrooms, Cat's Claw, Chamomile, Cardamom, Cayenne, Cinnamon, Clove, Chaparral, Devil's claw, Echinacea, Elderberry, Elecampane, Echinacea, Fumitory, Gentian, Ganoderma mushrooms, Garlic, Grapeseed extract, Graviola, Gentian, Goldenseal, Horseradish, Hyssop, Juniper berries, Lobelia, Milk Thistle, Myrrh gum, Neem, Noni juice, Olive leaf, Oregano, Papaya seed, Passionflower, Pau D'Arco, Raspberry, Reishi, Sage, Shiitake, Suma, Thyme, White Willow bark, Wormwood, Valerian.

Assisting: Siberian ginseng, Ginger, Galangal, Ginkgo, Fennel seeds, and Fenugreek seeds. Mucopolysaccharides in Echinacea have been found to strongly stimulate T-lymphocyte activity, macrophage and T-killer cell activity and host cell production of interferon. Sarsaparilla root has been shown to attack microbial substances in the bloodstream, thereby neutralizing them.

Herbal extracts of Samento and Banderol. Banderol is produced from the bark of the Otoba parvifolia, a tree that is found in Peru. The Cat's Claw and Banderol dissolve biofilms as well when taken along with the enzymes Lumbrokinase or Serrapeptase. Medicinal mushrooms (this includes Birch bracket, cordycep, reishi and maitake mushrooms) promote an adaptive immune system which helps control autoimmune reactions. Mutamba with Devil's Claw and Myrrh gum powder helps reduce the candida, insulin resistance, prediabetic foundations of Metabolic X that undermines sexual and creative potency. Cat's claw has demonstrated a capacity for flushing out pathogens and irritants from the gastrointestinal tract. Somebody mentioned success with a warm version of the master cleanser—lemon juice, cayenne, raw honey drink and 50 mcg zinc twice a day.

ANTIVIRALS

Monolaurin ($C_{15}H_{30}O_4$) is a chemical made from lauric acid, which is found in coconut oil and breast milk is effective in fighting viruses, bacteria and fungi. Monolaurin is used for preventing and treating the common cold, flu, herpes, shingles, candida and other infections. It is also used to treat chronic fatigue syndrome (CFS) and to boost the immune system. Monolaurin works by binding to the lipid-protein envelope of the virus, thereby preventing it from attaching and entering host cells, preventing infection and replication. Monolaurin also destroys the viral envelope, killing the virus. Monolaurin shows some ability of breaking down biofilms, but is more effective when taken along with enzymes such as serrapeptase. The enzyme serrapeptase, originally derived from silkworms, digests non-living tissue, including blood clots, cysts, scar tissue, arterial plaque and reduces inflammation. The combination of **Monolaurin and Serrapeptase** may be especially effective to take when under a saturation spray assault, or for anyone living in heavily chem-sprayed cities.

One cure which beats all cures for the C-Flu is 1-3 tsp of cayenne pepper per day in capsules, juices or in soups like spicy onion soup and Thai Tom Yum made with a medicinal mushroom base. The pineapple enzyme (bromelain) eats the spikes off the viral coat, and nettle leaf prevents the manufacture of prostaglandins, also useful for coughs. Lemon balm is a viricide and soothes nasal passages; skullcap is anti-inflammatory, and antihistamine, aids in treating allergies or allergic rhinitis, particularly when used with stinging nettle. The combination of Elder Flowers and St John's Wort is a traditional two punch against viral infection. Spike your green smoothies and vege juices with fresh ground pepper and turmeric to cut down inflammation

NATURAL ANTIVIRAL CURES:

Apple cider vinegar, Dimethyl sulfoxide (DMSO), Vitamin B-12 injections, IV Vitamin C, Zinc, L-Lysine, Helichrysum. Polygonum cuspidatum or Hu Zhang in Chinese contains resveratrol, a powerful antioxidant found in red wine and in the skin of grapes. Other virucides include Clove, Garlic, Ginger, Goldenseal, Echinacea, Star Anise, Astragalus Root. Olive Leaf, Oregano, Licorice, Cat's claw, Marigold, Sweet basil and Wormwood. Aloe vera possesses antiviral activity, preventing virus adsorption, attachment or entry into the host cell. Elderberry and St. John's Wort combined act as an antiviral. It is thought that hypericin, pseudohypericin, and other chemicals in St. John's Wort may stick to the surfaces of viruses and keep them from binding to host cells. Use Zinc-Propolis Lozenges against viruses.

Medical Mushrooms: Reishi, Cordyceps and Maitake have antiviral properties, and can inhibit the C-Flu. Also Turkey Tail Mushroom and Birch Bracket Mushroom. Mushrooms such as Reishi, Shiitake, Chaga and Sang Hwang mushroom boosts the immune system due to two polysaccharide-protein complexes, Beta D-Glucan and Lectin, which control the immune system.

ANTIVIRAL DIET

Fat burning, ketogenic metabolism or the ketogenic diet can be useful for treating viral and bacterial infections, because viruses and bacteria have no mitochondria, which means that the ketogenic diet starves them of their ideal food source, "glucose." An antiviral diet is similar to an anti-candida diet. The main thing to remember is that sugar is the main food of bacteria, viruses, fungi, yeast and cancer.

To eliminate viruses that cause Flu, Herpes, Hepatitis, HIV, Shingles or EBV etc… avoid foods **high in the amino acid arginine**, which can encourage the growth of viruses in the body. You can strengthen your body's natural defense by reducing arginine intake while increasing the intake of another basic amino acid called lysine which is needed for the skin, epithelial tissue and bones. Lysine suppresses the metabolism of Arginine, and helps keep outbreaks under control. Viruses loves arginine, and they are discouraged by lysine!

Eating foods with highest ratio of Lysine to Arginine can discourage viruses. Arginine competes with lysine for absorption so avoid arginine rich foods during flu season—like onions, Brussels sprouts, turkey breast, pork, chicken, pumpkin seeds, soybeans, peanuts, spirulina and dairy. I think it is a numbers game—obviously nuts and seeds are healthier than cereals. Remember right-spin molecules such as synthetic sugars and processed carbohydrates feed cancer. If someone has a particular preference for foods within the Arginine group they could still eat them, but balance that with plentiful Lysine rich foods. Lysine rich foods include bee pollen, brewers yeast, tempeh, quinoa, black beans, lentils, mung bean sprouts and seeds of sunflower, chia and hemp. The point is, ensuring that the body's collagen is strong so that the pathogens cannot easily dissolve tissues and slip between epithelial cells.

An antiviral, high lysine diet can help to strengthen immunity and protect against viral outbreaks by penetrating viruses from entering our surface "barriers." Because our body doesn't make L-lysine on its own, you must get this amino acid from foods or supplements. A good maintenance dose for the chemtrail holocaust would be between 1-3 g L-lysine per day, however, to treat an active viral or bacterial outbreak, lysine dose may reach as high as 9 grams in a single day. One rounded teaspoon is around 2 grams Lysine in weight.

Dr. Linus Pauling recommended Vitamin C=3g / L-lysine=6g daily. Starting off at 1 gram each and slowly increasing dose over time as my body acclimates. The Linus Pauling Institute also recommends a daily dose of 200-400 mg/day **Alpha Lipoic acid** (ALA) for generally healthy people. ALA improves skin texture, protects the skin from sun exposure preventing the inflammation and the generation of free radicals in epithelial tissue.

BOOSTING IMMUNITY: Infections reduce glutathione levels, as does poor diet, mitochondrial dysfunction, and stress. The key to avoiding infectious diseases is to keep a good supply of electrons in the body through antioxidant foods, supplements and grounding. Plus adequate methylation via the cabbage family, Folic Acid, Vitamin B12, Vitamin B6, Choline & Green Tea. Glutathione, most important antioxidant, is synthesized by most cells in the body, particularly those in the liver. The body makes N-Acetyl-L-Cysteine (NAC) into cysteine and then into glutathione, a powerful antioxidant. N-acetyl cysteine can neutralize toxins in the liver because of its ability to boost glutathione and is an unbelievably effective asthma remedy—draining sinuses and clearing the bronchioles and lungs. Also magnesium, zinc and selenomethionine (a source of selenium and methionine).

GUT IMMUNITY: Around 80% of the immune system's white blood cells reside in the gut's lymphatic and mucosal tissue. Since many pathogens enter the body via the intestinal mucosa, it is vital the gut-associated lymphoid tissues can provide effective immune responses when necessary. In addition to probiotic foods there is EpiBiotics that improve your digestion, strengthen your immune system, and restore healthy bacteria in your gut: Pau D'arco, Kiwi fruit, Purple Grape powder, Beets. Ginger Root, Fennel Seeds, Licorice Root, Chicory Root, Chamomile, Slippery Elm, Acemannan, Chinese Yam, Black Cumin Seed. Intestinal immune enhancing activities of macrophage colony-stimulating factor was triggered by the polysaccharides in Korean brown rice vinegar and apple cider vinegar. Diluted apple cider vinegar acts as an effective mouthwash or oral spray.

IMMUNITY HERBS: Calendula, Astragalus Root, Cat's Claw, Olive Leaf, Oregano, Thyme, Echinacea, Garlic, Aloe, Shiitake mushroom, Sarsaparilla, Suma, Barberry, Basil, Boneset, Chamomile, Ginger, Goldenseal, Licorice, Marshmallow, Mistletoe, Star Anise, St John's Wort, Astragalus, Ligustrum, Chaparral, Pau D'Arco. Hyssop is antibacterial, antiviral, antifungal and anticancer. Herbs that help neutralize toxins: Echinacea, Elecampane, Garlic, Fennel, Neem, Plantain. Oregano oil can be used to beat a really bad chest infection including bronchitis. Either diffuse or rub diluted on bottoms of feet for 3 days.

MEDICINAL AMPLIFIERS: You can amplify the positive effects of any herb or supplement by using flushing Niacin (50mg), Cayenne, Ginger and Ginkgo leaf, as these open the cardiovascular system. L-Arginine is also a powerful medicinal amplifier due to increase nitric oxide, which opens up blood vessels and capillaries. Arginine also decreases insulin resistance and advanced glycation end products (AGEs), and lowers oxidative stress, improves endothelial cell function, decreases peripheral vascular resistance and is effective in lowering blood pressure. Deficiency of Selenium (Se) results in oxidative membrane damage as it is contained in the body's main antioxidant enzyme glutathione peroxidase and heme oxidase which catabolizes heme. Everything that increases glutathione in the body such as selenium will be vitally important to maintaining cellular integrity against oxidation and mutation. Asparagus is the highest dietary source of glutathione.

THE THYMUS GLAND: The thymus responds to the negative vibration of harmful chemicals and produces thymosin, which stimulates the maturing of lymphocytes into T-Cells. Thymus Gland hormones have been shown to enhance, restore, and balance; by improving the immune system you enhance your ability to make DNA, to have normal cell division, to have normal insulin sensitivity, and to have normal thyroid levels and other things. Thymus Gland hormones prevent the bone marrow injury and subsequent reduction in white and red blood cell production. Inner Arts for the Thymus include beating your chest like a gorilla, tapping your thymus and the Light Sword Meditation. Low toning while holding an imaginary egg in your mouth, while putting your thumb and index finger either side of your Thymus (sternum) stimulates your thymus gland. Lack of sunlight and Vitamin D deficiency is behind the increase in conditions such as MS, diabetes, autism, dementia, schizophrenia, Crohn's, autoimmune conditions, arthritis and asthma.

THYMUS HERBS: Alfalfa, Echinacea, Horsetail, Licorice, Stinging Nettle, Chaparral, Pau D Arco. **Vitamins**: Niacin B-3, B-6, A, C and E. **Minerals:** Potassium, Sodium, Selenium and Zinc. Like vitamin C, the mineral zinc can help rev up your immune system. Zinc deficiency reduces T-lymphocyte cell numbers, thus low zinc levels weaken the immune system which makes us binge in an attempt to gain energy. This further damages the immune system so that we gain weight and fall even further into a lower zinc deficiency zone. Spirulina is very useful for thymus, which is the university for the immune system. Bee Propolis stimulates and normalizes the Thymus; L-Arginine must be balanced with L-Lysine; L-Phenylalanine, L-Tyrosine.

PROTECTIVE ANOINTING OIL: Massage the back of the neck, temples and occiput with an essential oil mix such as red sage, thyme, hyssop, rosemary, savory, dragons blood, along with black seed oil or jojoba. Massage your shins with this aromatic oil as well. Such strong aromatic oils can be used to help burn body fat between the thighs, under the upper arms and on the belly, while simultaneously assisting the immune system. Helichrysum essential oil on the neck under the ears rapidly supports the immune system, and dropped around the gum line, reduces oral inflammation and infection.

OZONE OR HYDROGEN PEROXIDE FOOT BATHS: Cure your head cold and lungs through your feet by using herbal foot baths, ozone or hydrogen oxide foot baths, plus thorough scrubbing and pumicing your feet. The best pumice to use for defoliating feet is the big one used for cleaning toilet bowls. After foot baths spray your feet with Apple Cider Vinegar and once they are dry rub castor oil or blackseed oil mixed with essential oils on the feet and put on cotton or wool socks.

INFRARED SAUNA: For throwing off chemtrail pathogens and heavy metals an infrared sauna may be of great assistance as infrared saunas remove 85% more toxins than regular saunas, and infrared saunas are said to alleviate the Flu, Morgellons and Mycoplasma symptoms. Morgellons sufferers report that a 30 minute infrared sauna will reduce disease symptoms for a day. Sauna, sunbathing and grounding will also aid immunity and detoxification.

MASTER TONIC

The Master Tonic effectively treats the most severe infections, strengthens the immune system, and acts as an antiviral, antibacterial, antifungal and antiparasitic medicine.
- 24 oz /1.5 pints organic apple cider vinegar
- ¼ cup finely chopped garlic
- ¼ cup finely chopped onion
- 2 chopped fresh Hot peppers.
- ¼ cup grated ginger root
- 2 Tbsp grated horseradish root
- 2 Tbsp turmeric powder or 2 pieces of turmeric root

Combine all the ingredients in a Mason jar and pour in the apple cider vinegar filling it almost to the top. Put the lid on, close well and shake. Keep the jar in a cool, dark, dry place and shake well several times a day for 2 weeks. After 14 days strain the liquid through a cotton cloth and squeeze out the juice. Put the juice into an amber glass bottle. You do not need to keep the tonic in the fridge. Use the Master Tonic undiluted but beware it is very strong and hot. Take 1 tablespoon every day to strengthen the immune system and fight colds. Gargle and swallow for greater effect and put a slice of lemon, orange or cucumber in your mouth directly afterwards to stop the burning. Mix a little with some olive oil and use it in making salad dressings.

Wearing a shungite pendant over the Thymus gland helps improve the body's immune system so that within several months the itchy chembug sores are likely to reduce or disappear.

3

RESPIRATORY SYSTEM

BREATHING PROTECTION: During heavy chemtrailing or the firestorm terrorism of Operation Torch California use a Half Mask Respirator and goggles when outside, and shower on coming inside. To modify the air in your house so that the toxic particles fall to the ground use a humidifier, negative ion generator, salt lamp or indoor fountain this will help drop the particles out of the air. Also bring whatever plants you can move inside your house and close up all your windows. If you don't have a humidifier, set up flat dishes of water inside a window in the sun. Steaming the face will help to clear the nose, bronchial tubes and lungs, put a drop of antiseptic oil like tea tree or eucalyptus oil in the water. When under chemotoxic skies it is a good idea to steam your face and blow your nose prior to sleep. Are air purifiers that remove up to 99.97% of all airborne particles, as small as 0.3 microns. These are expensive, but a regular Hepa filter would be better than nothing.

NOSTRIL LESIONS: Lesions typically occur just inside the nostrils from breathing in the chemtrail aerosol particulates and pathogens. It is almost as if one was breathing in fiberglass. Wash your nose out after you have been outside, and use natural antiseptic sprays like a few Thieves oil drops in a bottle of water or Colloidal Silver in the nostrils. Carry an oral spray containing such ingredients as clove, cinnamon, wintergreen, tea tree oil, oregano, Thieves, and colloidal silver. Clarkia, Medical Mushroom MycoShield spray or Zinc Oral Spray and spray your nose, mouth and neck under your ears several times an hour. Clove has an ORAC (Oxygen Radical Absorbance Capacity) of 1,078,700, while Oranges are only at 750. The Thieves Spray blend which includes Clove, Cinnamon Bark, Rosemary, and Eucalyptus has been found to be highly effective against airborne bacteria. Schisandra berry soak water helps heal the nostril lesions and chembug skin sores.

CLEARING THE SINUSES: Sinus remedies are the same as for bronchitis, the common cold, influenza and lung disease. The sulfur containing amino acid N-Acetyl Cysteine (NAC) thins and drains mucous, especially in the lungs and sinuses; and can prevent asthma attacks when inhaled. It also helps the body make its most important antioxidant, a substance called glutathione, which is everywhere in the body, but especially important in the liver and lungs.

Elderberry lessens swelling in mucous membranes, like the sinuses, and help reduce nasal blockage. Use colloidal silver in water (or Philosopher's Water) in a neti pot or nasal spray for sinus issues also. Colloidal silver makes vaccination intoxication and antibiotic poisoning unnecessary. Shungite water has strong antibacterial, antiviral ability.

Chronic bronchitis or any other infection is a sign of a weakened immune system. Make a big pot of Chaga Tea in a slow cooker, on low heat as this medicinal mushroom heals bronchitis and other lung diseases and can inhibit proliferation and induce the apoptosis of lung cancer cells. Chicory Chaga Coffee: You can also add roasted chickory to your chaga if you prefer to make more of a coffee-like brew.

Also in your arsenal of antimicrobials: Elecampane, echinacea, garlic, olive leaf, lobelia, mullein, thyme, cayenne, black radish. Mullein is a specific remedy for earache, bronchitis, coughing, sinus congestion, chest congestion and wheezing. Kelp broth made into a spicy Thai soup like Tom Yum with basil will clear the sinuses. Kelp remineralizes, detoxifies and increases blood oxygen. One tsp of Black seed oil (cumin seed) per day quenches infection, antiasthmatic and anti-histamine thus quenches sinus infection. Honey, bee pollen and propolis fight sinus infection. A homemade tea for sinus may include mints like peppermint or catnip, ginger, turmeric, black pepper, lemon zest, nettle, and elderberry. Studies have found that elderberry eases flu-like symptoms such as fever, headache, sore throat, fatigue, cough, and body aches. Vary your antimicrobials every few days.

*Black Seed Oil, Serepeptase, CBD oil, THC oil, N-Acetyl Cysteine and Turmeric for asthma, fibrosis, lung cancer etc… from chemtrail nanoparticulate inhalation.

NASAL AND ORAL MISTERS: Use of a colloidal silver atomizer is an easy way treat a sore throat and to disinfect the air to clear the lungs use a humidifier with colloidal silver in the water or silver with an ultrasonic nebulizer. For head and throat cold symptoms use Oral sprays of Medical Mushrooms such as Reishi, Cordyceps and Maitake. Oral sprays can be used for fever, colds, flu and bronchitis — Make up a bottle containing colloidal silver, salt solution, a drop of Lugol's and antiseptic essential oils such as Echinacea, Helichrysum, Oregano, Myrrh, Basil, Hyssop, Lavender, Marjoram, Sage, Clove and Tea tree. Careful not to overdo the oils, it has to be palatable and can also be used as a mouthwash. Artemisia lavandulaefolia has proven results against oral-esophageal cancer due to the induction of cell-apoptosis.

Mechanical means of clearing the sinuses include rebounding, vibe machine, alternating sauna/cold shower. Pinch the top of the nose and sniff-breathe; and tap fingers around the eye sockets and down the side of the nose and around the jaw. Occipital massage at the back of the neck helps to drain the sinuses. Apply finger pressure directly on the indentation of the eye sockets.

The Inner Art exercise called "**Clearing the Attic**" works to drain the sinuses by unclogging the brain's glymphatic system. This entails simply rolling the top of one's head on the carpet along the central "Mohawk" line, while sniffing to unblock the sinuses. This is similar to the rabbit yoga pose and praying to Mecca, but the cranium is gently pressed into a soft carpet. Sinuses also drain when the occipital ridge at the back of the head is massaged.

STEAMING: Steam the Face with Essential Oils with a humidifier/vaporizer, or put your head under a towel over a steaming saucepan. Cedar, myrrh, frankincense and Palo santo volatile essential oils will help to prevent the beta-amyloid protein plaques and tangles from Alzheimer's — caused by aluminum poisoning from chemtrails. Other essential oils and herbs for steaming include helichrysum, tea tree oil, eucalyptus oil, calendula, oregano, savory, fennel, hops, lemon balm, catnip, peppermint, sage, thyme, rosemary, valerian, wormwood, yarrow. A few drops of DMSO and colloidal silver in a nebulizer or steamer allows medicinals to penetrate deep into lung tissue to kill lung infections.

FACE STEAMING FOR THE LUNGS: 1 tablespoon each of dried herbs of choice: Eucalyptus, Peppermint, Oregano, Lungwort, Plantain Leaf, Elecampane Root, Lobelia, Chaparral Leaf, Cat's claw, Mesquite leaf or bark, dried root of Pleurisy-root or Butterfly Weed, Mormon Tea (Ephedra viridis) and Osha Root are herbs for respiratory relief. Heat a pot of water till boiling point, add herbs and put pot on a folded towel on a table. Lean your head over the pot of steaming water under a towel tent, and inhale slowly and deeply through your nose, exhaling out through your mouth for at least 10 minutes. Make fresh tea with ginger or other herbs and steam your face over the saucepan of tea with your head covered with a towel. Then drink the tea.

LUNG CLEANSING HERBS

The expectorants mullein and chickweed aid the lungs in expelling mucus and phlegm by loosening it from the walls of the lungs and allowing it to be coughed up. Make a tea of Chickweed, Fenugreek, Ginger, Licorice root, Mullein, Rosehips, Cardamom, Guayusa and Elderflowers. Lemon/honey/cayenne in water. Ginger tea. Tom yum soup. A tea made of Elderflowers and St John's Wort has been used to alleviate lung infections.

Rosemary Leaf - An aromatic herb used to promote increased blood and lymph flow while helping to reduce mucus production (congestion). If you have rosemary or lavender in the garden, put some in a pot of water on low on the stove, or in a crockpot to infuse the air in the house with antiseptic aroma.

Skullcap - This herb contains the flavonoid *baicalin* which is a powerful immune booster, especially for the upper body, even protecting against lung cancer. Traditionally used to treat inflammation, cancer, and bacterial and viral infections of the respiratory tract and gastrointestinal tract.

Honeysuckle Flowers - This herb has broad-spectrum immune system supporting properties. Wonderful for nourishing the lungs and spleen. Drink a couple of cups of honeysuckle and chrysanthemum flower tea every day to clear mucus from the lungs.

Chamomile Tea Steam - To keep the lungs clear and offer anti-inflammatory action is a small piece of the protective strategy, because the mucosal linings of the lungs are a part of the immune mucosal barrier. Chamomile contains anti-inflammatory bisabolol, and is mildly anti-microbial, helps to clear the lungs and is a restorative tonic.

Chrysanthemum Flowers - The genus Helichrysum has antimicrobial, anti-inflammatory, antioxidant, anti-allergenic properties and has excellent immune system supporting properties. A great herb for nourishing the lungs. Most effective when combined with Mulberry leaves and twig which strengthen the bronchial tubes and counteract insulin resistance. Helichrysum oil is used for treating wounds, fever, chest complaints, sores, coughs, teeth and beauty.

Alfalfa - Alfalfa means *father of all foods,* as it is one of the richest sources for nutrition and very nourishing to the blood. Hawthorn, cayenne and ginkgo improve peripheral circulation and body's ability to utilize oxygen. Dong quai, Dandelion, Yellow dock root, Nettle leaf, Raspberry leaf, Oatstraw and Burdock root have been reported to help in the treatment of anemia. Alfalfa (means "father of all foods") is one of the richest sources for nutrition and very nourishing to the blood.

Immunomodulators to help maintain the integrity of the body's connective tissues are Lapacho (Pau d'Arco), Echinacea, Astragalus, Yerba mate, Licorice root, Ginseng, Chaparral, Echinacea and Sarsaparilla. These would help oxygenate cells and help them burn calories. Other oxygen supporting herbs include Holy basil, Reishi, Rhodiola, Cordyceps, and Ginger. **Saffron** as blood purifier helps increasing the oxygen content of the blood, increases oxygen diffusion from the red blood cells, discourage uric acid buildup, and also inhibits the accumulation of lactic acid. Saffron also removes aluminum from the brain! The *crocin* pigment in saffron blocks Alzheimer's tangles and reduces Beta-amyloid plaque formation. Iran grows 90% of the worlds saffron and is doing fabulous scientific research on its benefits.

Cedar Berry or Juniper Berry has antiseptic, expectorant and mucus clearing properties helpful in treating a number of respiratory conditions, such as coughs, pulmonary catarrh, sinusitis, colds, chronic bronchitis, tuberculosis, and asthma. It is beneficial in breaking down mucus, reducing congestion and relieving respiratory infections. As for lung congestion an indoor fountain or negative ion generator will ease breathing—**the more positive ion rich the environment or proton rich (acidic) the metabolism, the less oxygen is absorbed and transported.** The buffeting of the magnetosphere and ionosphere is no doubt causing positive ion cascades into the atmosphere which make it hard to breathe—so you need to counter that with grounding, raw-green juices and negative ion solutions.

OTHER LUNG HERBS INCLUDE: Borage, Chamomile, Elderberries, Schisandra Berries, Lemon balm, Marshmallow, Ginkgo biloba, Rosemary, Comfrey, Eucalyptus, Lungwort, Oregano, Plantain leaf, Elecampane, Chaparral, Coltsfoot, Osha root, Thyme, Sage and Peppermint. Eat bioflavonoid rich foods such as spinach, berries—think max color. Sophora Flavescens Root (Ku Shen) improves lungs, clears damp heat and is used for lung cancer, bronchitis, the common cold, sinusitis, influenza and lung disease. New Zealand researchers found that an extract of the common edible seaweed Undaria pinnatifida (wakame) killed up to 80% of human lung cancer cells in the lab. The same extract also potently suppressed breast cancer, ovarian cancer, colon cancer, skin cancer, and neuroblastoma cells. New-study-found-seaweed-kills-80-percent-of-lung-cancer-cells! Kelp remineralizes, detoxifies and increases blood oxygen.

SUPPLEMENTS SPECIFICALLY FOR THE LUNGS: Vitamin D, Alpha Lipoic, L-carnitine, Essential Fatty Acids, N-Acetyl-Cysteine (NAC), Daily multivitamin, B complex, mixed carotenoids including beta-carotene, Vitamin C, Coenzyme Q10, Cordyceps, reishi mushrooms, Zhu ling (Polyporus umbellatus). Selenium is effective at reducing the incidence and severity of cancers, including lung cancer. Low levels of zinc ions contribute to the accumulation of thick mucus in the lungs in cystic fibrosis, respiratory diseases with chronic airway inflammation. Zinc supplementation also tempers the inflammatory response to common allergens. It goes without saying that smoking and breathing in toxins is not in the best interest of health as it toxifies the body and damages the lungs. We may not think of this, but drinking alcohol also damages the lungs. Increased protein levels and deficiency of pulmonary glutathione in the epithelial lining fluid of the bronchioles of individuals who chronically abuse alcohol signifies abnormal lung epithelial barrier function that does not readily reverse after a period of abstinence. Thyme destroys strep throat, flu virus and fights respiratory infections.

34

LUNGS AND OXYGEN

Chemtrails represent such a massive respiratory challenge and public health hazard that we must preemptively troubleshoot and raise our resilience against so that we can become immune to whatever pandemic the psychopaths choose to liberate on the masses. The nanometals and chemicals in chemtrail irritate the tissues and directly cause ongoing inflammation, thus leaving the respiratory system more susceptible to other irritants such as pollen, pollution, dust, household cleaners and industrial chemicals.

This constant histamine and free radical production lowers the blood's oxygen carrying capacity and leaves the body more susceptible to infectious and degenerative diseases. Nature cleans and revitalizes the air with negative ions, while cities are lower in oxygen, and higher in positive ions. Human activity tends to ionize the air positive, which makes for anger, disease and madness. Nature's negative ions draw out radiation, charge and hydrate cells and flush toxins, hence the need for grounding and nature. It is therefore a good idea to grow lots of houseplants, have an indoor waterfall and a lush garden.

Regular deep breathing of clean air helps keep the lungs clear and quickly removes damaging toxins from the body. Two pounds of carbon dioxide is expelled from our lungs per day, that is, 70% of the body's toxic load. To undertake this respiratory detoxification 35,000 pints of toxin laden blood pass through our lungs every day. When oxygenation is insufficient this leaves toxins in the blood that get recirculated, and hypoxia encourages pathogens and cancer. Clean blood carries more oxygen, increases energy and vitality, lowers appetite and burns fat. In Ayurveda, Indian Madder Root is one of the most popular blood purifiers that has been used to support the lymphatic system allowing nutrition to feed the cells and wastes to be removed from the body in an optimal fashion.

Because oxygen is key to brain energy, clarity, detoxification, and the balance and resetting of neurotransmitters, we could say that oxygen is the master orchestrator of our sovereign potential. The complexity, depth, span and connectedness of consciousness ie: the efficiency or speed of consciousness is reliant on the efficient use of oxygen in binding spent neurotransmitters, while sopping up free radicals. We eat 4 lbs of food a day, and 4 quarts of fluid, but we take in 7.5 lbs of oxygen a day. There is a tendency to oxygen deprivation in the current age because of our acidity, positive ion exposure, sedentary lifestyle, oxidation/inflammation of tissues and glycation of hemoglobin, coupled with the volatile phenolic compounds and alcohol given off by pathogens.

Oxygen and alkalinity need to be increased through the normal means of remineralizing the tissues, a low glycemic raw diet, superfoods, green food, aerobic exercise, breathing practice and neutral pH drinking water. To increase the oxygen saturation of the blood and tissues eat smaller meals that nutrient-dense, low fat vegetarian and alkaline, for overeating causes oxygen deficiency. Vitamin F and Vitamin K2 increases the oxygen carrying capacity of the hemoglobin in red blood cells. Vitamin E helps transport oxygen to the blood cells. The B12 and folic acid are necessary for the production of red blood cells. Cordyceps mushrooms increase ATP production and improve endurance during exercise, as does Creatine. Both help with cell's ability to use oxygen.

A high enzyme diet means maximizing ATP production with a minimum of exhausting the body's resources for digestion, maintenance and repair. Mega greens in the form of salads, green smoothies, wheatgrass juice to provide minerals, iron and oxygen. Lots of sprouts for salads, seed cheeses and pates are necessary for a high enzyme diet. Sprouted greens have thirty times the nutrition of other fruits and vegetables. Foods rich in photo-reactive enzymes and natural minerals are high in biophotons: sprouts, young spring grown produce, garden ripened food, bee pollen and royal jelly (fresh), fish and seafood and seaweed.

To improve hemoglobin and the oxygen carrying capacity use chlorophyll from sprouted greens such as wheatgrass, alfalfa, sunflower, buckwheat greens and pea greens. Increasing the iron in the hemoglobin requires iron rich foods such as dark green leafy vegetables, molasses, lentils, mushrooms, sunflower, kidney beans, B12, Folic Acid, alfalfa, beet juice, prunes, Goji berries, raisins, apricots, nettles, rehmannia, astragalus, cardamom. Vegetarian sources of foods containing iron are better absorbed when eaten along with foods containing Vitamin C. Magnesium enhances the binding of oxygen to heme proteins and gives red blood cells the flexibility to enter tiny capillaries. Magnesium deficient diet leads to significant decreases in the concentration of red blood cells hemoglobin and eventually a decrease in whole blood iron.

HYPERBARIC OXYGEN: Hyperbaric Oxygen treatments to help boost the immune system, rid the body of parasites and fungus and to help repair damaged organs, reduce scarring, improves eyesight and eliminates cancer. HBOT also curbs infection by providing a hostile environment to anaerobic bacteria, which thrive in the absence of oxygen. It promotes the growth of new capillaries and blood vessels to areas with poor circulation for cardiovascular support and boosts collagen formation for faster wound healing. It also mobilizes rejuvenating stem cells. Studies show that after just one HBOT treatment, concentrations of circulating stem cells doubled, and after a full course, there was an eight-fold increase.

The pressurized hyperbaric oxygen delivers 15 times more oxygen than normal breathing. The increased oxygen tension is a major controlling factor in killing bacteria, improving resistance to infection, increasing the strength of collagen, stimulating new blood vessel growth, and promoting skin regeneration. Angiogenesis, or "new blood vessel growth," generally occurs around 20 the twentieth HBOT treatment, thus it can rectify and regenerate necrotic lesions in the brain caused by vaccines, stroke, traumatic brain injury. HBOT is a broad-spectrum treatment for a collection of symptoms and causes such as candida and brain lesions from falling out of a cot in as a baby, environmental deprivation in early childhood, vaccines, fluoride, sex abuse, and excess kundalini.

Hyperbaric Oxygen has been known to regenerate gray-matter tissue in the brain that has been damaged from drowning or vaccines. Hyperbaric Oxygen is useful against Chemtrail Flu, Lyme bacteria, MS, Alzheimer's, ALS, Parkinson's, glioblastoma, dementia, and even Morgellons. It also helps with Stroke, Traumatic Brain Injury, Post Concussive Syndrome, Post Traumatic Stress Disorder, Seizures, Tinnitus, Wound Healing, Skin Disorders, Spinal Injury, Sports Injury, Radiation Necrosis and more.

Inversion therapy for good for draining fluid from the lungs, making breathing easier, moving lymph and increasing oxygen circulation around the body.

CHEMTRAIL ALLERGIES

An antigen is a molecule that stimulates an immune response, by activating lymphocytes, or the infection-fighting white blood cells. Antigens are "targeted" by antibodies. Viruses are among the simplest of such antigen structures, with most of the antigenic specificity residing in their coats. Allergens are antigens that cause allergic reactions either of the immediate or delayed type. They may be of widely different origins such as dust, fungi, hair, pollen, bacterial proteins, food, vaccines or drugs. Although metals are not allergens in themselves, their ions can bind to biological protein molecules and convert them into proteins which have greater allergenic potential. Sometimes antigens are part of the host itself as in autoimmune/inflammatory diseases like rheumatoid arthritis.

The nanometals and chemicals in chemtrail irritate the tissues and directly cause ongoing inflammation, thus leaving the respiratory system more susceptible to other irritants such as pollen, pollution, dust, household cleaners and industrial chemicals. This constant histamine and free radical production lowers the blood's oxygen carrying capacity and leaves the body more susceptible to infectious and degenerative diseases. When aluminum is in nanoparticulate form it is infinitely more inflammatory, and also more easily penetrates the brain by a number of routes, including the blood and olfactory nerves in the nose.

Aluminum is an adjuvant that increases the inflammatory response, amplifying allergic reaction and promoting autoimmune problems and creates such inflammation in the brain that it leads to ischemia, autism and dementia. The reason so many children in the US today have allergies is due to their mother's exposure to antibiotics and vaccines during pregnancy. Vaccines deliver 4925 mcg of aluminum by 18 months, while the safe limit is 25mcg. A saner way to go is to support the immune system don't cripple it with toxic adjuvants.

MELBOURNE ASTHMA STORM

An unprecedented freak thunderstorm asthma event kills eight people in Melbourne November 26 2016. Over 8,500 people were hospitalized with breathing difficulty, cardiac and chest pain. While folks in New Zealand reported aluminum/barium dust deposits over their cars two days later. The official story for this phenomena was that during the thunderstorm, pollen and mold spores, are lifted into the atmosphere and rupture into tiny particles, which are small enough to enter the lungs.

The immune system identifies the allergens as dangerous invaders and produces protective antibodies, free radicals and histamine in an effort to destroy them, thus airways become inflamed and swollen, and airflow is restricted. Lungs already inflamed by chemtrail nano-particulates would greatly exacerbate the allergic reaction to any allergens in the environment. Rather than "thunderstorm asthma, this event was probably caused by another fake quake attempt on New Zealand—ionizing the atmosphere with nanometals in order to conduct the HAARP quake frequencies.

Both New Zealand and Australia were experiencing extreme HAARPing from satellites (seen on NASA Worldview) associated with the effort to break the back of New Zealand by triggering the unzipping of the fault line. New

Zealand was being geo-terrorized with earthquakes into awarding oil drilling contracts to American oil companies. The evil empire are after New Zealand's unobtainium. Trillions of dollars of oil and gas. The game plan, first shake up the locals, destroy infrastructure, weaken the economy and then extort deals to rape the resources of the country.

ANTIHISTAMINES for ALLERGIES: Antihistamines reduce or block histamines, so they work to relieve symptoms of different types of allergies. Wild oregano, rosemary and thyme (herb and oil) contains a substance called Rosmarinic Acid which is a powerful antihistamine and antioxidant. Turmeric inhibits anaphylactic shock (extreme allergic reaction), stabilizes mast cells and prevents histamine release.

Other Antihistamines Include — Angelica, Ashitaba, Watercress, Pea sprouts, Onions and Garlic, Moringa, Holy basil, Tarragon, Sage, Savory, Hyssop, Chamomile, Grape seed, Skullcap, Jewelweed, Catnip, Feverfew, Goldenseal, Stinging Nettle, Catnip, Cayenne pepper, Black Pepper, Peppermint, Black cumin seed, Galangal and Ginger, Lotus root, Pomegranate, Capers, Mangosteen, Rhodiola, Milk Thistle, Propolis and Pine bark.

A diet rich in the flavonoid luteolin has been shown to reduce mast cell activation. This is found in carrots, bell peppers, thyme, rosemary, peppermint, oregano, romaine lettuce, artichoke, pomegranate, rooibos tea, buckwheat sprouts and cucumbers among other things. Lemon balm is a viricide and soothes nasal passages; skullcap is anti-inflammatory, and antihistamine, aids in treating allergies or allergic rhinitis, particularly when used with stinging nettle. Beta glucans and N-Acetyl-Cysteine will reduce allergy symptoms. The fullerenes in Shungite have pronounced anti-inflammatory, antihistamine, analgesic, anti-allergenic, detoxifying, immune-enhancing effects, and can be ingested like activated charcoal. *Wear Shungite jewelry to reduce allergy symptoms.*

HELIOSPHERIC FLU: The "atmospheric headaches" which are becoming more common are partially due to the coronal holes in the sun buffeting the earth's heliosphere. These magnetofield storms have been occurring for many years now ever since the sunspots numbers dropped off as we go into Grand Solar Minimum. The headaches are likely due to the back-pressure we are seeing in the Heliosphere SWMF-RCM on the darkside of the earth, or due to the close proximity our binary twin star system. Keep an eye on the SWMF-RCM INDEX online and when the heliosphere on the *night side - away from the sun goes into the red,* sensitive individuals are likely to get headaches and difficulty breathing. Grounding, lots of water (Hydrogen water), Vitamin C, and silicon rich calming teas may help. It is advisable to detox and eat an alkaline diet, as an acidic congested system will carry less oxygen and make matters worst. When the Sun-Earth electromagnetics is "stormy," our circadian integrity and Nature Connection must be enhanced.

Chemtrailing kills all trees. We should heavily tax industries that destroy oxygen producers (trees and ocean). The lowering of the planet's oxygen levels is far more dangerous than the inconsequential increase in CO2 which has been used as a political football for tax hungry politicians.

CHEMTRAIL LOBOTOMY

Nano-particles are so toxic they can even damage cells without even entering them!

Brain inflammation and cellular inflammation caused by the chemtrails leads to depression, hopelessness and torpor...making populations more easily manipulated, and less likely to rise up in command of or in defense of their lives. Chemtrail poisoning and heavy metal toxicity basically wipes out the executive capacities of the creative, sovereign functioning adult through the increased cellular inflammation in the prefrontal lobes...as there is a direct connection from the nose to the brain via the olfactory nerve and blood supply. That means that once you get something in your nose, if it's small enough, it can pass into the nerve and make its way all the way to the brain. We must focus on cleansing, strengthen and fortify the nasal passages against nanometals and synthetic polymers, bio-nano particles, and infectious agents.

DIMETHYL SULFOXIDE: DMSO can be used as a vehicle for essential oils, Lugol's or colloidal silver; addition to exerting therapeutic actions on its own DMSO penetrates rapidly and will deliver other substances into tissues thereby enhancing their anti-pathogen or healing effects. DMSO can be mixed with aspirin and/or magnesium chloride sol and applied topically for pain. DMSO acts as a transporter to get anti-inflammatory, anti-Alzheimer's, antiseptic and antifungal agents into the brain. DMSO readily crosses the Blood-Brain Barrier thus can be used as an effective vehicle for transporting other substances that may not normally cross the Blood-Brain Barrier. Fulvic acid also acts as a transporter that goes through the blood brain barrier.

VITAMIN C: Vitamin C is a water-soluble anti-oxidant compound that protects living organisms against oxidative stress. Vitamin C is also essential for the synthesis of collagen, carnitine, neurotransmitters like serotonin and the catabolism of tyrosine, among others. Due to a genetic mutation in the L-gulonolactone oxidase (GLO) gene which codes for the enzyme responsible for catalyzing the last step of Vitamin C biosynthesis in the liver, human bodies do not manufacture Vitamin C. A defect in the gene for the synthesis of the active enzyme (GLO) occurred 20 million years ago thus humans lost the ability to synthesize Vitamin C. Surprisingly many species, have lost the capacity to synthesize Vitamin C such as humans and other great apes, guinea pigs, teleost fishes, as well as some fruit bats and "perching" bird species.

An interesting point is the primitive monkeys, such as lemurs have the intact GLO for the biosynthesis of vitamin C. While higher monkeys, apes, chimpanzees and homo sapiens do not. Evolutionary biologists explain this genetic mutation where we lost the capacity to manufacture Vitamin C by theorizing that during the course of evolution, the advantage of not having to produce something readily available in food results in a reduction in the net energy required, thus the organism can dispense with making the substance.

Inflammation (or free radical decay) is one of the major sources of inefficiency, "noise," or incoherence in the body-mind, thus a significant cause of our unenlightenment. Brain inflammation and cellular inflammation caused by the chemtrails leads to depression and torpor...making populations more easily manipulated, and less like to rise up in defense of their lives to challenge pathological authority. Inflammation (or free radical decay) is one of the major sources of inefficiency, "noise," or incoherence in the body-mind, thus a significant cause of our unenlightenment. Vitamin C provides the electrons to quench cellular inflammation thereby removing the static on the central nervous system, so that it is easier to focus our energy. This way we can get the clear energy necessary to change our world.

Bill Sardi in *"The New Truth About Vitamins and Minerals"* mentions that a 160 lb mountain goat makes about 13g of Vitamin C a day, and even more when under stress. Vitamin C is an anti-stress vitamin and our need for it varies with our level of physical or emotional stress. Stress causes the adrenal glands to signal the release of sugars and fats into the bloodstream to prepare for a response to danger. In most other animals but humans and guinea pigs these sugars are converted to Vitamin C in the liver. Sardi suggests that if humans also manufactured Vitamin C, we would be immune to diabetes, heart disease, arthritis, cataracts, kidney stones and our lifespan would be more like 144-216 years. Sugar competes with Vitamin C at the cell receptor level!

Signs Of Chronic Vitamin C Deficiency—Signs of chronic vitamin C deficiency, commonly in combination with copper deficiency rather than just advancing age include: loss of hair color, gum disease, arteries that have lost their elasticity and are rigid and calcified, sagging breasts and enlarged prostates, aging skin, rigid arteries, aneurysms, varicose veins, and male-pattern baldness. Elevated glucose levels as in diabetes inhibit the cellular uptake of vitamin C, leading to greater degeneration of the blood circulation.

Vitamin C (L-ascorbic acid) is available in many forms, none is more effective than another, and natural and synthetic L-ascorbic acid are chemically identical. Mineral salts of ascorbic acid (Sodium ascorbate and calcium ascorbate, Magnesium ascorbate, Potassium Ascorbate) are buffered and therefore, less acidic to the stomach than ascorbic acid. Vitamin C plays an important role in the synthesis of the neurotransmitter norepinephrine, which might elevate mood. It is required for the synthesis of carnitine, needed for the transport of fat to mitochondria, for conversion to energy. Vitamin C is also needed for collagen, bile, an antioxidant, antimutagenic and for the regeneration of other antioxidants. Vitamin C may also protect from lead poisoning by inhibiting intestinal absorption or enhancing urinary excretion of lead.

The adrenal glands use more Vitamin C that any other organ or tissue in the body, so if you are stressed and/or have internal inflammation, you should be taking the bioequivalent of a Vitamin C-producing animal throughout the day. Chronic inflammation consumes vitamin C and eliminates production of vitamin D. All toxins and infections are pro-oxidant and need antioxidants to counteract them. High dose IV Vitamin C of up to 100g per day should be used for all infections, cancers, and acute poisoning conditions. The North pole of a magnet is a mechanic form of antioxidant that offers up electrons like Vitamin C.

Vitamin C makes the headlines when it comes to cancer prevention. Its antioxidant properties protect cells and their DNA from damage and mutation. It supports the body's immune system, the first line of defense against cancer, and prevents certain cancer-causing compounds from forming in the body. Vitamin C reduces the risk of getting almost all types of cancer. Levels of Arsenic in our environment are documented to be on the rise. As a result large doses of Vitamin C are an absolute requirement. Vitamin C has been proven to protect our cells from Arsenic toxicity which affects all our organs.

Benefits of Vitamin C have been show to include protection against immune system deficiencies, cardiovascular disease, prenatal health problems, eye disease, and even skin wrinkling. You can mix it with a little potassium bicarbonate to make a delicious fizzy drink. This way it is very easy to drink 10 or more grams a day. It is a good idea to do the bowel tolerance test to see how sick you are basically. When you take vitamin C tablets make sure they are not the chewable type or you will lose tooth enamel. Apparently you can store Vitamin C in the freezer — stock up on Vitamin C, Alpha Lipoic and Glutathione in order to macro-dose on high chemtrail days. See: Thomas Levy, MD on Vitamin C on YouTube

LIPOSOMAL VITAMIN C

Besides liposomal Vitamin C, it is advisable for those undergoing chemtrail attack or stress to take L-carnitine and alpha-lipoic supplements as well as adopt a low glycemic diet. Liposomal-C uses Vitamin C (ascorbic acid) powder and lecithin for a lipid delivery system, by encasing nano-particles of nutrients (herbs, too) in a phospholipid membrane or "liposome," allowing safe passage through the gastrointestinal tract without degradation. Thereby avoiding the destructive forces of the gut so that Liposomal-C can be directly absorbed into the bloodstream. The Liposomes of C because of their nano size and composition, provide the perfect transport system.

When it is Lypo-Spherically coated in Lecithin 90% of the Vitamin C gets absorbed into the cells, because cell walls are made of fats and normal Vitamin C is water soluble. In comparison regular vitamin C is only absorbed around 19%. The traditional form of Vitamin C, in tablet or capsule, is subject to a host of factors that can oxidize it, neutralize it, adulterate it, and even expel it before it ever gets to the cells that need it. When encased in liposomes Vitamin C is claimed to approach or exceed the absorption of intravenous Vitamin C, but it is less expensive than IV-C treatments.

Phospholipids are the primary building blocks of biological membranes that provide barriers to compartmentalize cells and their components. These membranes are dynamic and fluid in nature, incorporating proteins that perform critical functions including solute transport, signal transduction, and ATP synthesis. The best known phospholipid is phosphatidylcholine (aka lecithin). Because it's structure allows it to be an interface of water-lipid environments, there are two main functions of phospholipids: A key component of the cell's lipid bilayer, and emulsification. Foods rich in phosphatidylcholine include: egg yolks, liver, soybeans, wheat germ, and peanuts. Lecithin is a similar phospholipid to our cell walls so the liposomal material is assimilated by the phospholipid-craving cells that need phosphatidylcholine and the Vitamin C.

Vitamin C filled liposomes disperse in water or beverage and quickly navigate through the digestive system, requiring no digestive activity prior to assimilation. They rapidly absorb in the small intestine and are transported intact throughout the bloodstream to release the powerful, non-degraded Vitamin C for use throughout the body as the liposomal material is metabolized by the cells requiring repair. Liposomal-C can be made at home by blending solutions of Vitamin C powder and Sunflower Lecithin (from Swansonvitamins. com) and vibrating the mixture in an ultrasonic cleaner.

LIPOSOMAL-C RECIPE

• Soak and dissolve 3 Tbsp. of "Sunflower Lecithin" in 1 cup of distilled water.

• Dissolve 1.5 Tbsp. of pharmaceutical grade Vitamin C powder in 1 cup of distilled water. Then mix in a bullet mixer or blender for several minutes.

• Pour both solutions together in the ultrasonic cleaner bowl and turn unit on. With the lid open use a plastic straw to slowly stir the contents. This will take about 30 minutes or so. When done you will have a mix that is about the color of milk with no foam.

• Therapeutic dose can be 1/3 cup Liposomal-C, 3 times a day. This cuts inflammation, oxidation, pain and aging.

NB: Buffered vitamin C powder will NOT go into a liposomal state. It looks OK for a little while, then it separates. This system works to encapsulate 70% of the Vitamin C.

www.swansonvitamins.com — 1 lb each of Swanson Premium 100% Pure Vitamin C Powder and sunflower lecithin

Check out YouTube videos on making Liposomal Encapsulated Vitamin C

www.HERBALCOM.COM and hardrhino.com

lpi.oregonstate.edu/ — Linus Pauling Institute

CHEMBUG SORES

After the initial flu-like respiratory symptoms the infection sets in and expresses as skin lesions, brain inflammation and fatigue. The Chembug Sores are an ongoing expression of the Chemflu bug spectrum of illnesses. These little sores occur mostly on the arms and upper back, which is strange in itself. They are small, dark red and produce an unrelenting itch. Because of the chronic, recurrent nature of the Chemtrail induced flu and consequent chembug sores, Pharma's antibiotics are out of the question! However a full on chemtrail protocol will cut down the ongoing infection, along with reinstating and reinvigorating the immune system by an ongoing series of 3 day water fasts. Water fasting for 3 days is enough to reset the immune system, and so help the immune cells to evolve and keep up with the ever evolving bacterial and viral load within.

Since I am a farm girl I never get flus or colds. One of the first full moons of 2015 for several days they were spraying over 50+ trails a day. During this 3 day saturation spray, even I got sinus and cold symptoms along with abraded ulcerated nostrils that lasted over a week. After a few days of saturation spraying my nostrils had what seemed like an ulcerated nostril edges felt like I had been breathing something caustic. I also had a spontaneous small hemorrhage (bleeding sore) on my ear. This was associated with a flu-like infection that went into my prefrontal lobes and felt like an alien invasion of a non-ordinary sort. I wondered if it is the nanometals, piezoelectric crystals or the sulfur coated fiberglass that causes eye, nose and throat problems.

Whether it was sulfur and fiberglass coated aluminum particles or some infectious agent my body reacted against it— my immune system cells produced protective lysosomal digestive enzymes, such that it felt like my cells were leaking. Whatever was in the chemtrail cocktail the first week of February 2015 felt in the body like an **unnatural, alien, robotic, mechanical and demonic force.** When the body "wept" from its own free radical attack on the infectious agent, the cell plasma formed a nano-crystalline crust around the nostrils, the weeping eyes and vagina labia. This crystalline crusting in particular made me realize that this was not a disease of nature, but was a construct of the devil Man.

The end result months after the initial chem-flu response was the persistent symptom of small red itchy spots (lesions), possibly from spirochetes dropped in the chemtrails, revealing a systemic infection that may never go away. I am still working on a cure for the chronic infection and topical treatments for the itchy spots. It is possible that hyperthermia in infrared saunas, and increasing oxygen in hyperbaric chambers would be effective. Fasting and avoiding sugar, carbohydrates and alcohol help immensely, as the mycoplasma, Lyme bacteria or whatever is causing the itchy chembug skin lesions LOVES SUGAR!

I am not sure anything really works to eliminate the pathogens entirely other than periodic fasting, Ketogenic diet and EMF therapies. Whether it is Morgellons or Chembug Sores if you drink alcohol or eat bread or sugar then there is increased infection rate. Eliminating the pathogen entirely may be nigh impossible without change of lifestyle and location, and change of diet. A pristine tropical island with lots of sun and ocean water may be the best medicine.

QUENCH THE ITCH

The itchy chembug skin lesions and/or Morgellons sores respond to all substances that strengthen collagen and reduce inflammation. One remedy I found is the first tannin rich soak water of Schisandra berries. This can be run through a coffee filter and put into a spray bottle. It helps heal Morgellons lesions and the rashes and abraded nostrils and stops the itchy back. **Chamomile/Onion skin Infusion Spray** helps immensely to both heal the micro-lesions and to ease itchiness of the chembug lesions. Spray the affected area several times a day, and keep the spray bottle in the fridge.

Other skin healing allies are Gotu Kola and coconut oil mixture, fresh Aloe vera juice, Neem Oil, Black Seed Oil. Charcoal soap and sulfur soap and sulfur ointment help to soothe the itching. Wearing a shungite pendant over the Thymus gland helps improve the body's immune system so that within several months the itchy chembug sores are likely to reduce or disappear.

Silicon and colloidal silver (Philosopher's water) and the amino acid Lysine have a significant effect. I put 1 tsp of Lysine and 1 tsp of D-Ribose in 10 oz of Philosopher's water and take ½ a pill of Niacin B3 (50mg). However, you still need to avoid things that feed the (spirochete) infection such as bread and cereals in general, alcohol and sugar. I probably could have gotten rid of the pathogens with a series of 3 day fasts started immediately after infection to boost the immune system. By stimulating Natural Killer cells Beta 1, 3D-Glucan may be one of the best solutions to the chembug itch as well as fighting the chemtrail flu. Pau D' Arco and Chaparral internally and topically may be a primary remedy to the spectrum of Chembug infectious diseases.

 Medical mushrooms that grow on trees such as *Phellinus Linteus* (Sang Hwang), Turkey Tail, or Burch Bracket are ideal to be used in association with **Andrographis** as a primary defense against chem-bugs, colds, flus and skin infections, herpes, aids digestion helps relieve stressed skin from inflammation by boosting skin immunity and cures skin cancer. Apply *Andrographis Bianca Rosa* salve morning and evenings. You will have to make your own as they are very expensive. growforagecookferment.com/how-to-make-an-herbal-salve.

An **Andrographis leaf** water infusion made in a slow cooker, sieved and run through a coffee filter and then put into a spray bottle may be ideal for spraying on the skin for itchy lesions and Morgellons. Use the combo of Andrographis and Tree Mushrooms in sprays, salves, poultices and capsules. Grow these in your garden if possible, so you always have some on hand.

Antiseptic Spray: A topical spray of Colloidal silver and Apple cider vinegar is invaluable to chemtrail symptoms by supporting the skin immune system.

Schisandra Spray: The first tannin rich soak water of Schisandra berries sprayed on the skin are a few remedies for infections, lesions and rashes on the skin.

Onion/Chamomile spray: In a crock-pot on "low" heat 1/3 cup of ground chamomile flowers and skins of 1-2 onions in 3 cups of water overnight, sieve then fine-strain. Put infusion in a spray bottle with the rest in a glass bottle and keep in the fridge. Spray back arms and other affected areas several times a day to reduce itching and heal the chembug lesions, (and as hair spray for golden blond hair.)

Allantoin is a compound that softens and protects while actively conditioning and soothing skin. It also stimulates cell regeneration promoting healthy skin. It is extracted from mulberry tree root, comfrey root, sugar beet and wheat sprouts.

TOPICAL ESSENTIAL OILS: You might try Helichrysum, Oregano, Savory, Hyssop and Clove oil in Black Seed oil. If applied topically these oils will be absorbed and improve the immune system. Mix essential oils with colloidal silver and water-Himalayan salt solution and put in a spray or dropper bottle to use orally. Protective anointing oil can be massaged into the back of the neck, temples and occiput with an essential oil mix such as red sage, thyme, hyssop, rosemary, savory cut with black seed oil or jojoba. Massage your shins with this aromatic oil as well. Such strong aromatic oils can be used to help burn body fat between the thighs, under the upper arms and on the belly, while simultaneously assisting the immune system.

BLACK SEED OIL: Black Cumin Seed (Nigella sativa) is anti-inflammatory, neuroprotective, nephroprotective, antimutagenic, anticarcinogenic, and anticonvulsant activities. Moreover, Black Cumin Seed oil is known for its hypotensive, anti-spasmolytic, bronchodilator, hepatoprotective, antihypertensive and renal protective, and immunomodulatory effects. Black cumin seed oil was also shown to be antimicrobial, inhibiting the growth of microorganisms such as candida, bacteria, fungi, and protozoans. It is an exceptional oil for oral health, as well as skin cracking and rashes and gut lining protection. Blackseed oil is the perfect oil for "oil pulling" to keep down the bacterial overgrowth in the mouth.

ECZEMA CURES: Infrared light, Vitamin D, Vitamin E, , Omega 3, probiotics, Coconut oil, Fresh coconut water, Meditation, Witch Hazel Salve, Aloe vera, Basil, Calendula, Chamomile infusion spray, Licorice root, Burdock root, Comfrey, Borage Leaf, Cat's Claw, Dong Quai, Ginseng, Gotu Kola, Echinacea, Milk Thistle, Myrrh, Parsley, Purslane, Plantain, St John's Wort, Yarrow, Yellow dock, greens, Wheatgrass juice, Lavender essential oil, Activated Charcoal, Clay, Dead sea salt Baths, raw Shea butter, Rosehip oil.

COPPER: The trace mineral Copper is needed in a very small quantity. Its primary role is to help form hemoglobin and collagen in the body. A deficiency in copper results in poorly formed red blood cells, otherwise known as anemia. It also is an antioxidant, helping to eliminate free radicals. *Copper is used as a modulator of spontaneous activity of developing neural circuits.* Copper also assists the synthesis of phospholipids that are essential for the formation of these myelin sheaths, thereby, making your brain work much faster and more efficiently. Phospholipids are also the main component of cell membranes, and copper and sulfur-rich foods are essential in forming connective tissue.

In his YouTube videos **Harald Kautz-Vella** says that when you are copper deficient mercury strips the nerves leading to the dissolving of the nervous system, and the growth of these piezo-crystal prion proteins that act as antennas to electromagnetic signals. It was found that aluminum accumulated in the pituitary glands and testes when dietary copper levels were suboptimal.

Copper deficiency can manifest in parallel with vitamin B12 and other nutritional deficiencies. Copper deficiency symptoms can include increased parasitic infections, weakness from anemia and leaky gut. Copper must stay in balance in association with zinc and iron in the body, for if you consume too much of one it can throw the others out of balance. Zinc naturally balances copper and keeps it from building up in the tissues. People are losing their hearing perhaps due to the chemtrails exhausting the zinc and selenium levels in the body, and the nano-metal inflammation lowers all brain function including sensory acuity. If you are not eating much in the way of meat and eggs, you will develop copper excess problems because zinc is the natural antagonist to copper.

Vegetarian diets are very high in copper because the vegetable foods are a great source of this mineral. People report results with monoatomic copper and CBD's against the spirochetes; but you still have to give up the sugar medium they feed on…cereals, bread, alcohol and all forms of sugar. Fruit doesn't seem to feed the spirochetes, unless it is dehydrated fruit. You can also make your own colloidal copper and grow mustard sprouts with it, as an anti-fungal and to protect neurons in the brain from breaking down and building plaque. Colloidal copper and silver can be sprayed onto sprouts grown in trays of soil. This kills fungal growth on the sprouts and the plant uptakes the metal and it chelates it for you, thereby assisting assimilation.

Copper food sources include Black cumin seeds, Beef liver, Sunflower seeds, Lentils, Almonds, Dried apricots, Dark chocolate, Blackstrap molasses, Asparagus, Mushrooms, Turnip greens. Pure copper wire in a glass bottle of Fulvic Acid and/or Apple Cider Vinegar will help take copper into the brain to prevent Alzheimer's, Lyme and Morgellons from dissolving neurons. The RDA for copper is 900 mcg/day. Due to genetics and other factors some people may already have an excess of copper in the body.

The book *"Nutrient Power: Heal Your Biochemistry and Heal Your Brain,"* by William J. Walsh Ph.D., emphasizes the importance of taking into account biochemical individuality and how we should get to know our own signature and optimize factors in our life such as nutrition, relaxation and exercise accordingly. The extreme conditions we are face with regarding the toxic aerosols, polluted water and other environmental stressors including weather extremes and high UVC mean that we have to increase the integrity of our food supply and diet to that which is far superior to the ambient Borg culture.

DISSOLVING BIOFILMS

Bad bacteria, viruses, parasites, or fungus that make a home along the walls of the stomach and intestines releasing toxins directly into the bloodstream, creating inflammation and interfere with proper immune function. These contribute to things like leaky gut, autoimmunity and **brain fog**. The amount of biofilm and toxic waste from pathogens in the blood reduces, reducing sludgy blood and improving the blood's oxygen carrying capacity.

Microorganisms commonly generate biofilms held together by a matrix of hydrated extracellular polymeric substances. Pathogenic bacteria, yeast and fungi like candida create these biofilms to protect themselves and their colonies inside the body. Regular bacteria form a self-produced matrix of extracellular polymeric substance or "slime," which is a conglomeration generally composed of extracellular DNA, proteins, and polysaccharides. In addition to the glycoproteins and polysaccharides, these matrices may also contain material from the surrounding environment, including but not limited to minerals, and blood components such as erythrocytes and fibrin.

To address this, first you use fibrinolytics to help dissolve the fibrin, then you use EDTA to chelate out the minerals. When these biofilms are broken down the body starts dumping toxic metals that were accumulated in the biofilms. The Heavy Metals are all positively charged cations, that is why EDTA is able to chelate them well. As part of the anti chemtrail protocol you have to breakdown the biofilms in your existing pathogen load in order to release the heavy metals during a specially designed cleanse.

Biofilms adversely affect the body in unknown ways. The list may include fetal development, autism, depression, chronic fatigue, Lyme disease, cognitive impairment, etc. Chronic Lyme/spirochetes may play a role in the development of dementia and Alzheimer's. *Bovine spongiform encephalopathy* (BSE), commonly known as mad cow disease contracted from eating contaminated meat is implicated Alzheimer's disease. Many stealthy infectious agents have been identified (e.g: Borrelia, Mycoplasma, Bartonella, Babesia, Rickettsia), but some are still unknown or poorly understood. Chronic inflammation from infection + biofilm can lead to cancer, cardiovascular disease, dementia, and other debilitating conditions.

Biofilm or Microbial slime is a forerunner to calcification and the encasement of heavy metals in mineral plaques in the body. In the biofilms they sequester calcium, magnesium, iron and heavy metals to help build that matrix. Within a biofilm candida can become completely resistant to all antifungal agents, however if treated with EDTA first, this pulls out the calcium, magnesium and iron and destroyed the structural integrity of the biofilm allowing it to be dissolved. Dental plaque is an oral biofilm that adheres to the teeth and consists of many species of both bacteria and fungi (such as *Streptococcus mutans* and *Candida albicans*), embedded in salivary polymers and microbial extracellular products.

Colloidal silver ions — attack bacterial cells in two main ways: It makes the cell membrane more permeable and interferes with the cell's metabolism. It also ionically tears apart biofilms allowing anti-pathogen medicinals to get at the disease pathogens. ACS 200 Silver Gel and Colloidal silver ionically breaks down biofilms. Some other substances that have been found to be effective against biofilms include clove, lemongrass, serrapeptase, nattokinase, lumbrokinase, and a variety of other enzymes, as well as NAC (n-acetyl-cysteine), and apple cider vinegar. During the cleanse you want the GI tract to be loose and open so released heavy metals are not uptaken into the kidneys. Taking high doses of buffered Vitamin C helps to protect tissues while the heavy metals are being escorted out of the body. Colonics or enemas in the beginning weeks might be useful, if you do not have leaky gut syndrome.

The presence of metal cations has been reported to be required for biofilm formation as indicated by the reduced ability of bacteria to produce biofilms in presence of chelators like EDTA. Both chelation and antibacterials are used to get rid of nano-bacterial, viral and mycoplasmal plaques, but before an intensive chelation regime you have to remove your silver amalgams first to prevent them leaking mercury.

ANTIBIOFILM AGENTS

Biofilms are a matrix composed microbial cells encased within a matrix of extracellular polysaccharides, proteins, lipids, and extracellular DNA.

NAC and α-amylase, ACZ-nano Zeolite, Zeo-Gold. N-acetyl-cysteine (NAC) is an amino acid, a precursor to glutathione which disrupts biofilms, drains mucus and clears the sinuses! One study found that NAC reduced biofilm formation by 62 percent. The allicin in garlic has been shown to disrupt the bacterial communication process called quorum sensing thereby preventing biofilm development. Cat's Claw and Banderol dissolve biofilms when taken along with the enzymes Lumbrokinase or Serrapeptase. Jiaogulan, Dong quai (Angelica sinensis). Tree Peony, (*Paeonia suffruticosa*) and White Peony Root, (*Paeonia lactiflora*) blocks how bacteria are able to make biofilms by inhibiting the production of nitric oxide synthase. Oregano's active constituent "carvacrol," has long been used to naturally eradicate unwanted pathogens and inhibits the release of harmful toxins and biofilms released by these pathogens. Berberine found in Oregon grape and goldenseal is a potent anti-microbial with anti-diabetic and anti-cancer properties.

Researcher and educator Tony Pantalleresco suggested this volatile formula to break down and excrete the biofilm, nano-technology and metals in our bodies. You can try for five days on and then take a break. One ounce of brandy or whiskey plus one drop each of the Essential Oil's of Mountain Savory, Thyme and Oregano. This is an antibacterial, anti-fungal, antioxidant oil used to treat arthritis, stimulate the immune system, and is most often as a digestive remedy. I think that propolis added to brandy along with essential oils, and taken as an aperitif may be an ideal addition to methods of stripping the black tar biofilm off of the lining of the GI tract. This remedy may be too extreme for most people.

LEMON WATER—Lemon juice has a pH between 2 and 3. Systems in your body carefully maintain normal blood pH levels, which fall between 7.35 and 7.45. Because foods are not known to alter the pH of your blood or body, lemons won't acidify you either. Drinking lemon juice with water may increase the acid level of your urine, however, which is a sign that your kidneys are doing their job -- ridding you of excess acid. Lemon juice and apple cider vinegar help break down the biofilms and plaques, whereby pathogens, heavy metals and acids can be removed by the body.

SAPONIN CLEANSERS — Plants rich in saponins make a luxurious soapy lather and can be useful for breaking down biofilms as well. Plants containing saponins include jiaogulan (Gynostemma), Yucca root, Devil's Claw, Burdock Root, Sheep Sorrel, Red Clover Blossom, Licorice Roots, Slippery Elm Bark, Queen's Delight Root, Prickly Ash Bark, Turkey Rhubarb Root, Cat's Claw Root, Bladderwrack, dandelion, hawthorn, thyme, calendula, comfrey and fenugreek. Consuming dandelion greens and roots can help to detox the body due to their high levels of antioxidants but also help to support liver lung.

ACTIVATED CHARCOAL — When biofilms are broken and unwanted pathogens in the gut are killed, a massive toxin load is unleashed which could lead to a Herxheimer reaction. To avoid this autotoxemia activated charcoal is useful for absorbing the toxins from pathogen die off and passing them through the stool.

ENZYMES

Enzymes do all the "work" in the body. Enzymes recharge the body's electricity and only live-foods are rich is oxygen and enzymes. Therefore it becomes apparent that live-food is a way to impart more consciousness, mind and morphic integrity into the body. Cooked-food creates blockages which obstruct the life force and creates conditions of acidity, cell suffocation, reduction in bio-charge and enzyme depletion which radically reduce the body's conscious potential.

Enzymes are catalysts critically necessary for transforming minerals into alkaline detoxifiers that neutralize acid and balance pH. In 1902 Dr. John Beard proposed that the pancreatic enzyme trypsin provides the primary defense against cancer. He theorized all cancer grows from misplaced placental stem cells that migrate to all tissues of the body and grow tumors under the right conditions…ie: acidity, low oxygen, toxins, mineral and enzyme deficiency.

After adulthood we need very little food as long as it is enzyme and nutrient dense, and full of lifeforce — like right out of the permaculture garden. Many foods contain an abundance of antioxidant enzymes. A daily smoothie with fresh aloe gel, papaya, banana, and greens will lessen the gaunt look. Plant-based enzymes (bromelain, lipase, catalase) can be added to ensure optimal utilization of all of the above nutrients and assist in the breakdown and removal of plaques. A pesto of soaked raw pumpkin seeds and cilantro is a standard in the chelation diet, as are all colorful fruits and vegetables, raw juices and sprouts.

Taking enzymes in your drinking water all day allows a deeper cleansing of the body. The enzymes prevent the stagnation and fermentation of food in the GI tract which prevents the conditions that foster yeasts and parasites, as well as bad bacteria and viruses in the bowel. With the extra enzymes food is digested, assimilated and eliminated faster and so the immune system is stronger and helps to maintain ecological balance. Best things for lymphatic drainage is rebounding, alternating hot and cold, enzymes such as bromelain and papain and plenty of water for making lymph less morbid and sticky. You can also mix the enzymes with water or aloe and put on your face overnight for a deep cleanse and exfoliating resurfacing of your skin.

Papain (papaya) and Bromelain (pineapple) enzymes can be brought from herbalcom.com. Proteolytic enzymes serrapeptidase, lumbrokinase, nattokinase. Pure powders are better than pills as they don't have fillers, sugar or flavoring. Put the enzymes in a salt-shaker to sprinkle on food; put into herb, detox and chelation formulas for better assimilation. These enzymes fight inflammation, heal fibrosis (scar tissues), and viruses; modulate the immune system; and cleanse the blood. First do the enzymes along with EDTA.

KIWIFRUIT—Raw kiwifruit is rich in the protein-dissolving enzyme actinidin, (in the same family of thiol proteases as papain), which is commercially useful as a meat tenderizer. Health properties of actinidin include anti-inflammatory, anticancer, anti-calcium and mucoid plaque, digestive aid. Consuming two to three kiwifruit daily for 28 days significantly reduced platelet aggregation and blood triglyceride levels, potentially reducing the risk of blood clots. Kiwifruit could be a good source of proteinases in countries which do not grow papaya and pineapple. An 8-10 Kiwi fruit smoothie is an excellent internal cleanse.

FIBRINOLYTIC ENZYMES—Dissolve Biofilms With Fibrinolytic, Proteolytic Enzymes that break down proteins. In particular serratiopeptidase and trypsin have been studied for the ability to mitigate the formation of biofilms. Enzymes, like DNase I, α-amylase and DspB are biofilm-dispersing agents that degrade the biofilm matrix, permitting increased penetration of antibiotic herbs. **Banana tree stem juice** is one of the best dissolvers of fibrin.

Biofilms almost always consist of a mixture of microbes including many different species of Candida, fungi, bacteria, protozoa, and parasites. For example, more than 500 different species of bacteria have been found in dental plaque biofilms. Protease enzymes cut through biofilms: bromelain (pineapple enzyme), papain (papaya enzyme), ground papaya seed, Kiwifruit, and Serrapeptase (silkworm"enzyme) and Nattokinase derived from Natto. Another enzyme that cuts through biofilms is lumbrokinase, which is derived from the common earthworm, Lumbricus rubellus. Lumbrokinase or earthworm fibrinolytic enzymes (EFE), is a more potent enzyme preparation than nattokinase.

Chitosanase breaks through the exoskeleton (called Chitin), or outer wall of the fungi in our gut, attacks it and is thereby able to kill yeast. Enzymes strip the off protective protein coating so that the underlying positive charged cancer cell is exposed—whereupon the immune system can recognize and target the cancer cell. Remember the same terrain conditions that foster candida foster cancer! Take Candex and other biofilm/candida enzymes between meals.

NEUROENDOCRINE INTERRUPTERS

We are under daily assault by the deliberate use of endocrine disruptors and immune-depressants by desperate governments acting under the direction of the United Nations and its agencies and aided by the military-industrial complex for the sake of preserving international peace by controlling population growth and ensuring citizen compliance (dumbing down). The endocrine disruptors in the chemtrails not only impair consciousness and increase aging and disease symptoms, they also reduce fertility.

We can now see how the chemo-industrial culture has set up a perfect storm of eugenics and depopulation; reducing fertility on every possible front from spermicidal corn and endocrine disruption chemicals throughout agriculture, to aluminum rich Gardasil vaccines, to plastics and nanometal aerosols from the skies. Even if there were no chemtrails, we would still be undone by the inescapable chemo-toxic environment of so called modern civilization.

Atrazine is an endocrine disrupter that the abominable Monsanto advises farmers to mix in with their Roundup herbicide. Atrazine, commonly found in the water supply.causes a kind of "chemical castration" that is one of the factions leading to a precipitous drop in birth rate, and the birth of male babies as atrazine is a androgen blocker, ie: it reduces testosterone. This leads to the rise in transgender and gay numbers, which again reduces breeding rates. The lowering of neurohormonal potency and psychosexual development decreases the maturation and realization of the fully actualized HUman. This metabolic chaos lowers our spiritual empowerment and executive function necessary to "get us out of this mess."

The delicate protein structures of enzymes do all the work in the body. The 55,000 to as many as 75,000 thousand different enzymes in the human body not only break down food, they are biocatalysts critical for transforming minerals into alkaline detoxifiers that neutralize acid and balance pH. The enzymes require the correct bioavailable minerals without competition from toxic and radioactive minerals from chemtrails and other pollution sources.

Much of the world, are being poisoned since 1945 with endocrine disruptors that are inserted in water, food, beverages and dental as well as cosmetic products so as to turn the basic elements of life into weapons of mass sterility, while immune-depressants delivered through vaccines, drugs and GMOs increase morbidity and mortality, and in this fashion bring the number of births and the number of deaths in equilibrium, which results in stable populations. And it is this hypocrisy that gave rise to the concept of "plausible deniability," a defense strategy term that like nuclear deterrence makes the civilian population the target of military operations.

The human brain's preservation and evolution represents the only possible of survival for mankind. Thus we must directly address the chronic assault of breathing/absorbing billions of tons of hazardous aerosolized chemicals and heavy metals over more than a decade without our informed consent. Heavy metals in our air, water, and topsoil lead to a rise in chronic diseases, learning disorders, cancer, dementia, and premature aging. The poisoning starts from before conception.

Heavy metals poison us by disrupting our cellular enzymes, which incorporate nutritional minerals. Once in the body, they compete with and displace essential minerals such as iodine, zinc, copper, magnesium, and calcium, and interfere with organ system function. Toxic metals kick out the nutrients and bind to their receptor sites, causing diffuse symptoms by affecting nerves, hormones, digestion, and immune function.

The reason why people age is that they accumulate greater toxicity over time causing more damage to the mitochondria and less energy is produced for detoxification, metabolism and repair. Toxins, such as mercury and other heavy metals, can severely damage the mitochondria and prevent them from receiving the nutrition they requires to function, in turn causing us to have less and less energy throughout the years as we accumulate more and more toxins. Magnesium is present in all cells of the body and is involved in over 300 enzymatic processes, including energy production. A magnesium deficiency may be responsible for more diseases than any other nutrient.

"Magnesium and potassium are mainly intracellular ions, sodium and calcium are mainly extracellular ions. When cells are excited, stressed, or de-energized, they lose magnesium and potassium, and take up sodium and calcium. The mitochondria can bind a certain amount of calcium during stress, but accumulating calcium can reach a point at which it inactivates the mitochondria, forcing cells to increase their inefficient glycolytic energy production, producing an excess of lactic acid. Abnormal calcification begins in the mitochondria." Raymond Peat, PhD.

Calcification is a component of thousands illnesses and is a component of "all" degenerative disease. Magnesium inhibits hydroxyapatite formation in the extracellular space, thereby preventing calcification of vascular smooth muscle cells — magnesium can help clear out arterial calcification while reducing damage to the vascular system.

Since the brain uses 20% of the body's energy, when energy generation is impaired that is when we start getting depression, poor cognitive function, dementia and fatigue. Heavy metals such as those from chemtrails (aluminum, barium, strontium and titanium) exhaust the body's antioxidant system promoting the terrain for cancer, fungi and other pathogens. The opportunistic fungus Candida albicans takes advantage of an immunosuppressed state and increases the risk of cancer genesis and metastasis via the production of carcinogenic by-products and triggering of inflammation.

Fluoride, microwave, WiFi and cell phone radiation increase the permeability of the blood-brain barrier (BBB) allowing more aluminum and other toxic heavy metals into the brain. Microwave pollution as well as the Glyphosate in Roundup produces leaky gut as well as leaky Blood Brain Barrier, which increases the assimilation and damage from harmful chemotoxic agents and poisons from opportunistic pathogens that thrive in an immunosuppressed body. Avoiding gluten and cereals in general and drinking bone broth on a regular basis help to restore the GI lining from leaky gut.

Fungal disease now represents 12-15% of all hospital-acquired infections The 10,000 years of agriculture and cereal production has led to the fungal takeover of the body and brain by candida and to general dysbiosis which contributes to our insanity as a culture. As a consequence of cooked food Western culture, most of us have an orgy of fungi, parasites, and other opportunistic organisms in our brain and our body waiting to be fed by sugar.

Childhood trauma, current trauma, abuse, deprivation, insufficient novelty, lack of change, boredom and plain old self-abuse and addiction all make us crave bad sugars, bread and alcohol...in order to feed candida fungi and make us go more unconscious. The trick is to be compassionate about our suffering, to sit with it and feel it, to cherish it and to find healthy ways to destress and grow. If we cannot deal with the slings and arrows of this world we use self-damaging methods to zone out and avoid the integration of our suffering, then rather than growing to a level of self-resourcefulness where we can avoid harmful situations before they happen, or quickly recover when they do, we end up with a life of endless suffering and very little pleasure, satisfaction or mastery.

The more we abuse ourselves, the more others abuse us. If we are slave to life harming compulsions we remain a slave. We give up being a slave when we become our own beneficent master. I was wondering why we reach for sugar and carbohydrates when fear increases. I assume that after shock, trauma, attack, abuse...or in anticipation of danger, we reach for "quick fuel" in case our animal body needs quick energy to fight or flight. Thus, the way to get around this biological programming, would be to self-soothe in healthy ways in which you get adequate exercise and oxygenation that meets the intensity of the level of distress. After several times of doing this...acknowledging the stress response and Meta-adapting by going running/jumping jacks/calisthenics, and doing something positive like sungazing, yoga or meditation etc... we will no longer use life-harming means to deal with distress in our lives. It is then we will begin the path of accruing self-mastery, emancipation, sovereignty and Spirit.

Most people with high levels of heavy metals also have a high load of candida (which is also called fungus or yeast), parasites, viruses and bad bacteria. The heavy metals will severely weaken the immune system, making it easy for infections and opportunistic organisms like candida and parasites to multiply and overgrow. These organisms will ferociously feed on sugars, specifically glucose, fructose, and sucrose, and it is extremely more challenging to get rid of them without quitting sugar. Quitting sugar is essential to detoxification, and it is something you can do for free. That includes all "natural" sugar, from fruits, honey, agave cereals and carbohydrates.

Aluminum poisoning causes candida to flourish, because heavy metals collect in the biofilms and shelter Candida making it harder to get rid of. Yeast and candida are now recognized as an immune system response against lead, aluminum, excess iron, and especially mercury. They also will use these metals to transport their spores throughout the body. If you do not cleanse yourself of the heavy metals and you do have excess metals in your system, you will not be able to get rid of your yeast infections and candida. When the candida population reaches a certain point, it suppresses the production of neurotransmitters such as serotonin, thus leading to depression, anxiety, and other mental health problems.

Sovereign empowerment requires a strong neuroendocrine and immune system. Heavy metals like aluminum, lead and mercury deplete magnesium, and magnesium deficiency has been proven to be a direct cause of premature ejaculation, erectile dysfunction, and is associated with poor sexual health and lower testosterone levels. Toxins reduce the connectivity between the sex organs, heart, the brain and the spirit. Toxins in the brain can hinder our intelligence, lower our IQ, make us stupid, impulsive, reactive, irrational, emotional, needy, unfocused, unable to concentrate, easily distractible, irritable, forgetful, indecisive, and less resourceful.

Thrival involves promoting the organism's strategic adaptation to different kinds of environmental assaults. Ultimately our thrival as individuals necessitates that we live in an ecologically sane culture. Healing the environment and restoring ecological function is essential to maintaining a sustainable and evolving socioeconomy and to eliminate war. The people need to demand permaculture and land restorative experts come in and design systems for preventing effluent and toxic seepage from farmland, by increasing permacultural methods such as mulch, ground cover, soil organic matter, creating marshland filter systems from farms, gravel beds, and methane plants with fertilizer byproducts. The more sensitive and vulnerable the landscape, the more intelligent the land management systems need to be. Only laziness and stupidity leads to the collapse of environmental systems — we humans are actually smarter than that.

See YouTube *Healing the Earth* by John D. Liu

4

OPERATION INFLAMMATION

ATTACK ON GAIA'S IMMUNE SYSTEM

Inflammation is the immune system's defensive response to injury. Inflammation is a process by which the body's white blood cells produce cytokines and free radicals to protect us from infection with foreign organisms, such as bacteria and viruses. During chronic inflammation and autoimmune diseases the body's normally protective immune system causes inflammation damage to its own tissues. But chronic inflammation can also occur in response to unwanted substances in the body, such as nanometals from chemtrails, toxins from cigarette smoke or even excess of fat cells (especially fat in the belly area). Inside arteries, inflammation helps kick off atherosclerosis, and tumor proliferation and metastasis may occur when inflammatory cytokines create a microenvironment conducive to cancer progression. Chronic inflammation leads to cognitive decline, digestive dysfunction, muscle loss, weight gain, accelerated aging, joint pain and loss of mobility.

Aluminum is one of the only elements which has no positive biological function. Which is unusual for one of the main principles of nature is that of using everything available in a "positive" sense. Aluminum is an adjuvant that increases autoimmune problems and allergies and creates such inflammation in the brain that it leads to ischemia, autism and dementia. The reason why aluminum is added to vaccines as it has the remarkable ability "to turn the body's own defensive resources against itself!" An adjuvant is a substance (like mercury) that is added to a vaccine to increase the body's immune response to the vaccine.

The geoengineers are dumping 20 million tonnes of Aluminum Oxide into the atmosphere annually which will make one out of two kids born have Autism within ten years and a large majority of the adults will have dementia. Nano aluminum from chemtrails is inhaled and goes through the nasal passages and into the bloodstream of the brain, thereby contributing to brain fog and Alzheimer's. In the USA Alzheimer's is up almost 90% since the year 2000.

The aluminum in the chemtrail aerosols acts like an adjuvant to the bacteria, fungi, and viruses in the air, prolonging the body's inflammatory response to pathogens. Thus everyday as we breathe nanometals taken directly into the brain's blood supply through the intranasal passages, we are being vaccinated without our consent!

Humanity is obviously engaged in a war-without-end against itself, and all life on earth! We must ask ourselves why we are all getting arthritic inflammatory pain? For the answer we must look to the skies. The intranasal route of exposure makes spraying of massive amounts of nano-aluminum into the skies especially hazardous, as it will be inhaled by people of all ages, including babies and small children for many hours. We know that young and older people have the greatest reaction to this airborne aluminum. Because of the Nano sizing of the aluminum particles being used, home filtering system will not remove the aluminum, thus prolonging exposure, even indoors. Exposure to aluminum stops the maturation of eggs in the ovaries and may be a significant factor in falling sperm counts and reduced male fertility.

If we don't put a stop to the chemtrail nonsense, aluminum poisoning may be the death of us all!

INFLAMMATION & EUDAIMONIC HAPPINESS

Chemtrails are both inflammatory and infectious both leading to dysregulated cytokines and inflammatory-stress response. Inflammation in the body and brain represents static, interference or "Noise" that reduces the clarity of our consciousness, deflates our "Presence" and undermines our charisma, will and our influence. The inflammatory response and cellular inflammation basically translates as intracellular stress and oxidation, which ultimately damages our mitochondria and reduces our ATP energy production. Numerous stressful conditions activate kinases that activate a gene expression program known as the integrated stress response.

Besides a stress reducing, anti-inflammatory diet and lifestyle, perhaps the principal way that we hold ourselves together against the aging effects of inflammation is focusing on the apex of Maslow's Hierarchy of Needs pyramid, that is on improvement of the self, with self-actualization being the apex of self-improvement. Research is finding that happiness that is derived either by the **hedonic approach**, or pleasure attainment and pain avoidance, is surmounted or the **eudaimonic approach**, which focuses on meaning and self-realization and defines well-being in terms of the degree to which a person is fully functioning.

We reduce the psychoneuroimmune, inflammatory stress response by actualizing our potential and becoming all we can be by engaging in artistic, creative long term goals and engaging in compelling a philanthropic purpose that is "larger" than our personal sphere. Thus increase neurogenesis, hormonal fitness, cognitive optimization and longevity when we substantiate and become fully HUman by amplifying self-actualization.

Presence, charisma, a soul-fulfilling lifestyle, along with good circadian and hormonal health including the capacity for deep restorative sleep requires our body to have a low level of inflammation. Once you come ALIVE, you magnetize or hypnotize your audience to come alive also through quantum resonance, which acts at the scalar level. A sympathetic resonant entrainment that includes the electromagnetic spectrum, but goes beyond it and spreads out like a radiant sun to influence consciousness around the globe. We reduce the psychoneuroimmune, inflammatory stress response by actualizing our potential and becoming all we can be by engaging in artistic, creative long term goals and engaging in compelling a philanthropic purpose that is "larger" than our personal sphere. We thrive and youthify by following our eudaimonic muse and establishing a creative lifestyle along with an anti-inflammatory diet, based on the rawfood and Mediterranean diets. We are what we eat! That which is living, with a high vibratory rate, greatest strength and resilience is the best food for supporting the evolutionary force.

Know Thyself and Become What You Are: A Eudaimonic Approach to Psychological Well-Being, Carol D. Ryff and Burton H. Singer

• *How of Happiness,* by Sonja Lyubomirsky thehowofhappiness.com/

• Love 2.0: How Our Supreme Emotion Affects Everything We Feel, Think, Do, and Become, by Barbara Fredrickson

IMMUNE-INFLAMMATORY-STRESS RESPONSE

Nano-sized aluminum and other nano metals from chemtrails etc... greatly increases inflammation and oxidation, that is rusting of the body! It is interesting how the heavy metals, aluminum and pathogens offer a 1,2,3 punch against us. Fortifying ourselves from this chemo-toxic culture requires a new approach to existence and the re-evaluation of our own lives. We intuitively feel, we have to get over our wounds and addictions and to strengthen our immunity, our collagen and our minds and hearts. Never before has Mankind had to deal with such clandestine deadly forces and foes. Only by caring for and cherishing our own lives, can we care for and support the whole. Let us take up this fight not with fear, but with the staunch power of the righteous.

Connective tissue is the structural matrix of the organs. Its main protein is collagen, which may thus be 30-40% of all the proteins of the body. Even the scaffolding matrix for the bone is 90% comprised of collagen protein. Since the body is essentially built from collagen, maintaining our youth and vitality is reliant on building and maintaining strong, elastic collagen. Inflammation releases proinflammatory cytokine proteins, which destroy collagen. Cytokines are a large group of proteins, peptides or glycoproteins that are signaling molecules that mediate and regulate immunity, inflammation and hematopoiesis.

Proinflammatory cytokines are produced predominantly by activated macrophages and are involved in the up-regulation of inflammatory reactions that inhibit collagen production and breakdown existing collagen. What is more inflammatory cytokines stimulate cells to synthesize other inflammatory cytokines...fueling the inflammatory fire. These inflammatory, degrading, and catabolic processes lead to the progressive degeneration of the connective tissue resulting in osteoarthritis of the joints, osteoporosis, spinal degeneration, aging skin and degenerating the structure and function of the organs.

When you eat sugar, it triggers the release of pro-inflammatory molecules called cytokines that rev up the fire inside you. To prevent this inflammation choose to avoid sugar and certain inflammatory foods like gluten and dairy products, processed meats, artificial sweeteners, trans fats, fried foods, soybean oil and vegetable oil, processed soyburgers, snack foods, such as chips and crackers. To maintain strong, elastic and youthful collagen include plenty of these anti-inflammatory foods in your diet: tomatoes, virgin olive oil, green leafy vegetables, such as spinach, kale, and collards, nuts like almonds and walnuts, fatty fish like salmon, mackerel, tuna, and sardines, raw organic fruits such as strawberries, blueberries, cherries, and oranges.

Inflammation generated by the immune cells occurs across the board in all degenerative diseases including cognitive dysfunction including autism, depression and schizophrenia. Autism and Alzheimer's = inflammation. Leaky Gut and gut inflammation leads to brain inflammation and leaky Blood Brain Barrier. Also, the microbiome has been shown to alter brain development and modulate behavior and cognition in animals through gut-brain connections. Microorganisms make up 90 % of the human body, and they contain around 100 times the number of genes in the human genome, cumulatively weighing approximately the same as a human brain.

Stress proteins (heat shock proteins) are a diverse group of proteins that are synthesized at increased levels by cells exposed to a variety of stressful stimuli and which have a protective effect against the stress. Cytokines release a chemical signal to the immune system to fight against the cause of the damage or threat. Cytokines are produced by a broad range of cells, including immune cells like macrophages, B lymphocytes, T lymphocytes and mast cells, as well as endothelial cells, fibroblasts, and various stromal cells; a given cytokine may be produced by more than one type of cell.

Cytokines act through receptors, and are especially important in the immune system; cytokines modulate the balance between humoral and cell-based immune responses, and they regulate the maturation, growth, and responsiveness of particular cell populations. Some cytokines enhance or inhibit the action of other cytokines in complex ways. They are important in health and disease, specifically in host responses to infection, immune responses, inflammation, trauma, sepsis, cancer, and reproduction.

In many cases, inflammation is your body's response to stress. Therefore, reducing "fight-or-flight" responses in the nervous system and lowering biological markers for stress can also reduce inflammation. Engaging the **vagus nerve** and improving "vagal tone" can be achieved through daily habits such as yoga and meditation. Deep diaphragmatic breathing—with a long, slow exhale—is key to stimulating the vagus nerve and slowing heart rate and blood pressure, especially in times of performance anxiety.

Civilization has increased the pro-inflammatory omega-6 fatty acid found in cereals, most vegetable oils, baked goods, and margarine triggers an inflammatory cascade...which is one of the key reasons why the 12 thousand year agricultural basis of civilization is degenerating humanity in body, mind and soul. We would be further along in our evolution if Homo sapiens had not eaten meat (putrefaction), had not grown cereals and made sugar (fermentation and fungi), had not cooked food (lack of enzymes and nutrition), had not worn shoes (lack of grounding), had not demineralized the soils and had not fluoridated the water etc... Now we must develop lifestyles that rectify the inflammatory assaults so that we can regenerate our "whole" being.

Inflammation lies at the heart of the degenerative Metabolic X Syndrome by causing oxidative stress-related DNA fragmentation, receptor damage, insulin resistance, microvascular degeneration and ossification of the tissues. A general loss of energy, numbness and corresponding nihilism, inability to focus ie: discombobulation, cognitive dissonance—combined with a "follower," herd or crowd mentality—means that the majority of the world's population are sitting sheep for the globalists evil plans.

ANTI-INFLAMMATORY LIFESTYLE

CEASE AND DESIST: To establish an anti-inflammatory lifestyle you need to drop the inflammatory foods including wheat bread, refined flour, fried foods, processed oils, dairy, sugar, artificial sweeteners, artificial additives and establish an anti-inflammatory diet, learning from both the rawfood and Mediterranean diet.

GRASS FED ANIMAL PRODUCTS: Avoid "grain" fed industrial animal foods as they are high in Omega-6 which creates inflammation in the body.

LIVER: Improving liver function promotes the effective detoxification of heavy metals and other toxins, thereby lowering inflammation. Raw Thistle Seed porridge, milk thistle extract, chicory leaves and root, dandelion root, garlic mustard and other cabbage family, and NAC.

DHA Omega-3 is anti-inflammatory, with Ratfish Oil being the single most antioxidant oil. Krill Oil is a good second. Oily fish and fish oil (from cold water fish such as salmon, herring, cod, trout and sardines. Super antioxidants, chlorophyll and colorful plant pigments (phytochemicals) and olive leaf will protect the Omega-3 and allow its healthy incorporation into cells. Dr Jack Kruse says vegan supplements of DHA Omega-3 are contaminated with aldehyde.

EXTRA VIRGIN OLIVE OIL: Extra virgin olive oil, has been shown to lower the number of chemicals in the body that cause inflammation, in much the same way that ibuprofen does. Oleuropein present in olive oil and olives has major anti-tumor activity. Olive Leaf contains phenolic compounds that are anti-inflammatory, antibacterial, antifungal, antioxidant, anti-atherogenic, activity; anti-hypertensive and anticancer.

HUMAN BLOOD ACID: Alkali ratio needs to be at pH 7.365. Anything below 7 (acidic, anaerobic) = inflammation and disease. Pathogens thrive in oxygenless (hypoxic) environments. The same, unnatural, oxygenless cardiovascular environments of those who've been duped into consuming the cooked/processed Standard American Diet suffer chronic dehydration, chronic inflammation, acidosis, lack of oxygen, telomere-shortening, and poor DNA repair. High sugar/carb diet feeds low-grade infections such as Candida yeast and bacterial overgrowth in the gut; a low-grade infection slowly drains the body's energy by repeatedly tapping into your immune-inflammatory and stress response system. You can control and eliminate infections in the body by eating fermented foods and drinking probiotic beverages.

ALKALINIZE: Inflammation is an acidifying process so increase the raw greens, vegetable juices, sprouts and microgreens to counteract acid pH and remineralize.

OXYGENATE: Oxygenating alkalinizes the blood, thus chlorophyll, deep breathing, exercise and other methods help reduce acidification, stagnation and blockage of metabolism. Sulfur and selenium are oxygen carrying minerals that transport oxygen across the cell membrane. http://jana-sovereignstate.blogspot.com/2011/04/methods-of-oxygen-increase.html

GROUNDING: Lying on the grass and hanging out in negative ion environments like near waterfalls and moving water will reduce blood pressure and inflammation. The earth is the most anti-inflammatory source of negative ions; an endless supply of antiaging healing. Make sure you get grounding/earthing—as it is needed for immunity and bone/teeth health.

HABITAT MODIFICATION: Plants, negative ion generator and indoor water fountain, along with amber lighting and alpha frequency music will help make the home environment more fitting for Thrival.

BLOOD CLEANSING HERBS: Burdock Root, Basil, Burbur (Manayupa), Dandelion, Garlic, Guduchi stem, Kawakawa, Manjistha root, Milk thistle, Neem leaf, Reishi Mushroom, Red Clover, Stinging nettles, Turmeric.

FRUITS AND VEGETABLES: Fruits and vegetables contain antioxidants that can help reduce inflammation. Specifically, green leafy vegetables rich in vitamin K like spinach, kale and broccoli dramatically reduce markers in the blood that indicate inflammation. Research has also shown that kiwifruit, cherries, strawberries and other red and purple fruits have an anti-inflammatory effect.

ENZYMES: A raw colorful enzyme rich diet is the foundations of the anti-inflammation lifestyle. Fermented vegetables, Miso and GcMAF Bravo yogurt both reduce your appetite and lower inflammation. Enzymes are anti-inflammatory if taken away from meal time. If taken with meals they act as digestive aids. Take Betaine after meals for better absorption.

VITAMIN D: Vitamin D3, K2 and sunshine reduces inflammation and pain, builds bones and operates at the DNA level to regulate genes that reduce inflammation.

METHYLATION: Garlic Mustard (Alliaria officinalis) a weed from the cabbage family, is the most nutritious plant on the planet, especially for methylation of toxins in liver and brain, DNA methylation, anti-inflammation and regeneration.

IODINE FOR THYROID: An anti-inflammatory lifestyle is critical for full recovery from autoimmune hypothyroidism. Most of us are deficient in iodine, needed for metabolism, cardiolipin, hormones, antioxidant, antibacterial, antifungal, anti-radiation functions and to reduce candida and prevent cancer. Iodine and kelp is anti-cancer and anti-inflammatory. Buy Lugol's tincture and Norwegian kelp (Southern Hemisphere Kelp if possible). David Brownstein, author of "Iodine: optimally he recommends 50mg of iodine/potassium Iodide (Lugol's or iodoral) per day; at 2%, then 1 drop Lugol's is about 5 mg. Lugol's can be used on toenails for fungi and mixed with topical remedies for absorption through the skin. (See Dr. Robert Cassar's YouTube videos).

STRUCTURED WATER: Aging and disease is accelerated by dehydration and dead stagnant body fluid, and the wrong types of cooked and rancid fats in the cell membranes. The younger our food, the younger our cells…as the energized structured water in young living things is the most life giving (fructifying). Therefore living sprouts and microgreens, and plant shoots are the most youthifying of foods. Silicon rich Philosopher's Water and Shungite charged water is highly anti-inflammatory. I think it important to drink "hungry" water while removing heavy metals and other toxins from the body, thus drink distilled, but charging with shungite and adding a little Himalayan salt. Low Deuterium water is highly anti-inflammatory!

DETOXING FROM SUGAR: Epsom salts and baking soda baths, spray skin with Magnesium chloride topical sol in water, chromium, cinnamon and devils claw to adjust insulin chemistry, ginger root tea to reduce GI inflammation, sunbathing to increase energy and cleansing, raw-greens to detox and rebuild, spirulina/kelp to remineralize. You can use either coconut oil, or Vitamin C as a glucose fuel substitute as they are similar molecules and the Vitamin C will not only help you detox and give you energy it also fills up opiate receptors thereby reducing detox pain. B-complex and magnesium to assist in energy and mood. Sugar substitutes for Lyme and Morgellons: Stevia, Mesquite Flour and Lucuma. Bitters tincture helps to train the pallet off of sugar. Bitters, lemon juice and ginger tea are fantastic allies in overcoming a sweet tooth.

ANTI-INFLAMMATORY LIST

Astaxanthin, a red carotenoid from algae, has super star status as a painkiller, antioxidant and anti-inflammatory. Other inflammation quenchers are Angelica, Artemisia, Astragalus, Avocado leaves, Bromelain, Boswellia (frankincense), Basil, Black haw, Black Cumin Seed Oil, Bone set, Bupleurum, Cat's Claw, Celery seed, Cordyceps, Chamomile, Chaparral, Echinacea, Fenugreek, Flaxseed, FoTi, Frankincense, Myrrh, Gentian, Ginger, Goldenseal, Grape Seed extract, Green Tea, Horsetail, Juniper, Larch, Licorice root, Lion's mane mushroom, Marshmallow, Meadowsweet, Mistletoe, Plantain major, Raspberry Leaf, Rehmannia, Red Sage, Rhodiola, Rosemary, St John's wort, Sarsaparilla, Skullcap and Schisandra berry, Turmeric, White Willow. NAC and Epigallocatechin gallate (EGCG), Royal Jelly.

Drinking 6 cups of homemade ginger tea, ginger beer, or ginger-lemonade Master Cleanser per day should quickly eliminate cranky joints and aching muscles. It will cure the fuzzy head by settling the stomach and cutting inflammation in the brain. Combine turmeric, ginger and black pepper to reduce inflammation. Astaxanthin is an anti-inflammatory red carotenoid pigment from algae that is one of the world's strongest antioxidants; it's 5,000 times stronger than vitamin C.

He Shou Wu is anti-inflammatory and helps maintain the strength and stability of the lower back and knees. FoTi is shown to significantly increase levels of SOD (Superoxide Dismutase) and protects DNA from damage. If everyone took FoTi and looked after their adrenal glands, liver and kidneys they would not feel the need to extort or parasitize energy from others.

Polyphenols and flavonoids within avocados have anti-inflammatory properties. Avocados contain the antioxidant glutathione that can be absorbed into our mitochondria and then neutralize the free radicals, prevents heart disease, cancer and slows the signs of aging. The super antioxidant-rich red berry of the coffee bean plant has an **oxygen radical absorption capacity** of 16,000, compared to the ORAC of blueberries which is only 2,400. Horsetail is known for its anti-inflammatory, antibacterial, anti-hemorrhagic and analgesic properties.

PULSATILLA KOREANA: The Pulsatilla Koreana is a hairy, flowering perennial herb native to Korea. A member of the buttercup family Pulsatilla shows high concentrations of an active compound called Saponin. Saponins possess incredibly high anti-inflammatory, anti-parasitic and eliminating infections. Pulsatilla saponin D also shows potent antitumor effect by inhibiting DNA polymerase.

WHITE PEONY ROOT: White peony (Bai Shao Yao) is thought to be the oldest and most important herbal remedy in traditional Chinese medicine (TCM) to help nourish and regenerate the blood, which frees up the spirit, inducing a more restful sleep and relaxed mind. White peony also has anti-inflammatory and analgesic properties and is often used to treat chronic painful autoimmune diseases such as rheumatoid arthritis, lupus and psoriasis. White peony cleans and builds the blood and calms the liver, also for pain, headache and dizziness.

SOPHORA ROOT: Sophora Root (Ku Shen or Shan Dou Gen) can be used both internally and externally. Internally, it can kill some parasites, treat dysentery and some bacterial infections, and promote the production of urine. Externally, it can be applied to the skin to improve blood flow, treat scabies, eczema and other skin ailments. Sophora Root is used in formulas for painful swelling in the throat, mouth, and gums, to clear lung heat, to alleviate constipation, and to resolve masses (including carcinoma). Sophora Root removes toxic materials in many herbs, stops pain, reduces inflammation, soothes the lungs and stops cough. It cures pharyngitis when sucked, eliminates abdominal distension when ground and taken orally, when taken with red wine it relieves female abdominal distention due to blood stasis, and treats baldness, squeezed to get juice it is applied to wounds, bites and infections. For esophageal cancer and pharyngeal cancer, Sophora Root is ground with ginger for sucking.

LOTUS LEAF: Lotus leaf extract, when combined with L-carnitine, may offer some relief for obesity-related diseases. The mixture was shown to prevent the formation of fatty tissue (adipogenesis). Lotus leaf slowed the absorption of fat and carbohydrates, increased energy expenditure and accelerated fat metabolism. Lotus leaves contain high concentrations of phytochemical compounds (flavonoids and tannins and isoquinoline alkaloids) that have antioxidant, sedative, antipathogen and antispasmodic properties, which aid digestion, weight loss and cardiovascular health.

GINGER ROOT: Ginger root in combo with Turmeric root has been shown to inhibit cancer growth, be anti-inflammatory, anti-arthritic, effective against asthma and allergies. One of the best supplements you can take for all health ailments. Ginger Root Supplement administered to volunteer participants reduced inflammation markers in the colon and nausea from chemotherapy within weeks. Ginger contains a chemical that is used as an ingredient in antacid, laxative and anti-gas medications. Daily ginger tea reduces muscle, joint, digestive and neurological pain. Homemade ginger beer is another way to get ginger in your diet.

TURKEY TAIL MUSHROOM: Coriolus versicolor (Trametes versicolor) or Yun Zhi. Turkey Tail has been used as a tonic in Chinese Medicine for centuries. This well-researched medicinal mushroom is a biological response modifier. Turkey Tail Mushroom suppresses inflammatory bacteria while enhancing good bacteria, thereby greatly enhancing the body's immune system. Studies show that it improves cancer survival rates and acts an immune modulator with immune stimulating and anti-tumor properties. Use of Turkey Tail mushroom for breast cancer can enhance the effects of chemotherapy cancer treatment and reduce the side effects of radiation therapy.

ALLANTOIN: Asian medicine has made use of yams (Dioscorea spp.) for eons. Yam tubers contain allantoin, vitamins, polyphenols, flavonoids, mannans, fibers and three enzymatic hydrolysates (pepsin, trypsin and papain). Antioxidant rich Chinese yam (Dioscorea oppositifolia) significantly increases superoxide dismutase and contains chitinase so can be used as an antifungal. Raw yam contains highly viscous manna-protein molecules, and can be used to enhance the growth of Lactobacillus acidophilus. Uric acid has an antioxidative effect, producing allantoin in a nonenzymatic reaction with uric acid as the level of free radicals in the body increases during exercise.

Allantoin is one of the active principles contained in yam that is said to extend life of rats by more than a fifth, according to one study. The 'miracle' ingredient, allantoin, is also found in comfrey root (knit bone), tobacco seed, chamomile, wheat sprouts, the cabbage family, plus the root bark of Birthwort, Virginia snakeroot, and Uva Ursi. The compound promotes skin cell growth and encourages skin to regenerate and is added to many moisturizers and anti-aging creams. Chinese yam can also help with diabetes, by decreasing plasma glucose, and modulating oxidative stress, antioxidant activities, and lipid profiles. Antioxidant rich Chinese yam contain maximum allantoin in tubers after 170 days growing. See YouTube videos by **Dr. John Bergman**

OLIGOMERIC PROANTHOCYANIDINS: OPC's are a set of bioflavonoid complexes that perform as free radical scavengers in the human body. These polyphenols are found in a variety of plants such as citrus skin, grapeseed, pinebark, cocoa beans, apples, cinnamon, Aronia berries, and sea buckthorn berries. They have many healing properties such as improved Vitamin C utilization, skin hydration, UV protection, strengthening blood vessels, improving eyesight and supporting the collagen and elastin of the skin.

PYCNOGENOL is a water extract from the bark of the French maritime pine. Pycnogenol contains bioflavonoids that stimulate the cells to produce more anti-oxidative enzymes and free radical scavengers and protects endogenous vitamin E and glutathione from oxidative stress. It also protects the nerve cells against beta-amyloid and glutamate induced toxicity, accelerates wound healing processes, reduces scar formation, decreases histamine release from mast cells, inhibits pro-inflammatory cytokines, and protects DNA against oxidation.

MUCOPOLYSACCHARIDES: Glycosaminoglycans (GAGs) are endogenous organic compounds synthesized in most tissues of human body that play important roles in fundamental biological processes, mostly by binding to variety of proteins. Special nitrogen containing polysaccharide carbohydrates called mucopolysaccharides and Beta glucans prevent bacteria and viruses from finding binding sites. In fact, they literally trap and destroy them along with antibodies, thus halting infection caused disease and autoimmune diseases, while promoting growth and enhancing the immune system. Mucopolysaccharides are found in many of the foods including: Aloe vera, nutritional yeast and medicinal mushrooms (reishi, maitake, yucca root, okra, cordyceps, oysters, oats, Irish moss, mussels). The active polysaccharide fractions in aloe galactomannans or beta-glucomannans act as a bridge between foreign proteins (such as virus particles) and macrophage cells in the human body, facilitating the destruction of the invading the protein by the macrophage. Activating the receptor sites of the macrophages is also a key to the overall boosting of cell-mediated immunity. Mucopolysaccharide polysulfate (MPS) is used topically for the treatment of inflammatory disorders.

ACEMANNAN: Acemannan is a mannose rich polysaccharide which is found in the inner leaf gel of aloe vera plant. Acemannan is one of the major constituent groups of hemicellulose in the wall of specialized cells called a leucoplast. It's composed of mannose, glucose, and galactose monomers making it into a linear polysaccharide. This carbohydrate component of Aloe vera gel is a long chain sugar that gets incorporated into our cell membranes. This results in an increase in the fluidity and permeability of the membranes allowing toxins to flow out and nutrients to enter the cell more easily. Acemannan enhances the entire immune system, detoxify the body, repairs tissues and organs, improves digestion and helps with the destruction and elimination of invading bacteria, viruses, and parasites.

Aloe gel is best fresh from the plant and can be taken in smoothies. Acemannan upgrades the immune system by accumulating in, and nourishing, our large white blood cells called macrophages. Aloe vera gel contains only about 1% acemannan, and extracts are very expensive, so it would be preferable to eat the live gel by growing lots of Aloe vera in volcanic soil with rockdust, magnetite, shungite, etc... to increase the ORMUS factor.

The Most Important Paragraph in this book:

We can still thrive in the chemtrail holocaust if we adopt a stress reduction lifestyle, preemptively prevent the Chemtrail-Flu and assist in detoxification and rapid recovery. The first step of heavy metal cleansing is to remove your amalgams, increase your methylation (cabbage family), raise glutathione levels, and use broom fibers, clays, zeolite, algae-seaweeds and chelating foods like chlorella, spirulina and strawberries. The body's antioxidant system, immune and lymphatic system and detoxification organs must be up and running to a high degree of functioning before heavy metals can be safely and quickly escorted out of the body. Only then you can start with heavy metal chelating agents. All healing is kicked off with saunas, infrared red saunas, running, rebounding, skin brushing, colon hydrotherapy, coffee enemas, relaxing herb/Epsom salt baths, grounding, Nature, sunshine, natural diet, conscious breathing, right livelihood and spiritual "connection" practices.

Self-destruction, body-mind suppression and devitalization feeds the roots of fascism. The eugenics agenda demands that you must brain damage the slaves so you can feed on them without them squealing. Time to wake up people!

5

BIOLOGIC CHEMTRAILS

"There are hundreds of thousands of microbes surrounding us, but they cannot harm us unless we become weak, until the body is ready and predisposed to receive them." Vivekananda

The chemactivist Will Thomas, has reported findings of over 300 types of virally mutated fungi in the chemtrail fallout. It is suggested that the fungi and bacteria living in the upper atmosphere, mutated by the high UV levels, might piggy back to earth on the chemtrail chemicals. The Aluminum and Barium in chemtrails form a semiconductor (diode) plasma layer in the upper troposphere. This 800 foot high blanket of chemtrail particulate blocks microbes from the ocean from passing through to higher reaches of the troposphere and consequently atmospheric fungi, bacteria and viruses actually drops back down onto the earth (and us). The disruption of the jet streams and the raising and lowering of the atmospheric layers with atmospheric heaters (HAARP) may also create such turbulence that the upper atmospheric microbes are brought down to earth and represent a health threat in the form of "Thunderstorm Asthma" and virulent flus and sinus infections etc…

BUGS IN SPACE

According to a paper in the International Society for Microbial Ecology Journal a new study by scientists in Canada, Spain and the U.S. shows that viruses are swept up from the Earth's surface largely from sea spray into the free troposphere, beyond Earth's weather systems but below the stratosphere where jet airplanes fly. The viruses can be carried thousands of kilometers there before being deposited back onto the Earth's surface via dust storms from the Sahara, rains from the oceans and [chemtrails].

Everyday around 800 million viruses fall from the sky onto each square meter of the planet. The viruses are swept into the upper atmosphere from the ocean waves, and coast back down to earth on organic molecules, pollution or chemtrail aerosols. The deposition rates for viruses were up to 461 times greater than for bacteria, because viruses tend to hitch rides on smaller, lighter, organic particles suspended in the air so they can stay aloft in the atmosphere longer. See: *Deposition rates of viruses and bacteria above the atmospheric boundary layer.* The ISME Journal, 2018.

Viruses play a huge part in the regulation of the biosphere and even in evolution itself. In fact 40-80% of the human genome is said to be of viral origins. The fact that mutated pathogens naturally fall from the upper atmosphere obfuscates the fact that chemtrollers are spraying us with laboratory designed bioweapons. Regardless of whether it is incidental or intentional, chemtrails greatly increase the disease burden due in no small measure to the toxic burden and immune suppression.

UV mutated fungi spores naturally in the upper atmosphere taxi down to earth on the chemtrail aerosol particles. Plus chemtrails are said to contain many types of fungi, perhaps because fungi are used in the micronizing production process of the nanometals. Fungi secrete extracellular proteins which have been used to turn metal ions into metal nano-particles. If metal ions are mixed together with fungal hyphae rich in nitrate reductase enzyme and an organic carbon source, the metallic ions accrue and will eventually form nano-sized particles.

With cross-genera disease agents and nano machines that build fibers out of the elements of living creatures we are entering an experience of the world, which no previous generation of humans ever had to endure. Transcending the fungal aspect of chemtrails is fundamental, due to the loss of immune strength from heavy metal exposure and the fact that candida and other fungi collect and store heavy metals in their structures, preventing their elimination from the body. The infection of the brain with candida sp. etc... in association with heavy metal and radionuclide sequestration in the beta-amyloid plaque formations and other biofilms makes recovery from chemtrail fallout the most pressing health crisis we face in the world today, especially so since fungi are an intrinsic component in the concoction of the chemtrail formulas.

The chemactivist **Will Thomas**, has reported findings of over 300 types of virally mutated fungi in the chemtrail fallout. It is suggested that the fungi and bacteria living in the upper atmosphere, mutated by the high UV levels, might piggy back to earth on the chemtrail chemicals. The disruption of the jet streams and the raising and lowering of the atmospheric layers with atmospheric heaters (HAARP) may also create such turbulence that the upper atmospheric microbes are brought down to earth and represent a health threat in the form of "Thunderstorm Asthma" and virulent flus and sinus infections etc...

They manufacture **New Flu's** in order to sell their vaccines, which in turn damage people, then they need antibiotics which do further damage, weakening folks for the next round of fake flu. According to the government, their estimates call for a minimum of 2 million dead and 5 million hospitalizations should a viruses such as the H7N9 flu strain or a respiratory coronavirus (MERS-CoV) mutate into a more deadly and contagious form.

They have been trying to get a good pandemic going for years, but nothing really takes off. Remember the (H1N1-2009) bird flu scare — Bill recalls the expensive "medicine" they were peddling was actually star anise, and Rumsfeld was involved in the scam. H3N2 was manufactured at Fort Detrick Naval Base by the US army as a bioweapon — combining deadliest swine/avian flu with common cold put into the aerosol nasal vaccine (chemtrails) and sprayed over entire countries. It might be a good idea to invest in a particle mask just in case to wear on heavy spray days. Cambridge Mask Company Anti Pollution Mask, Military Grade N99 Washable Respirator. I even bought some sunglass swimming goggles, because I found out in 2015, that even I can get infected by their high tech bugs.

The chemtrailers like to spray a big fat chemtrail really low over town centers in the middle of the night, especially on full moon. You can be sure that it is a disease delivery laden with a pathogen mix for generating chemtrail flu in the population. They spray the biologic chemtrails at night because the low temperature makes the disease agents more effective. For maximum killer effect they spray when there is no wind, lower temperature and no rain.

This night spraying is obviously not geoengineering, it is bioengineering. There is NO other reason why they would undertake such a mission. Communities that show signs of being able to "think for themselves," ie: a spark of personal sovereignty, would be the hardest hit by these night escapades. I saw such a trail being laid down in Boulder CO, full moon January'15, when they sprayed heavily during the day for 3 days, creating mass respiratory illness in the population. One of the disease agents they used can leave a semi permanent infection of small itchy lesions on the upper back and arms, which still persist today 3 years after.

THE FAKE FLU SEASON—The chemtrailers like to spray populations heavily during the winter months, especially January and February in the Northern Hemisphere in order to spread the C-Flu. The Chemtraitors find that January and February are the best flu seeding months for the fake flu season—to make the most of the strategic genocide measures and generate the highest medical and pharmaceutical profits. The chemtrail spraying causes respiratory illness and influenza symptoms from the mycoplasma, bacteria and viruses that infect the nose, throat, and the lungs. This Fake Flu Season increases the number of people being herded into the predatory medical industry to get flu shots that contain cancer causing chemicals, neuro toxins and chemicals that cause sterility. Then like a good little citizen you go to your doctor for the "cure" and now you get hit with a course of antibiotics which destroy natural immunity. Avoid walking outside without a mask under heavy spray days. The bugs they spray on us are chimeras, and our immune system is not geared to deal with them.

The antibiotics kill off your intestinal bacteria, thereby promoting dysbiosis, maldigestion and tooth decay, and cause your body chemistry to go acidic, lowering your immunity and making you more susceptible to ongoing and repetitive infection. Then to kill the pain of tooth decay, respiratory congestion, skin lesions, inflammation and migraines you trot off to your doctorer again for opioid compounds such as morphine, fentanyl and codeine that produce powerful analgesic effects and interfere with the immune response. Finally at least you can die pain free and happy in ignorant bliss.

Not all spray days would be infection runs, but specific 3 day heavy sprays on low wind days may be for spreading the Flu, mycoplasma, Lyme-type bacteria, Morgellons etc... Also, UV mutated fungi, bacteria and viruses naturally in the upper atmosphere are known to taxi down on the charged particles of the chemtrails. The viruses, fungi, bacteria and mycoplasma could actually be in the chemtrail cocktail mix, or these mutated pathogens may be brought down to earth on the chemtrails as they descend from 35,000 feet? The very young, the very old, those individuals who are weakened by a chronic illness, and the immunocompromised or immunosuppressed will be more susceptible to developing severe illness from viruses, fungi and bacteria in the environment. Fungal (mycotic) disease now represents 12-15% of all hospital-acquired infections.

Chemtrails are said to contain many types of fungi, perhaps because fungi are used in the micronizing production process of the nanometals. The biologic chemtrails that smell like rot or fungi may be specifically formulated to create illness (and death), or fungi could be used along with the carbon black to create nano-particles of aluminum, barium, strontium, and mercury. Fungi secrete extracellular proteins which have been used to turn metal ions into metal nano-particles. If metal ions are mixed together with fungal hyphae rich in nitrate reductase enzyme and an organic carbon source, the metallic ions accrue and will eventually form nano-sized particles.

Regardless of whether the biologic chemtrails are sprayed with the intent to do grievous harm to populations or not, the effect is widespread flu symptoms, inflammation, respiratory illness and immunosuppressive effects over the long term; not to mention dementia. The fungal aspect of chemtrail survival is a serious health risk, due to the loss of immune strength from heavy metal exposure and the fact that candida and other fungi collect and store heavy metals in their structures, preventing the elimination of heavy metal from the body. The infection of the brain with candida sp. etc... in association with heavy metal and radionuclide sequestration in the beta-amyloid plaque formations and the biofilms of pathogens, makes recovery from chemtrail fallout the most pressing health crisis we face in the world today. Especially so since fungi are an intrinsic component in the concoction of the chemtrail formulas, and the cooked food human populations are already suffering from candida overgrowth.

The 82,000 synthetic chemicals, combined systemic electromagnetic assault (cell towers, G-5, wifi, etc) dampen the cosmic energetic effects, and essentially deaden human DNA, disrupt coherent light (superluminal communication) and block DNA from receiving vital messaging and stimulus necessary for ascension and evolution. Heavy metals and aluminum in the body form an "antenna" to pull radio frequencies into the body, whereas normally the bodyfield will form a protective field to resist the EMFs. An environment high in wifi, cell phones and 5G frequencies when our bodies are laden with nanometals is likely to act like **Magnet Assisted Transinfection (MATra)** technology to transinfect cells. Magnet Assisted Transfection (MATra) is a highly efficient technique in which nucleic acids are tagged with specific magnetic nano-particles then a magnetic force is applied to delivered into the target cells leading to efficient transinfection without disturbing the membrane architecture.

We have to wonder about the combination of indiscriminate aerial spray of infectious agents and nanometals coupled with our highly EMF polluted environment. We know that radio frequencies in general weaken cell membranes, and create leaky gut and a leaky blood brain barrier, thereby making the body more permeable by pathogens of all kinds. Whether it is intentional or not the chemtrail assault appears to be a method of collapsing the immune system of organisms and the environment and threatening the food supply to prepare for letting loose a series of pandemics. I think they tried to get an epidemic going during Obama's reign—hence the H5N1 bird flu scare of 2006, however it was a dud as far as global pandemics go. There was a second swine flu pandemic in 2009 caused by a new H1N1 strain that purportedly originated in pigs in Mexico. The fact that 300 million people have died from Smallpox was not enough to stop scientists from using "CRISPR" DNA editing technology to bioengineer the killer virus – and then tell the world how they did it. Wonders never cease!

1918 Spanish Flu—The US Centers for Disease Control and Prevention has succeeded in reconstituting the full RNA segments of the 1918 Spanish Flu H1N1 virus by using reverse genetics. First known as trench fever, the "Spanish Flu" pandemic of 1918-1919 at the end of WW1 killed between 60 and 100 million people. The Spanish flu a unique event due to its short incubation period, and the extremely high number of deaths. The disease course was frequently less than 5 days, but sometimes it killed within a matter of hours, often with either massive acute pulmonary hemorrhage or pulmonary edema. Approximately 30% of the world's population (500 million people) is thought to have been clinically infected with the 1918 pandemic.

The 1918 pandemic virus killed quickly and directly with a violent viral pneumonia caused by the H1N1 virus, the so-called "swine flu" that also affects pigs. However, most deaths were caused from secondary bacterial pneumonia due to a lack of antibiotics. During that epidemic symptoms included hemorrhaging from mucous membranes, especially from the nose, stomach, and intestine. Bleeding from the ears and **petechial hemorrhages** (tiny pinpoint red marks) in the skin caused by a minor bleed from broken capillary blood vessels also occurred. IV Vitamin C would have saved millions of lives.

The countries involved in the war censored news about flu cases in their own countries. Arbitrarily it was called the Spanish Flu to pin the blame on Spain as it was a neutral country in WWI and had no wartime press censorship so people in Spain were hearing about the pandemic while the rest of the world was oblivious. The first mild wave of the disease occurred in the spring of 1918, with a more severe wave happening later in the year. Troop movements and other war-related disruptions played a role in its rapid transmission.

The more virulent disease appeared almost simultaneously in Sierra Leone, France, and Boston. Hardest hit were young, healthy adults, invading the lungs and causing suffocation via edema. Mostly people aged 18 to 29 died of the Spanish flu apparently because they had not been exposed to anything resembling the H1N1 strain of the Spanish flu and so had no immunity. However that doesn't explain why Greece - the one country in Europe that escaped the Spanish Flu, was also the one country which was not vaccinated against it.

MONBAYERSATAN: Bayer AG, the chemical and pharmaceutical giant founded in Barmen, Germany in 1863 by Friedrich Bayer and Johann Friedrich Weskott trademarked acetylsalicylic acid as aspirin in 1899. Twenty years after Bayer contributed to the largest number of deaths in human history by disease during the Spanish flu epidemic as aspirin produced by Bayer apparently stopped people's lungs from draining by lowering blood pressure and suppressing the immune system leading to pneumonias and death due to overdosing with aspirin. Bayer (of Bayer-Monsanto) was a primary funder of Hitler and helped run the basic operations of the war, including the concentration camps.

We might ask was Bayer a financial backer of the German military during WWI as well? Now Monsanto and Bayer are united! Monsanto, the GMO giant, was originally a chemical company founded in 1901, besides many genetically engineered species of crops, Monsanto may have let loose on humanity a pestilence which has the ability to change our DNA. ***See Dastardly Plot below.

The soldiers at Fort Dix, near Trenton New Jersey, who were said to have had Swine Flu had been injected with a large variety of vaccines like those that caused the 1918 flu epidemic. These soldiers may have been the first guinea pigs to the vaccine induced pandemic that then took the world by storm in several waves of infection.

They may go straight for a **prion pandemic**, however that is something of an unknown entity, and uncontainable. Apparently the cattle mutilations are due to their experiments with observing the range and physiological effects of spreading prions in the environment. That is, assessing the use of prions as a weapon of war.

Dr Wil Spencer and Patrick Jordan talk about how prions or lab modified proteins have been spread through the environment from GMO foods such as corn. These prions mutate the candida albicans yeast/fungi within our body to create diseases such as Mad Cow Disease—essentially making zombies out of humans. This explains the cattle mutilations, as the military go to great length to collect samples to study the effectiveness of their experiments to spread the prions out in the ecosystems.

In his YouTube videos **Harald Kautz-Vella** talks about the piezo-crystal seed form of the prion protein of mad cow disease and Alzheimer's being barium/strontium based from the "smart dust" from chemtrails. Apparently the phenomena of cattle mutilations are due to the US military's experiments with observing the range and physiological effects of spreading prions in the environment. That is, assessing the use of prions as a weapon of war.

DEALING WITH AERIAL ASSAULT

Our immune systems are not designed for the manmade preternatural organisms combined with the mutated pathogens that coast down to earth on the chemtrail particulates from the upper atmosphere. Rather than getting stronger with this "aerial vaccination," it is more likely that after years off chemtrail assault the immune system of the biosphere will become exhausted. The main point is to hit the chemflu hard right off and treat it as a serious threat...BEFORE it can infiltrate systemically in the body! You've got to fight those elusive buggers FAST before they insidiously entrench themselves in the remote cul-de-sacs of the body—and hide behind their biofilm barriers that are concealment devices for their covert operations.

When we see the **3 day 50-plus trail** days we ideally need to wear a face mask, steam the face with antiseptic herbs, use herbal-saline -silver nasal sprays, beef up Vitamin C + Alpha Lipoic to medicinal levels 6 gms for women, 9 gms for men of Vitamin C. Chances are if we can resist being exposed to the initial inoculation spray, and establish a full on antiflu protocol including infrared sauna, we may be strong enough to resist subsequent infection from others in the community that are infected. Maintaining an antiviral raw diet with strong detox pathways and high glutathione levels should allow us to live through a pandemic, as long as we refuse vaccination.

Flu shots inhibit the immune system so people who get flu shots are setup to become flu dupes, carriers and casualties. Flu vaccine contains nagalase, a cancer causing enzyme that interferes with GcMAF (Globulin component Macrophage Activating Factor), an immune system protein. (See more on GcMAF and Bravo yogurt in ***Biologic Chemtrails). With the cancerous component of chemtrails there is a need to change the body's terrain from being mutagenic by detoxing, raising oxygen levels, eating a raw diet, getting grounding, sunlight and exercise.

Vitamin C fills up the opiate receptors so take up to 6000 mg/day or more. Take 1 Alpha Lipoic pill to every 2 Vitamin C for a synergistic effect. 50mcg Niacin and D-Ribose once or twice per day flushes your system and amplifies all other medicinals. Using Niacin and D-Ribose would have a similar effect to Elysium, in raising cellular energy production especially when reinstating circadian atunement, and sungazing/grounding.

The less sun energy you get (physically or by consuming real food grown in the sun) the more spiritually dark you will get and the earlier you will become diseased and die. Go barefoot, get grounding and sunbathing every day, sungaze and get some sunshine on the skin each day, especially morning light. Avoid blue light from computer screens. Get amber incandescent light bulbs for your house. Toning or humming all day is also useful for relaxation and cleansing brain and blood. Green salads with lots of colorful fruits and veggies, and nice salad dressing. Up to 1 gallon of good water per day, and Herbal Tea with some local herbs. Do lots of heavy deep outbreaths during the day...this turns on the Off Switch to the nervous system and is relaxing and cleansing.

If a pandemic is underway it is best to get whatever food you can and get out of towns and cities. This is the kind of circumstance where a gas mask is advised.

For more on the disease aspects of the eugenics program read: *"Chemtrails, HAARP, and the Full Spectrum Dominance of Planet Earth,"* by Elana Freeland

Spirochete Warfare - Borrelia and other spirochetes were weaponized, by Elena Cook www.elenacook.org/spirowarfare.html

See YouTubes: "Sofia Smallstorm (Pt 1-6) at Consciousness Beyond Chemtrails 2012" on the EMF killing fields; Sofia Smallstorm on DNA manipulation through geoengineering!; The ĒLite are manipulating human DNA through chemtrails! www.aboutthesky.com

For more on this see YouTube Videos: Dr. John Bergman, *"Truth Vs Lies About Flu Vaccines *Updated*"*

And *"The Exploding Autoimmune Epidemic* - Dr. Tent - It's Not Autoimmune, you have Viruses." Dr Tent talks about how the attempts to build a weaponized cancer virus is central to the historical events involving of Castro, JFK and Oswald.

EUGENICS SPECTRUM COMPLEX

The six genera or kingdoms of organism are: Plants, Animals, Protists (algae, slime molds, and amoebas), Fungi, Eubacteria and the extremophile Archaebacteria. The weaponized pathogens in chemtrails are best thought of as "**biotech chimera**," that is part virus, part bacteria and part fungi, with multiple morphological stages including spores, capable of generating cognitive, neurological, meningeal, digestive pathogenic, endotoxemic, inflammatory and autoimmune effects as well. Lyme bacteria was engineered to use magnesium rather than iron in its metabolism. Lyme also changes natural Vitamin D to be immune inhibitory rather than immune enhancing.

This is a spiritual war against all living creatures of the earth—and requires a comprehensive rethinking of our place, purpose and actions—as individuals, communities and as a species. Modern humans like to identify and name specific disease agents, as it gives them a sense of control and agency over illness. However, we are going to have to ease off knowing the name and even the genera of the pathogenic agents because the interaction with the eugenic chemtrails and microwave technology and the earth's natural mechanisms means that we are under attack by an entire spectrum of health destroying processes.

We could start talking in more general terms such as "Eugenics Spectrum Complex." Heavy metals, disease agents and collapsing environmental vitality lead to the complexification of disease, through the decline in the energy and resources needed to maintain health (wholeness). Lyme disease and coinfections (such as Human Herpesvirus 6, Epstein–Barr virus, chlamydia, cytomegalovirus, mononucleosis and candida) can activate other infections due to an compromised immune system and autoimmune state.

A great diversity of Lyme's bacteria (Borrelia burgdorferi) strains are sustained in the wild and enter the upper atmosphere along with other microbes where they mutate under the high UV conditions. Spraying nanometals and other toxic chemicals into the upper atmosphere, and charging it with microwaves, coupled with the UV from the sun can change those elements into even more biocidal isomers. And those same radical conditions could mutate the bacteria, viruses and mycoplasmas into aberrant, pandemic creating plagues.

Bacteria, viruses, mycoplasma and fungi in the upper atmosphere are thought to attach onto the chemtrail aerosols and thus taxi back down to earth. This is one reason why these pathogens always show up in samples taken for assaying the chemtrail contents from the environment. In cyst form bacteria can survive in extreme environments and conditions. Encysted lyme spirochetes survive freezing and thawing and can be viable for up to 2.5 years, plus the bacteria can survive over winter inside vectors.

There is an insect component to the chemtrails, perhaps as a vector for dispersing infection or in the production methods of the pathogens. Also pathogens and insect eggs naturally in the upper atmosphere can coast back down to earth by on the aerosols. Spirochetes and coinfections are spread not only by ticks, but by mosquitoes, mites, fleas and biting flies. Insects are the best vectors for dispersing multiple coinfections to populations targeted for extermination.

Why are red blood cells found in chemtrails? Accounts of chemtrail contents mention human red blood cells, but they don't mention white blood cells. In order to separate them, the blood would need to be centrifuged. Can we assume this phenomena is a type infection method, similar to giving smallpox infected blankets to indigenous folk? DNA is present in white blood cells of humans, but not red blood cells which lack nuclei. Dried red blood cells would be an excellent disease vector when breathed in. Spirochetes could be inside the desiccated red blood cells that are present in the chemtrails and hence could be breathed in. The body's response to this would first be flu, then rashes and ultimately for the unfortunate few...Morgellons.

If bacteria cysts, fungi and viruses rain down on us via chemtrails or the endemic upper atmosphere pathogen layer, then there is every possibility that we will breathe them in resulting in upper respiratory diseases, cardiac illness, and other chronic and multiple illnesses. Lyme bacteria could be easily distributed via chemtrail aerosols, and it must be noted that both insect proteins and dessicated red blood cells have been found in the chemtrail cocktail! If red blood cells in chemtrails are a vector, humans and other creatures would breathe in the red blood cells and thereby become infected with the syphilis-like Borrelia species — directly entering the brain through the nasal blood supply.

Rather than wait for the answer to this question, we should be amplifying our health and disease protective regimes to the full extent of our capacity.

Morgellons is likely an extreme expression of Borrelia burgdorferi, that affects certain individuals, of the same disease processes occurring in the general population exposed to these infectious agents sprayed on us from the sky. Spirochetes are very ancient bacteria consisting of 300 different species. "Spirochete" is any of a group of spiral-shaped bacteria, some of which are serious pathogens for humans, causing diseases such as syphilis, yaws, Lyme disease, and relapsing fever. Lyme disease is not a recent phenomena, even the Iceman who lived 5,300 years ago was infected with Lyme disease. Spirochete bacteria enter into red blood cells and reduce the oxygen carrying capacity of the blood.

Borrelia invade skin cells and change how they produce collagen, keratin and other proteins: Borrelia binds to collagen fiber producing fibroblast cells, invades them, and undergoes extracellular cystic transformation, becoming surrounded by a dense microfilament network. Borrelia attach to and transmigrate fibroblasts in the skin, and undergo cystic transformation outside the fibroblasts. Fibroblasts preserve their vitality and express a prominent granular endoplasmic reticulum, suggesting activated protein synthesis. Collagen growth factor mRNA which regulates collagen metabolism is significantly enhanced in **skin fibroblasts** cells infected with Borrelia. This is thought to be the main factor contributing to the production of "fibers" in Morgellons.

The official line is that Morgellons IS a climax condition of Lyme, but that may be because of a co-infection with Lyme from the same chemtrail cocktail. So it could be deliberate misinformation, because they could easily tell what is what with an electron microscope. If Morgellons is indeed nano-technology that causes the skin fibroblasts to over-produce cells creating the Morgellons fibers then Electromagnetic Pulse and other electronic healing devices may be the most effective remedy. Coat the body in neem oil as it is a natural pesticide.

Borrelia enter fibroblasts by forming tethers between the cell wall of the Borrelia and the cell membrane of the fibroblast, then transmigrate through these cells, and are continuously surrounded by the fibroblast cell membrane. Borrelia burgdorferi is able to invade different eukaryotic cells including endothelial cells, fibroblasts, neuronal, and neuroglial cells. Because the spirochete infection is "intercellular" you cannot treat it with antibiotics. Treatment with regular antibiotics for more than 2 weeks creates leaky gut, and leaky blood-brain-barrier! The tight junctions become porous allowing the leakage of fluids through the vascular walls, which overburdens the immune system and detoxification organs. Asparagus root, Licorice root, Slippery elm, Marshmallow root and Plantain leaf, MSM (*methylsulfonylmethane*), and zinc helps reverse leaky gut.

Borrelia pathogens thrive inside parasitic nematode worms, worm eggs or larvae, and tick bites deliver the nematode into the human body. The fact that there are red blood cells in the chemtrails points to a pathogen factory producing spirochetes and other infectious agents, incubated within mammals, and then the blood is harvested, separated by centrifuge, and freeze dried to be added to the chemtrail mix. Lyme is also transferred between hosts through sexual activity, kissing, as well as into babies in the womb and even via human breast milk. A third of people who get infected with Lyme show no bullseye rash.

If Lyme-type bacteria was spread on the population via the red blood cells from the chemtrails, the effects would not be the round bullseye target, but very small dark red itchy spots on back and arms. See ***"Quench the Itch."

See YouTube: "Dr David James Chemtrails GIVE YOU Lymes disease."

PARANASAL SINUS SPIROCHETE INVASION

When looking at chemtrails as a disease vector we must consider the connection between lyme disease and paranasal sinus spirochete invasion! Multiple sclerosis is thought to be caused by the CNS invasion by spiral-shaped bacteria (spirochetes) through defects in the wall of the paranasal sphenoidal sinuses and subsequently inducing an "anti self" autoimmune response. Evidence supporting this is demonstrated by the presence of Borrelia burgdorferi in the central nervous system in some patients with active MS. Multiple sclerosis is considered to be an autoimmune disease directed against oligodendrocytes in the CNS, its myelin, and to the underlying nerve axon. Oligodendrocytes are a neuroglial cell that creates the myelin sheath, or nerve insulating layer which is 80% lipid and 20% protein.

It is thought that T cells with a specificity for myelin basic protein (MBP), or another myelin protein, become activated as a result of a virus, or environmental stimuli. As myelin sheaths break down they release myelin basic protein, which the body perceives as a foreign agent, and so the T cells attack and damage the sheaths further. These activated T cells are thought to migrate to the CNS via the blood-brain barrier where they secrete cytokines which initiate an inflammatory cascade via molecular mimicry, leading to oligodendrocyte death, myelin sheath destruction, and damage to the neuron axons.

This mechanism of spirochete invasion via the paranasal sinuses and the consequent autoimmune and neurological deterioration presents clues as to why Borrelia spirochete species are found within chemtrail fallout. This alone, the breathing in pathogens could represent an ideal means of effectively rendering the global population sick, incapacitated, pliable and mentally incompetent to revolt or save themselves from the slow, silent holocaust. Spirochetes are constantly in flux and transform their genome to outwit the immune system. They enter the brain through the meninges in 12 hours causing inflammatory cytokines that weaken the tight junctions of the Blood Brain Barrier. CD40 cytokine receptor activation is associated with the beta-amyloid plaque build up of Alzheimer's.

Flu-like symptoms are the body's first response as phagocytic cells produce hydrogen peroxide to attack the invading pathogen. Then 48 hours after infection the spirochetes get inside the cells and start replicating, consequently releasing new bacteria into the extracellular fluid. Inflammatory activation of defense systems in the glial cells inhibits neural-repair and neurogenesis, while creating glial scars or lesions in the brain. This produces impaired cognition, memory loss, emotional volatility or flatness, diminished mental complexity, and this culminates in reduced direction, Presence and Meaning in our lives. The spirochete generated cytokines, immune response cytokines and antibodies cause massive brain damage over time, and even if Borrelia is killed with antibiotics the bacteria fragments continue to cause inflammation.

Pharmaceutical antibiotics do not work against viruses, and generally cause bacteria to form cysts (round bodies) and thus reduce the symptoms without curing the disease. They revert to helical swimmer populations that grow vigorously when conditions are right with regards to low oxygen, salt, food, temperature, acidity, media viscosity and other factors are adequate. Thus Pharmaceutical antibiotics are the very worst thing in response to US chemtrail warfare as it drives Lyme into cyst form, and creates dead spirochetes to which the body still responds with inflammation. The only way is through a holistic healthy lifestyle, raw diet, detoxification, boosting immunity, adaptogenic and anti-pathogenic herbs, and regular periodic water fasting to reboot and update immunity. That is 3 days per week water fasting, intermittent fasting or calorie reduction lifestyle.

***Antibiotics and hospitals may be necessary during cases like acute bacterial pneumonia, but only with consideration of the intensive repopulation of the GI microbiome after coming out of danger to repair the body's immune system.

BRAIN FOG: The reason we get brain fog and lose our sense of selfhood and sovereignty from the chemtrailing is largely due to brain inflammation and consequent nerve damage from the heavy metals and infectious agents in the chemtrails. Dementia and anemia have been linked to exposure to nanoparticulates in that aerosols which inhibits the cholinesterase of the brain, liver and red blood cells. Cholinesterase is a family of enzymes present in the central nervous system, particularly in nervous tissue, muscle and red cells, which catalyze the hydrolysis of the neurotransmitter acetylcholine into choline and acetic acid, a necessary reaction that allows cholinergic neurons to return to resting state after activation. Cholinesterase enzyme inactivation leads to acetylcholine accumulation, hyper stimulation of nicotinic and muscarinic receptors, and disrupted neurotransmission. Remedies for brain fog include: Dandelion, Ginger, Cinnamon, Forskolin, Rhodiola, Vacha, Rosemary, Tulsi, Bacopa, Ginkgo, Ginkgo nuts, Ginseng, Gotu kola, Lion's Mane Mushroom, Maca, Ashwagandha, Huperzine, L-Theanine, NAC, Phenylalanine, Phosphatidylserine.

The Exhaustion Phase pages on biologyofkundalini.com are a synopsis for nervous system recovery. Olive leaf is one of the best things for your nerve sheaths.

CAT'S CLAW: *Uncaria rhynchophylla* has remarkably inhibitory effects on the formation of fibrils and beta-amyloid protein thus is a principle therapeutic agent for the prevention and/or cure Alzheimer's disease. Cat's Claw also is useful for inflammation in the brain due to spirochete, candida and other infections, and it is also antiseizure.

DAGINGYE: Chinese Woad (*Isatis indigotica*) is considered powerfully antibacterial, antivirial, anti-inflammatory, cathartic, diaphoretic, diuretic, emetic, purgative, stimulant, and vasoconstrictor. It is also called indigowood root, because the roots are used for indigo colored dye. As a top antiviral herb, woad root has a very broad spectrum of antimicrobial activity. Banlangen is an Isatis root beverage used for malaria and encephalitis. Applied topically for herpes or venereal disease sores or blisters.

HYDROGEN PEROXIDE (H202): Fred Vandenberg of morgellonsmisery. blogspot.com/ says not to use Hydrogen Peroxide internally due to the fenton effect, where it makes more hydroxyl free radicals in the body that enhances the iron peptide bonds of the morgellons pathogens. See Fred's article *"Morgellons Misery -Fred's Morgellons-Lyme Protocol."* 3% Hydrogen Peroxide can be used on the Chembug itchy sores and dropped in the ears with an eye-dropper. *"The One-Minute Cure : The Secret to Healing Virtually All Diseases,"* by Madison Cavanaugh.

OVERCOMING ANTIBIOTIC RESISTANCE

There is a worldwide pandemic of Chemtrail Lung occurring due to the chemicals and infectious agents in chemtrails, and we can no longer depend on antibiotics to save us, because of the ongoing nature of the cause. We must therefore turn to natural solutions such as Propolis, as antibiotics often do not work anymore due to bacteria developing antibiotic-resistance, and due to the multiple-coinfections.

MANUKA HONEY AND PROPOLIS: Combating Antibiotic Resistant Bacteria—In recent years a marked increase in antibiotic resistance by certain pathogenic bacteria has been seen, thus we cannot rely on antibiotics to save us from drug-resistant bacteria. Pathogens cannot develop resistance against bee propolis! Propolis has antibacterial effect against both Gram-positive and Gram-negative microorganisms including multidrug-resistant bacteria such as Escherichia coli, Salmonella, or Staphylococcus aureus (MRSA).

Propolis is a resinous natural substance produced by honeybees from plant exudates, beeswax, and bee secretions. Propolis is composed of 50% resin, 30% wax, 10% essential and aromatic oils, 5% pollen, and 5% other substances. Propolis has wide range of biological activities which include antimicrobial, antioxidant, anti-inflammatory, anaesthetic and anticancer properties.

The antimicrobial properties of propolis are related to the synergistic effect of its various compounds. The antibiotic effect of propolis arises from its action on the bacteria's cytoplasmic membrane plus inhibiting motility, enzyme activity, cell division and protein synthesis. The galagin and caffeic acid in propolis inhibits the enzymes and RNA-polymerase in bacteria, thereby inhibiting protein synthesis. Turmeric in honey potentiated its antimicrobial effect, destroying every bacteria or pathogen scientists tested it on.

The antimicrobial property of propolis varies with its geographical origin. It was found that honey collected from United Arab Emirates inhibits polymicrobial cultures as well as single microbial culture. Honey increased nitric oxide end products in various animals and humans' biological fluids and decreased prostaglandin concentration.

PROPOLIS TINCTURE: Always have some Propolis Tincture on hand. To make Propolis Tincture freeze raw propolis pieces to make it brittle and then grind up (in a bullet or coffee grinder). Put this in an amber glass bottle and cover with 40% brandy or vodka by 1 inch. Shake and store in a dark place. Shake once a day for 2-4 weeks. Then strain and put tincture in amber dropper bottles. The propolis tincture residue (oleoresin or balsam) may be reused for another tincture or mixed with honey. This balsam can also be used on gums overnight to reduce inflammation from periodontal disease. The propolis oleoresin in manuka honey can be used to make the Master Cleanser: A hot or cold cleansing drink comprised of fresh lemon juice, water, honey and a pinch of cayenne pepper. This is the perfect drink to both prevent and treat Chemtrail Flu!

YUNNAN BAIYAO: Yunnan Baiyao is an old Chinese herbal medicine that is know as Chinese penicillin. This therapeutic mixture would be good to have on hand during the chemtrail holocaust as an alternative to pharma-antibiotics, as an effective remedy for respiratory infection, chem-Flu, mycoplasma, fungi etc... It is a potentially new application in inflammatory bowel disease and leaky gut. It speeds healing, reduces pain, inflammation, infection and swelling of injuries, wounds and surgery. Yunnan stanches bleeding, and can be used to arrest hemorrhaging, prevent blood clots and potential strokes and post-concussion syndrome. It enhances circulation and "resets" the brain at a higher frequency...by "electrifying" the blood. This formula is traditionally used for everything from wounds, joint aches, tinnitus, to serious trauma and diminishes itch and swelling due to mosquito and insect bites. It reduces pain and numbness associated with arthritis, backache, strains, bruises, frostbite, and joints. The Yunnan Baiyao may make you dizzy initially if you have high blood sugar, high pathogen load, but it quickly holts fermentation and purification in the body. The powder can be rubbed into skin lesions and cuts.

Yunnan Baiyao Ingredients: Ginseng root, Chinese Yam, Myrrh and Dragon's blood, Camphor, Boea clarkeana Hemsl, Sheep's Ear, Ground Cedar, Galangal, Cranebill, Calcium Phosphate. Alcohol is used in the preparation of the extracts.

WEAPONIZED MYCOPLASMA

"Mycoplasma is not really a fungus, it's not really a bacteria, it's not really a virus. It has no cell wall. It goes deep into the cell nuclei thereby making it very difficult to mount an immune response against it. It's a man-made biological weapon. The patent report explains how it causes chronic upper respiratory infections that are virtually identical to what's going on right now." unifiedserenity.wordpress.com/tag/slow-kill

Pathogenic Mycoplasma used to be very innocuous, but biological warfare research conducted between 1942 and the present time has resulted in the creation of more deadly and infectious forms of Mycoplasma such as genitalium, fermentans, salivarium, hominis, pneumonia, incognitus, pirum, fucium etc...

Mycoplasma fermentans probably comes from the nucleus of the Brucella bacteria that is the cause of brucellosis. This disease agent is not a bacterium and not a virus; it is a mutated form of the Brucella bacterium, combined with a visna virus, from which the mycoplasma is extracted. Researchers extracted this mycoplasma from the Brucella bacterium and actually reduced the disease to a "crystalline form." They "weaponized" it and tested it on an unsuspecting public in North America.

The CDC has labeled Brucella species as highly weaponizable, as people may be infected by inhalation of contaminated dust or aerosols. Dr. Maurice Hilleman, chief virologist for the pharmaceutical company Merck Sharp & Dohme, stated that this disease agent is now carried by everybody in North America and possibly most people throughout the world. There has been an increased incidence of all systemic-neurological degenerative diseases since World War II, especially since the 1970s, with the prevalence of hidden bacterial infection diseases like chronic fatigue syndrome, fibromyalgia, cancer, multiple sclerosis, ALS, peripheral neuropathy, AIDs, cardiovascular disease and more. www.bettyelders.com/EBV.htm

MYCOPLASMA ERADICATORS: Natural plant antibiotics like Olive leaf extract, Neem, Cinnamon leaf, Uva ursi, Red Sage (Danshen), Cordyceps, Birch Bark Mushroom, Grapefruit seed extract, Pau D'Arco, Cat's claw are worth trying. Turmeric and Raw Honey, and IV Vitamin C.

"The Mycoplasma in chemtrails is not really a fungus, it's not really a bacterium, and it's not really a virus. It has no cell wall. It goes deep into the cell nuclei thereby making it very difficult to mount an immune response against it. It's a man-made biological weapon. The patent report explains how it causes chronic upper respiratory infections that are virtually identical to what's going on right now." Zen Gardner

MORGELLONS DISEASE

Morgellons disease is currently known to be a filamentous Borrelia dermatitis due to spirochete parasites.

Morgellons Disease is an all-inclusive term for numerous afflictions consisting of coinfections of Lyme spirochetes (Borrelia burgdorferi) and babesia (a malaria-like parasite). Candida, Epstein-Barr Virus, Cytomegalovirus, MRSA, Pseudomonas aeruginosa, etc... probably due to a weakened immune system. While analyzing correlations between Lyme Borreliosis and Alzheimer's, Dr. Alan MacDonald discovered Borrelia spirochetes in 70% of Alzheimer's samples in one study. There are 5 subspecies of Borrelia burgdorferi, over 100 strains in the us, and 300 strains worldwide, adding to the antigenic variability of the spirochete.

Morgellons disease (MD) is an emerging multisystem illness characterized by skin lesions with unusual filaments embedded in or projecting from the skin. Spirochetes genetically identified as Borrelia burgdorferi sensu stricto predominate as the infective agent in most of the Morgellons cases, is the same causative agent as Lyme disease. Lyme Borrelia spirochetes love feeding on collagenous tissues, so the stronger and healthier our collagen is the more resistant it is to being broken down by the spirochetes. Wherever spirochetes degrade collagen tissues is where our symptoms arise. Thus all of us need to be working on building and repairing our collagen. ***See Collagen

Morgellons disease (MD) is a skin disease characterized by multi colored filaments that lie under or project from skin. Morgellons fibers are predominantly composed of collagen and keratin and are produced by keratinocytes. Keratinocytes constituting 90% of the cell types in the epidermis, the outermost most layer of the skin. The unusual thread-like fluorescent fibers appear under the skin. The most common symptoms of MD are the presence of small white, red, blue, or black fibers under, on, or erupting from sores or unbroken skin and the sensation that something is crawling on or under your skin. Those with Morgellons may feel like something is crawling, biting, or stinging all over.

Morgellons is purported to be bio-engineered filaments of nano biological hybrid composites, that are cross-domain bacterial organisms. Morgellons is likely related to the fallout of fluorescent polymer fiber cobwebs, piezoelectric crystals, or the "Smart Dust" from chemtrails. Smart dust or programmable matter, could be associated with the self-assembling tubular fibers of keratin and collagen that has come to be known as Morgellons Disease. I am not going to attempt a definitive answer to what Morgellons Disease is because it is so mysterious and chemtrails contain so many components that may combine to create disease symptoms the likes of which we have never seen before. So rather than claiming that it is alien technology, genetically engineered chimeras or prehistoric pathogens from permafrost melt, I personally must defer to the future and admit a disturbing lack of understanding of this phenomenon.

Lyme is a weaponized spirochete bacteria which is being found in chemtrail residue assays. Lyme is also a coinfection with everyone who gets Morgellons. Once the truth gets out I think we will find that different Borrelia species are being dispersed through the air via chemtrails and these do not create the rash that forms a "bull's eye" shape, but rather creates small itchy lesions on the arms and back. The spirochete of Lyme can invade various parts of the body, including brain and spinal cord, creating Borrelia meningitis, and encephalitis. At first, patients might develop symptoms like encephalitis or meningitis, such as a loss of sensation, nerve pain and inflammation of the brain causing flu-like symptoms, headache, fever, confusion, a stiff neck, and vomiting. Complications may include seizures, hallucinations, trouble speaking, memory problems, and hearing loss.

Not all chemtrails would be infection runs, but 3 day heavy sprays on low wind days may specific be for spreading the Flu, mycoplasma, Lyme-type bacteria, Morgellons etc... All chemtrails would however pull pathogenic spores and organisms down from the upper atmosphere, as they ionically glom onto the aerosols and become heavy enough to descend to ground level. Morgellons may be a man made phenomenon or it may be created via UV in the upper atmosphere mutating fungi, bacteria and viruses which then taxi down on the charged particles of the chemtrails.

DASTARDLY PLOT

These aberrant diseases are something straight out of a scifi horror movie... and the plot line appears to be getting progressively worse.

The Morgellons story is the greatest science fiction horror story of the 21st Century...and it is true! The morphology of Morgellons appears to be a chimera of bacteria with a fungus-like aspect. Morgellons may not a single bacteria, but a mixture of different bacteria, with spirochete bacteria living in "intracellularly" symbiosis. The fact that most Morgellons sufferers also have an infection of the spirochete Borrelia (Lyme), points to the multi-pathogen chimeric nature of the original disease-causing microorganism.

Those with Morgellons first start noticing a subdermal itching which will not subside, feeling as if something is crawling beneath the skin. This then may progress to tiny fibers of various colors (red, blue, green, yellow) that push their way through to the surface of the skin. After which open lesions develop over the body where the fibers are most present. These Morgellons fibers are long, segmented strands or hollow polysaccharide filaments, made of polymer carbohydrates much like sugars except with a greater number of molecules in their chains.

Initially exhibiting similar symptoms to the chemtrail flu, Morgellons feels robotic, unnatural and alien, just as we can expect from experiencing self-assembling fibers from the body's keratin and collagen of our body. Electron microscopic imaging of Morgellons disease samples reveal that the filaments are composed of keratin and collagen and result from proliferation and activation of keratinocytes and fibroblasts in the epithelial tissue and hair follicles, that are predominantly populated by keratinocytes. There are also black spores which will disclose the genetic diagnosis of this crippling disease.

The encapsulating filament sheath is composed of keratin and is more fungal in nature, while the black and white specks that are inside of the sheath are more "bacterial-like" or "chlamydia-like." The term **"cross-domain bacteria"** (CDB) has been introduced by one of the principle Morgellons researchers, **Clifford Carnicom**, to describe the chimeric-like organisms he calls a **"baculovirus,"** that are comprised of an *encapsulating filament, bacterial hosts and biofilm.* Strong evidence now exists that an artificial or modified form of erythrocyte, or red blood cell is a dominant internal component associated with the Morgellons condition. The Carnicom Institute and its founder Clifford Carnicom have an extensive history of research on geo-engineering topics and aerosol research. See the online article: *"Cross-Domain Bacteria Isolation,"* Clifford E Carnicom, May 17 2014

When these fibers are analyzed they universally come back testing positive for the DNA of Agrobacterium tumefaciens, which is bacterium used in the genetic engineering of transgenic GMO crops to inject foreign genetic material into host cells. Argos Bacteria requires a carbohydrate energy source and would benefit from a polysaccharide enclosure. Even weirder than the debilitating lesions, Morgellons fibers have been found to actually produce foreign red blood cells that are not of the host body itself. It would seem the effect of causing the injection of foreign DNA into the human host is an intentional design of the product.

Because of the lack of nuclei and organelles, mature red blood cells do not contain DNA and cannot synthesize any RNA, and consequently no virus can evolve to target mammalian red blood cells. It appears that because of the gene splicing bacteria Agrobacterium tumefaciens the Morgellons fibers are producing red blood cells of a prior host organism. One can only imagine how the immune system reacts to this alien tissue.

Somehow mutated insect genes or insect eggs are associated with Morgellons symptoms and at some point in the future we may learn what is causing this very enigmatic disease. Bed bugs, ticks and mosquitoes make perfect vectors for deliberately spreading disease. The appearance of "insect-like components" seems to point to insect eggs or insect genes being in the mix as vectors or in the manufacture. It really is the most confusing thing — and I suspect that we cannot attribute the symptoms to simply being Lyme. So the Jury is Out, and the truth has been deliberately hidden.

***See information online on the strange case of the Bollworm and a possible Monsanto connection to Morgellons. Monsanto put an insect-selective scorpion toxin (AaIT) gene into transgenic crop — thus permitting the crops to express a scorpion neurotoxin that "makes a fungus hyper infectious to insects! This mechanism of genetically manipulating fungi to become hyper infectious, may possibly be genetically changing the candida that resides in all of our bodies.

MORGELLONS AND LYME DISEASE

Although the common denominator in the evolution of Morgellons lesions seems to be infection with Borrelia species, spirochetes the etiology of Morgellons disease is presumed to be multifactorial. Morgellons sufferers invariably test positive the Lyme bacteria Borrelia burgdorferi and exhibit constitutional, musculoskeletal and neurocognitive symptoms that are associated with Lyme disease (LD) and tick borne coinfections. Spirochetes (Borrelia burgdorferi or Lyme disease) were also detected, providing evidence that Morgellons disease is associated with an infectious process.

The **Chembug Sores** may be an outward sign of the same disease agents that create Morgellons disease (and coinfection of Lyme bacteria etc…), however the expression of Morgellons fibers only shows up in susceptible individuals. Our current understanding is that "Morgellons disease" is not a symptom of Chemtrail Flu, rather it is the full-blown disease process, which occurs in only susceptible individuals and usually takes years to manifest into its most serious forms.

I don't know the specific organism that causes the Chembug Sores but it is probably a spirochete such as Lyme...and Lyme is also attributed to Morgellons. The cocktail of chemtrail pathogens first causes the chemtrail flu symptoms and respiratory infection along with the chemtrail lobotomy as the organism(s) infect the brain, then inflammation of the joints and you end up with a semi-permanent rash of small itchy spots on the upper back and arms. After which dementia and other forms of organ failure would occur if the infection is not dealt with by lifestyle changes, detoxification and boosting of the immune system. Kris Kristofferson, has revealed that he was misdiagnosed with Alzheimer's when he actually had Lyme disease, and he subsequently reversed his dementia with Lyme-disease treatment.

Secondary contributing factors such as mineral deficiency, low antioxidant levels, genetic background, hormonal influences, immune status, and the presence of other co-infections appear to play a role in the full-blown development of the disease. Morgellons disease seems to be found primarily in people with RH negative blood type whose blood is typically more alkaline. Northern European ancestry, especially Basque ancestry, U5 Ursula gene - the most ancient European genome, Blue green or hazel eyes and/or an extra 1q42 12 gene.

Plasmafied isomers and mutated bacteria, viruses and mycoplasmas: Have you thought about how putting nanometals and other toxic chemicals into the upper atmosphere, and charging it with microwaves, and the UV from the sun can change those elements into even more biocidal isomers. And how the same radical conditions could mutate the bacteria, viruses and mycoplasmas into pandemic creating plagues? The species of microorganisms that naturally live in the upper atmosphere taxi down to earth on the chemtrail aerosols. With cross-genera disease agents that act like nano machines that build fibers out of the elements of living creatures, we are entering an alien experience of the world, which no previous generation of humans ever had to endure.

"There are myriad variations of infection patterns among family members present in the home. Most are just prone to Morgellons perhaps due to a immunocompromised immune system caused perhaps by latent or

already active infection by Borrelia bacteria which is causing Lyme disease, or Morgellons itself is transmitting Lyme bacteria and causing then an infection…most of the Morgellons afflicted also have bacterial coinfections, acquired probably by this fungus (vector)." Marc Neumann, morgellons-research.org

YouTube: *The Morgellons and Artificial Intelligence Connection*: Kandy Griffin @ Phoenix Rising
Listen to Rense Radio Program: Morgellons Special No. 26, Jan Smith
www.thecehf.org/morgellons-disease-fiber-analysis.html — The Charles E. Holman Morgellons Disease Foundation.

See YouTubes by the German researcher Harald Kautz Vella *"Speaks Morgellons-Watch"* and others on chemtrails, nano-technology, cluster piezoelectric nanocrystals.

Morgellonsexposed.com — Morgellons Research Foundation
www.stopthecrime.net/docs/SILENT.pdf

SPACE POX

The chemtrail particulates serve as taxis to mutated pathogens that naturally exist in the upper atmosphere, so life on earth has rarely had to deal with these "alien" diseases, except during major catastrophic events such as comets in which the natural order is thrown into upheaval.

Lyme, mycoplasma, candida, chemflu, nanobot dust, Morgellons and other biological weapons are sexually transmitted diseases (STDs). That means we have the potential of getting space pox from the chemtrail assault! The Lyme pathogen is a spirochete (spiral shaped) bacteria, is 40% genetically similar to the spirochetes that cause syphilis. Since Lyme is a genetically manipulated disease and Morgellons is associated with Lyme, we might consider whether the Lyme-Morgellons disease we are being sprayed with is a STD! The biological weapons of the eugenic genocide and sexually transmitted diseases (STD) like gonorrhea and Human papillomavirus, HIV and syphilis can be transmitted via kissing and other sexual activity.

This requires the discussion of a code of appropriate ethical social behavior. If you have been infected by chemtrails in your local environment that means most other people in that community are similarly infected and so the moral question of infecting others via sexual activity is less of an issue. It only becomes an issue when you move beyond the global net of bioweapon infection into territories that are not being hit with the chemtrails containing smart dust and infectious pandemic agents. Since each individual has a different level of resistance to bioweapons and infections in general some people could be harmed via transmission through sexual activity.

The psychological component to health is vitally important to our thrival. Focus on positive progress and optimism is vitally important to recovery. Pessimism raises our anxiety, decreases our happiness, saps our energy, lowers our immunity and resilience and makes us feel helpless in the face of the world's problems. Because the scientific community are still largely working for the dark side we are in this limbo state of not knowing the full causes and ramifications of our present bizarre circumstances of the Chemtrail Holocaust. Get informed, make connections and evolve solutions without rigid ideas.

Are we under attack by slow acting chronic infectious biological warfare agents? A **Mengele-style** silent World War 3 of weapons of mass degeneration! See the reading on YouTube: "*Silent Weapons For Quiet Wars Document*," through Deborah Tavares and Dr Edward Spencer. This NASA document was published May 1979 and is also in this document is in William Coopers book. "Behold The Pale Horse." See: fedgeno.com/documents/future-strategic-issues-and-warfare

COMBATING BIOLOGIC CHEMTRAILS
CHEMFLU~LYME~MORGELLONS CURES

Lyme symptoms flare up depending on our emotional state, how happy we are, our stress level, diet, exposure to environmental toxins and EMF pollution, our exercise and sunlight exposure and our commitment to maintaining an anti-infectious body terrain. Pathogens such as Lyme associated Borrelia burgdorferi require a toxic host with a weak immune system in order to survive. To eliminate Morgellons, you need to reinstate the immune system by doing a heavy metal cleanse, eliminate candida overgrowth, stop life-harming addictions and detoxify and regenerate the liver.

Symptoms increase when you drink alcohol, eat sugar or damage your immune system with processed and cooked foods etc… The first issue to address is backing off of sugar, alcohol, grains, coffee, smoking etc... Grains and all other dead/cooked sugars are fuel for candida, Lyme, Morgellons and other pathogens including the newfangled genetically engineered pathogens being sprayed on us from above via chemtrails. The Morgellons fiber growth feeds off of sugar, as does Lyme and Candida, and these also complex the heavy metals in their biofilms and structures, locking away the heavy metals in the body and preventing their elimination. When these pathogens establish themselves in the joints this leads of arthritic type soreness and in the brain, it leads to brain fog, memory loss and the loss of sensory acuity.

To deal with the chemtrail bioweapons a comprehensive program that needs to be undertaken that includes going on a ketogenic fast, and/or by eating 1 tsp of coconut oil every 2 hours, or monolaurin (for Lyme, bacteria, viruses, fungi) is the fastest way to remedy the situation. But we also have to increase cell voltage, remagnetize the body, do the heavy metal chelators, take antifungal and antiviral agents, break down the biofilms and do colon cleanses to eliminate the accumulated morbid mucoid layer in the GI tract. Mucoid plaque is a term was coined by Richard Anderson, author of "*Cleanse and Purify Thyself*," to describe what he claimed to be a combination of harmful mucus-like material and food residue that coats the gastrointestinal tract of most people. It is said that the black mucoid plaque must be removed to achieve physical, mental, emotional and spiritual health.

Lyme disease is exceedingly difficult to treat, due to its well-known shape-shifting (pleomorphic) abilities and biofilm, with conventional antibiotics often failing to produce a long-term cure. Whatever "cures" you employ you need to incorporate them as party of your diet and daily routine. Preventing and treating Lyme disease symptoms by improving overall immune system and cleanse your body of immune-compromising toxic heavy metals and other toxins. In order to minimize inflammatory cytokine cascades, you must have good gut health including strong digestive enzymes, good bacteria, and adequate stomach acid.

For those not already in a high fever, then heating the body helps to kill off pathogens. Hyperthermia treatment in a sauna or infrared sauna, steam room, and hot and cold while taking antifungal/antibiotic herbs like Cat's Claw, Olive Leaf and Stevia Leaf, plus Cayenne pepper to assist. Also whole-body hyperthermia makes other forms of cancer treatment work better.

If you have coinfections such as Lyme, Morgellons or Mycoplasma you need to adopt an anti-candida-type diet, and stay away from sugar, alcohol, cereals and life harming addictions like smoking. The anti-infection diet needs to be free of gluten/cereal, dairy, sugar and consist largely of fresh-raw fruit and vegetables, bitter herbs, non-damaged fats, plant proteins, and sprouts for enzymes. Due to the demineralized cooked food diet, the average human is overrun with candida sp. which makes us vulnerable to infectious disease, cancer and Morgellons. Both sugar, cereals and alcohol should be avoided as they feed pathogens.

People are finding probiotic fermented cabbage juice (not Jillie's Juice) beneficial to cleanse the liver and thus support resistance to Morgellons and Borrelia. Probiotic fermented cabbage and cabbage juice is a fast fix for inflammation pain. The Max Gerson method of cancer cure with fresh potassium rich juice (carrot, celery, beet, apple), in association with coffee enemas will stimulate the immune system to overcome Lyme bacteria and other infections. By detoxifying the liver and colon coffee enemas treat the emotional basis of disease, treating depression and mental illness.

COPPER: Copper deficiency reduces the elimination of iron and heavy metals. Colloidal Copper and Niacin + D-Ribose helps eliminate spirochetes and other pathogens and repairs DNA and repairs telomeres. Copper peptides help convert the amino acids to collagen. Taking copper rich food sources not only helps maintain healthy white blood cell numbers, but it also helps your cells better engulf pathogens. Copper Rich Foods: Beef liver, sunflower seeds, lentils, almonds, dried apricots, dark chocolate, molasses and asparagus. Many of the excellent food sources of copper are leafy greens, including turnip greens, spinach, Swiss chard, kale, and mustard greens, legumes, whole grains, nuts, and seeds. There is an inexpensive way of getting chelated copper into the body to reduce mycoplasma, Morgellons and Lyme infection. You can add copper sulfate to the soil when growing vege greens in the garden, or wheatgrass sprouts and microgreens. You can also spray colloidal copper on growing food so that it is absorbed and chelated.

THREONINE: A therapeutic dose of 8-15g/day of the essential amino acid Threonine supports thymus growth, is an immuno-stimulant and reduces inflammation. Threonine improves intestinal absorption, helps metabolize fat and prevents fatty liver. It also strengthens collagen, elastin and tooth enamel. L-Threonine is useful for improving mental stability, irritability and reducing spasms, as it increases glycine in the brain and acts as a calmative and sedative. 1g in the morning and evening reduces depression. Threonine also aids in the formation of B12, and needs to be taken along with B6, B3 and Magnesium. Threonine stabilizes Blood Sugar by improving gluconeogenesis (the creation of glucose) in the liver. Threonine and Lysine is found in cottage cheese and wheat germ, chicken, brewers yeast, eggs and other protein foods.

LYSINE: Lysine is the rate limiting essential amino acid necessary for the production of skin, bones, cartilage, connective tissue, nails and hair. The levels of the amino acid Lysine go down with stress, age and poor diet reducing epithelial collagen strength and leaving us vulnerable to infection by bacteria, fungi and viruses. Lysine along with cofactors B-complex and Vitamin C are involved in the production of the coenzyme acetyl CoA, and in carbohydrate metabolism. In fact Vitamin C increases Lysine strength and levels in the body. Lysine deficiency causes a loss of calcium in urine. For Herpes (and other viruses) take lysine, zinc, Vitamin C and bioflavonoids, and use Zovirax cream or 4% zinc sulphate topical solution for lesions and sores. Avoid foods high in arginine when taking Lysine therapeutically as it competes; and avoid copper as it degrades lysine. Lysine is a biosorbent that protects against heavy metal toxicity by chelating the metals so they can be removed from the body.

N-ACETYL CYSTEINE: The sulfur containing amino acid N-Acetyl Cysteine (NAC) can help with a diverse array of issues including mood disorders, brain issues, lung problems, sleep disorders, infections, and oxidative stress. NAC is more detoxifying to the body than Vitamin C, is a powerful liver-detoxifier and it can even offer protection against the flu. NAC aerosol nasal spray such as NAX (N-acetyl cysteine & Vitamin C) can help drain the sinuses and mucus burdened bronchioles, and helping to reduce fluid in the lungs. Nebulized glutathione or NAC is one of the most efficient antioxidants/anti-inflammatories used in treating conditions of the respiratory tract infections, pulmonary fibrosis, asthma, emphysema, and lung cancer.

GLUTATHIONE: The levels of the body's main antioxidant Glutathione reduce as we age. NAC increases glutathione levels which promotes the proper functioning of B-cells, T-cells and phagocytosis. In high doses NAC is anti radiation and anti-tumor, it chelates heavy metals, dissolves kidney stones as well as improving lung and skin conditions. Glutathione helps transport amino acids across membranes, including L-alanine and threonine, which are necessary for the production of lymphocytes (white blood cells) and macrophages, as well as red blood cells. Glutathione levels are high in the thymus gland; in fact thymus size increases when supported with supplemental NAC to boost glutathione levels, along with supporting cofactors such as Vitamin C, Zinc, Selenium, Beta Carotene and Alpha Lipoic acid. IV Glutathione has been found effective for treating Parkinson's. Cruciferous vegetables include broccoli sprouts, broccoli, cauliflower, Brussels sprouts, garlic mustard, cabbage and kale, and in addition to providing sulforaphane, they are some of the richest food sources of glutathione.

QUICK FIXES: Juicing a cabbage and putting probiotics in it, and drinking a shot glass every few hours should quickly reduce symptoms. Sore inflamed joints can be rubbed with DMSO, Magnesium Chloride Sol, Black Seed Oil or Castor Oil for immediate relief. A bath with Baking soda, Sea salt, Epsom salt and Borax will detox and alkalize your blood, providing immediate relief. For Lyme and other bacteria take 5,000iu vitamin D3 and 100 mcg K2 a day for 16 months to completely eradicate these infections. Omega 3-Krill oil, Magnesium, CoQ10, Turmeric, and Probiotics. Medical Mushrooms: Reishi Mushroom is known to digest or block the following pathogens: Aspergillus niger, Bacillus subtilis, Candida albicans, and Escherichia coli.

Other ingredients may be Hyaluronic Acid, Fulvic Acid, DMSO and MSM. Put in spray bottles and keep in the fridge, spray face, neck, chest etc… throughout the day, and especially just before bed. It reduces the stress lines in the face, and relaxes wrinkles…it also feeds and softens the skin. It would be helpful to heal the Morgellons/Lyme/Mycoplasma skin lesions caused by chemtrails. Itching stops within hours. Our bodies make Creatine from the amino acids glycine, arginine and methionine. Creatine may be key to turning the body toward anabolic building metabolism for it increases protein synthesis, especially within muscle fibers.

ARGIRELINE: (*Acetyl Hexapeptide-8)* is a peptide that visibly reduces wrinkles, scars and lesions. It relaxes the muscles in the face to promote a smoother, less wrinkled look. Argireline is a unique peptide composed of three amino acids: glutamic acid, methionine and arginine. Argireline is expensive, however you can make your own version of the anti-aging formula by mixing a tsp each of glutamic acid, methionine, arginine and magnesium chloride in a cup of special water (ORMUS Trap, octagonal, shungite water or high silicon spring water).

ANTI-INFLAMMATORIES: Some herbal remedies to reduce inflammatory cytokines and repair glial scarring are: Artemisia, Astragalus, Bromelain, Boswellia (frankincense), Capparis spinosa, Celery seed, Cordyceps, Ginkgo, Licorice root, Lion's Mane Mushroom, Magnolia, Olea europaea, Paeonia lactiflora, Propolis, Punica granatum, Japanese Knotweed, Banana Tree Stem Sap, Red Sage, Rhodiola, Skullcap and Schisandra berry, Turmeric, Green Tea leaf extract, NAC and Epigallocatechin gallate (EGCG), Royal Jelly, Yuan Zhi (Chinese Senega or Snakeroot). Grate some ginger root and make 6 cups of ginger tea per day; this will cure the fuzzy head by settling the stomach and cutting inflammation in the brain.

ANTIHISTAMINES: Antihistamines assist in the alleviation of symptoms from infection with spirochetes and other bacteria, viruses, mycoplasma and fungi. Wild oregano, rosemary and thyme (herb and oil) contains a substance called Rosmarinic Acid which is a powerful antihistamine and antioxidant. Turmeric inhibits anaphylactic shock, stabilizes mast cells and prevents histamine release. Other antihistamines include, Angelica, Ashitaba, Watercress, Pea sprouts, Onions and Garlic, Moringa, Holy basil, Tarragon, Sage, Savory, Hyssop, Chamomile, Grape seed, Skullcap, Jewelweed, Catnip, Feverfew, Goldenseal, Stinging Nettle, Catnip, Cayenne pepper, Black Pepper, Peppermint, Black cumin seed, Galangal and Ginger, Lotus root, Pomegranate, Capers, Mangosteen, Rhodiola, Milk Thistle, Propolis and Pine bark.

A diet rich in the flavonoid luteolin has been shown to reduce mast cell activation. This is found in carrots, bell peppers, thyme, rosemary, peppermint, oregano, romaine lettuce, artichoke, pomegranate, rooibos tea, buckwheat sprouts and cucumbers among other things. Lemon balm is a viricide and soothes nasal passages; skullcap is anti-inflammatory, and antihistamine, aids in treating allergies or allergic rhinitis, particularly when used with stinging nettle. The fullerenes in Shungite have pronounced anti-inflammatory, antihistamine, analgesic, anti-allergenic, detoxifying, immune-enhancing effects, and can be ingested like activated charcoal. Shungite charged water sprayed on the skin offers relief.

***Dr. Cass Ingram** has great home-cure books on all aspects of Chemtrail survival including "Natural Cures for Radiation and The Lyme Disease Cure."
Dr. Cass Ingram includes in his Lyme Protocol: Wild Oregano, Bilberry extract (25% anthocyanosides), Noni, Milk Thistle, Echinacea (purpurea & angustifolia), Goldenseal, Shiitake, White Willow (bark), Garlic, Grapeseed extract (min. 90% polyphenols), Pine bark, Black Walnut (hull and leaf), Raspberry, Fumitory, Gentian, Tea Tree oil, Galbanum oil, Lavender oil (plant & flower), Oregano oil (plant & flower). I would suggest a Tea made from Elderberry, Elder Flowers, and St John's Wort as an antiviral.

RAW COCONUT: Fresh raw coconut flesh contains high levels of lauric acid, a type of saturated fat that resists harmful viruses, bacteria, and fungi, and promotes brain health. The natural water from a young, raw coconut, for instance, is loaded with vitamins, minerals, and electrolytes, and is perfectly balanced to keep your body hydrated and nourished. Raw coconut can also help boost energy levels, promote healthy thyroid function and hormone levels, rejuvenate skin, and heal a damaged gut.

SPICY COCONUT CHAI: An antiseptic tea can be made with coconut milk, cinnamon stick, cardamom, clove, galangal, pinch of black pepper and turmeric and ginger root.

SYMBION FOR LIFE: This probiotic is especially formulated with three strains of lactic acid bacteria that have been proven to not only get the aggressive candida strains back under control and to prevent the overgrowth of the aggressive strains of candida in the future. Morgellons sufferers find it beneficial. www.symbionprobiotics.com

COLLOIDAL SILVER is a popular broad spectrum germ killer. Colloidal silver treatment protocol known to effectively disable the bacterial coinfections of Lyme disease. Colloidal silver works quickly — killing disease-causing organisms in six minutes or less and the pathogens cannot develop resistance to it.

DMSO/Ag/Si: The Philosopher's water works to reduce the Chembug, especially in association with intermittent fasting of 3 days, to reboot the immune system every week (for severe cases) or every month (for mild cases). Colloidal Silver, DMSO and Silicon may be a method of killing nano-bacteria, Lyme, mycoplasma and candida inside of cells in the body.

STEVIA LEAF TINCTURE: Whole leaf Stevia tincture absorbed sublingually may effectively kill Borrelia burgdorferi spirochetes and cyst forms. Stevia also effectively reduces the biofilm of B. burgdorferi by about 40%. Liquid Stevia made from alcohol extraction was most effective against Borrelia, while the powder form showed no effect. Alcohol extraction of whole leaf Stevia provides a safe and more effective means to combat Lyme spirochete infection. Stevia is three hundred times sweeter than sugar, has zero calories and does not raise blood sugar levels. To treat Lyme disease, the chemical compounds present in stevia must be absorbed through the intestines — but the reason it works so well as a sweetener is because these substances are not absorbed through the intestines. To get around this point a whole leaf stevia tincture used sublingually (under the tongue) may work to get the active anti-lyme ingredients directly into the bloodstream — and consequently into the brain

The Stevia/Propolis tincture is taken sublingually to kill the spirochetes, even those in the brain. *The whole leaf Stevia powder is so fine, the tincture doesn't need to be filtered and put into dropper bottles, instead the thick brandy/herb mixture can be put into a small amber bottle and applied under the tongue with the back of a small spoon.

*CAUTION: Although certain stevia preparations fall under the U.S. Food and Drug Administration's "generally recognized as safe" list, they may still cause mild side effects such as nausea. I think Whole leaf Stevia would only cause problems used in large quantities as a sugar substitute. Minute quantities as a sublingual tincture should be fine.

MULTI-TINCTURE: One possible tincture for chemtrail flu/Lyme/ Morgellons could be made of the leaves of Bilwa, Olive leaf, Cat's claw, Guava, Lemon, Graviola, St. John's Wort, Clove, Wormwood, Sida acuta, Cryptolepis, Andrographis, Stevia leaf, Turmeric, Galangal, Cardamom and Cinnamon sticks. Take directly sublingually or in a small amount of filtered water.

BILWA LEAF: The leaves of Bael patra is considered as one of the most important herbs in Ayurveda. The sacred tree can cure problems like inflammation, bleeding gums, constipation, dysentery, asthma, heart attacks, jaundice, anemia etc. It helps to regulate the digestive system, blood sugar & lipid levels. The extract of unripe Bael fruit can effectively treat hemorrhoids and vitiligo (discolored patches in different areas of the body). It is also used to treat anemia, ear and eye disorders. Extract of Bael fruit has antimicrobial, antiviral and antifungal properties that help in treating various infections in the body. The oil extracts from Bael can be used to cure respiratory disorders like asthma or cold.

BIOCIDIN: Biocidin® has broad reaching effects, including addressing biofilms. Ingredients Bilberry extract (25% anthocyanosides), Noni, Milk Thistle, Echinacea (purpurea & angustifolia), Goldenseal, Shiitake, White Willow (bark), Garlic, Grapeseed extract (min. 90% polyphenols), Black Walnut (hull and leaf), Raspberry, Fumitory, Gentian, Tea Tree oil, Galbanum oil, Lavender oil (plant & flower), Oregano oil (plant & flower).

PURGATIVES: The African plant medicine Iboga, is an alkaloid rich root bark that causes an intense psychological journey, and a serious detox of the body, mind and spirit. During a shamanic Iboga journey the powerful purgative effects can kill and expel viruses, parasites, harmful bacteria, other diseases and nano-fibers from the body. It is said that those who use Iboga would find strange fibers coming out of their stomachs in their vomit. Ayahuasca would have a similar healing effect.

ANTI-NANO-BACTERIA PROTOCOL: David Wolfe has a great Longevity NOW Program for changing the body's terrain to no longer support nano-bacteria, calcification, candida or cancer. This anti-nano-bacteria protocol is similar to that needed for the complex chemtrail syndrome that includes harmful agents as Lyme, Morgellons, and mycoplasmas and heavy metals. See YouTube Video: David Wolfe Educates About Arthritis, Calcium, Osteoporosis; and the book "Longevity Now: A Comprehensive Approach to Healthy Hormones, Detoxification, Super Immunity, Reversing Calcification, and Total Rejuvenation" (2013).

In the book *"Longevity Now,"* David Wolfe exposes the number-one cause of all degenerative illness and aging: calcification. Caused by an excess of calcium and the presence of nano-bacteria, calcification can be found in some degree in virtually every adult and even some children. It leads to a plethora of illnesses and manifests as achy joints, hardened arteries, cellulite, cysts, kidney stones, gallstones, dental plaque, cataracts, and bone spurs, among many other health problems. By breaking down calcification and removing parasites, heavy metals, and other "unwanted guests" from your system, you can reverse the aging process and eliminate the prospect of degenerative disease from your future.

ESSENTIAL OILS: Tea Tree oil, Galbanum oil, Thyme, Marjoram, Hyssop, Sage, Savory, Lavender oil, Oregano oil, Frankincense, Thieves, Neem oil and Tamanu oil. Applying an oil, like lavender, to your ankles, lower legs, waist, neck, and arms can repel them and prevent acquiring them and their bites. Lucuma nut oil promotes skin regeneration and wound healing and, thus, may a good base for topical Lyme/Morgellons treatment. The leaves are good for parasites. Cinnamon leaf oil has antiseptic, analgesic, antispasmodic, antibiotic, astringent, carminative, aphrodisiac, cardiac and other benefits. In a Johns Hopkins lab study, essential oils from garlic, myrrh trees, thyme leaves, cinnamon bark, allspice berries, ginger flowers and cumin seeds showed strong killing activity against dormant and slow-growing Lyme disease bacterium.

OXYGEN THERAPIES: Removes heavy metals and prevents pathogen overgrowth. Spirochetes can hide but must feed in plasma. But seem to love red cells at the non-oxygenated side of hemoglobin or in venous blood cells that are O2 deficient. When well oxygenated and the body's pH is alkaline and bacteria, viruses and fungi can't reproduce. Food grade Hydrogen Peroxide therapy, Ozone foot bath therapy, Ozone ear insufflation, Hyperbaric Oxygen Therapy. Ozone converts ammonia to nitrates.

BORON: Boron improves the natural ability of the human body to absorb calcium and magnesium. Boron significantly reverses arthritis and osteoporosis by improved calcium integration into the cartilage and bones. Boron is able to enhance the testosterone level in males and improves the production of estrogen in women. It increases the level of natural sex hormones and can bring back sex drive within a few days of treatment. Borax is taken throughout the day against Mycoplasma, Morgellons, Nano-bacteria. For internal use make up a recipe of 2 tsp Borax/Qt of distilled water, with 1 tsp to 1 Tbsp taken 3X per day. Borax in baths and footbaths is also recommended. Externally—soak in a hot bath for over 30 minutes with 1 cup of Epsom Salt, 1 cup of Baking Soda and ¼ cup of Borax; or a footbath with 1/4 cup of each, Epsom Salt, Sea Salt, Borax.

CLAY PACKS: Pure Calcium Bentonite Clay with a 100% negative ionic charge will rid the body of these positive ionic charged nano-particles, by pulling them out the like a magnet. It will also pull out at the same time all the toxins, poisons, heavy metals, unwanted bacteria, viruses, and radiation simply and easily without passing them through the bloodstream at all. Clay and activated charcoal is even stronger at drawing out toxins.

CHARCOAL SOAP: Activated charcoal soap binds to dirt and oil to cleanse your pores, while tea tree oil cleanses and kills bacteria and fungus. It is relief giving to the "itchies"when scented with peppermint oil.

SULFUR SOAP: Helps reduce itching and inflammation of the skin and speeds the healing of acne and infection lesions. Sulfur based Amino Acids Methionine, Cysteine, Homocysteine, and sulfur rich vegetables aid the detox necessary to fight infection. Regularly rub sulfur ointment onto your feet and onto bumpy areas of skin infected with candida.

CASTOR OIL PACKS: Castor oil contains a unique fatty acid that stimulates the liver, reduces inflammation, and increases lymphatic circulation and NK killer cell production (NK cells are lymphocytes that play a major role in deactivating viruses and combating tumors). Castor oil packs before bed can dramatically improve sleep. Packs may also be placed over the thymus gland (under the breastbone) to increase NK cells and over congested lymph nodes to help the lymph move.

REMINERALIZING TOOTHPASTE: A clay, charcoal peppermint toothpaste is great for cleaning the teeth. Make a toothpaste with bentonite clay, food grade calcium phosphate, activated bamboo charcoal mixed with water, ionic minerals and drop or two of peppermint or clove essential oil. Bamboo charcoal has more silicon in it than regular charcoal.

THE LEMON CURE: In case of itching, burning sensation or eczema apply lemon on the affected area. It is very good to cure any kind of skin disease. Cut open a squeezed lemon half and rub on your lesions, acne, scars and marks.

MORGELLONS LESION TREATMENT: Tony Pantalleresco offers a formula for a Topical Solution for Nano Poisoning/Morgellons sores on the face and body. What many are experiencing are sores on their scalp, forehead, jawline, back of ears, neck, back and chest. Mix into a paste and put on offending areas. 2-3 ounces of egg white, 10 drops of rosemary oil, 10-20 drops of iodine, 10-20 drops of colloidal copper.

Check out *Steve Beddingfield* and his parasite protocol for dealing with Morgellons and other Lyme induced conditions.

Dr. David James speaks about the correlation of Lyme's Disease and chemtrails. See YouTube: Dr David James: *Chemtrails cause Lyme disease.*

Healing Lyme: Natural Healing of Lyme Borreliosis and the Coinfections Chlamydia and Spotted Fever Rickettsiosis, 2015, by Stephen Harrod Buhner and Dr. Neil Nathan M.D. http://gaianstudies.org

How Can I Get Better?: An Action Plan for Treating Resistant Lyme & Chronic Disease, 2017, by Richard Horowitz, MD, president of the International Lyme and Associated Diseases Educational Foundation

Suffered Long Enough: A Physician's Journey of Overcoming Fibromyalgia, Chronic Fatigue, & Lyme, by William Rawls MD

In his book *"Boiling Point,"* Dr. Bill Rawls explores the connection between Lyme disease, Fibromyalgia, and Chronic Fatigue Syndrome, and how to overcome them.
www.lef.org/protocols/prtcl-143.shtml#whynot" —Fantastic Life Extension people on Gulf War Syndrome

NATURAL REMEDIES TO CURE SHINGLES

Besides lowering immunity, *Dr. Edward Group* found that the chemicals sprayed from chemtrails can "turn on" certain issues such as shingles (caused by varicella-zoster virus) within your body under certain circumstances such as prior infection with chickenpox. Immune suppression from prolonged chemtrailing may aggravate prior conditions. Anyone who has recovered from chickenpox may develop shingles. We know that a weakened immune system might wake the virus up, and risk increases as people age.

Natural shingles remedies include apple cider vinegar which provides relief from pain and discomfort when applied directly to the infected areas. Apple cider vinegar is a shingles remedy that helps remove the itching and burning rapidly and heal the shingles more quickly.

Dimethyl sulfoxide (DMSO) is another shingles remedy that helps stop the growth of the virus by penetrating right to the center of the infection. Dimethyl sulfoxide is a shingles remedy which helps you to get rid of the stinging and rash in three days, if applied to the affected areas twice daily.

Vitamin B12, an important nutrient for nerve health, is another shingles remedy that provides pain relief and helps rapid drying of the rash. Vitamin B-12 shows dramatic results in curing shingles, when 500 mcg of vitamin B12 is injected daily for three days. Sublingual or injection of B-12 is more beneficial than taking supplements, for it bypasses the digestive system. Vitamin B12, whether in supplements, fortified foods, or animal products, comes from micro-organisms, so maintaining healthy intestinal bacteria is advised.

Vitamin C (oral, liposomal and IV Vitamin C) is another shingles remedy that shows good results in curing shingles. The dosage of this shingles remedy is 2-3 grams orally every two hours. Vitamin C helps to relieve pain quickly and dries the blisters within a few days.

Vitamin E is another shingles remedy that is very effective in curing neuralgia, the advanced stage of shingles.

Applying a salve made by mixing a tablespoon of aloe vera juice and the contents of one 1,000 IU capsule of natural Vitamin E with zinc ointment on the blisters provides quick relief from pain.

Zinc is another shingles remedy commonly used to cure shingles.

Colloidal Silver applied topically has given AMAZING relief from the itching!

Natural antiviral cures include: Apple cider vinegar, Dimethyl sulfoxide (DMSO), Vitamin B-12 injections, IV Vitamin C, Zinc, L-Lysine.

Wear a shungite pendant over the Thymus gland to improve the body's immune system. Shungite ankle braclets assist grounding and prevent arthritis.

SHINGLES SKIN FORMULA: The healing comfort of Blue Tansy Essential Oil, Yarrow and Spikenard combines well with oils of Lavender, Geranium, Rosewood, Bergamot, Helichrysum, Carrot Seed, Tea Tree, Myrtle, Melissa, Thyme, Citrus and Palmarosa. Palmarosa oil is used to treat skin problems like eczema and psoriasis, as well as boils, abscesses and acne, as well.

VIRAL SKIN BREAKOUT TOPICALS: Zinc and castor oil ointment, Sulfur Ointments, Colloidal Silver applied topically gives relief from the itching! Calamine lotion, Chamomile Tea Infusion Spray, Vibrant Health Gigartina Red Marine Algae Ointment, Aloe gel, Manuka Honey, Chickweed Salve, Black Cumin Seed Oil, fennel seed oil, black caraway seed oil, Geranium oil. The following essential oils kill breast cancer cell lines: cinnamon, thyme, chamomile, and jasmine. Topical Colloidal silver treats bacteria, fungi, parasites, molds and fungi, burns, thrush, periodontitis, psoriasis and eczema.

THE VACCINATION SCAM

Mercury poisoning (from vaccines and amalgams) combined with microwave exposure leads to 100% autism in children.

In this sick culture the focus is on the questionable notion of vaccinating against illness, rather than on optimizing natural immunity and fundamental health. This is because the culture aims to promote sickness and disease as it is one of the greatest industries in the blind, ignorant upside-down world of the Borg.

The permanent and insidious damage from vaccines plainly reveals that they are a method of making lifelong customers for the medical mafia. Thanks to the faulty cut, burn and poison philosophy behind the allopathetic medicinal scam invented by Rockefeller et al to monopolize the "health industry," and make as many people as sick as possible, for as long as possible. The abominable Monsanto (glyphosate and GMOs) and vaccines cause brain damage, immune suppression, autism, chronic GI disruption and cancer.

Flu vaccines do nothing to address the underlying problem of Vitamin D deficiency, which is effectively hindering your immune system from working properly, nor can vaccines keep up with the rapidly mutating disease spectrum. Homo sapiens is already in degenerative free fall. The brain and immune damage from mercury and other vaccine contents, make populations vulnerable to mass pandemics. The answer is to heal from the original poisoning and nutritional deficiencies. See Don Huber on youtube.

VACCINES AND FACIAL ASYMMETRY

One of the main causes of Facial Asymmetry is brain lesion damage from inflammation in the brain due to vaccine damage. Lesions reduce nerve firing to various parts of the face causing atrophy, muscle prolapse, weak blood/lymph and lowered immune supply. Nerves feeding the mouth are also damaged leading to poor oral immunity, tooth decay and tooth death, which contributes to all aspects of degenerative disease, mental impairment and spiritual imbecility. Vaccine brain damaged parents go on to breed brain damaged children, both through the crime of vaccinating their children, plus nature deprivation and mal-nurture, *since broken parents cannot bring up whole HUmans,* as they have no idea what a whole, unwounded HUman is.

Apparently it takes a **20 session treatment in hyperbaric chamber** to reverse the brain lesion damage from vaccines, traumatic injuries and other causes. Once circulation to the brain areas are restored there would need to be simultaneous physiotherapy to the facial areas and other afferent tributaries of the nerves. Thus nerve growth factors and nervines in the diet would help along with therapies such as infrared wands, acupuncture, Transcranial Stimulation, electro acupuncture pens, electronic muscle stimulators, medical magnets, massage and massage tools, light and laser therapies, sound/maser therapy, hydrotherapy-water stream falling on the face, facial yoga and meditative breathing. Topical feeding/cleansing of the skin with things like wheatgrass juice/clay facial packs will also help provide the stimulation necessary. Royal Jelly may be one of the best substances to kick start brain lesion repair.

***This YouTube video explains this vaccine/brain damage connection with the highest degree of intellectual ethics: *Vaccine Injuries, Dr. Andrew Moulden, Conférence Liberté de Choix en Santé, Montréal, 12 sept. 2009.*

Besides the toxicity and immune impairment and genetic interference factors that are propagated by vaccines, parents brain damaged by vaccines then pass on their "brain damaged" condition onto their children through lack of health, wholesomeness and human-complexity. The vaccine damaged family exhibit effects are physiological, social, psychological, emotional and environmental. Both nature and nurture aspects must be investigated and exposed in the rape, torture and extortion of the gullible vaccinated population by the pharmaceutical industry.

"The combined profits for the ten drug companies in the Fortune 500 ($35.9 billion) were more than the profits for all the other 490 businesses put together ($33.7 billion) [in 2002]." ~ *The Truth About the Drug Companies: How They Deceive Us and What to Do About It*, by Marcia Angell

If vaccines make kids healthy, why are the kids receiving the most vaccines, the most sick? There is an ongoing study in Germany that compares the long term health of 17,641 vaccinated children with that of 15,320 unvaccinated children. **The study showed that vaccinated children are:**

- Twice as likely to have allergies
- 7 times more likely to have asthma/chronic bronchitis
- 3 and half times more likely to have hayfever
- 3.8 times more likely to have Hyperactivity
- 19 times more likely to have an Autoimmune disorder
- 10 times as likely to have Scoliosis
- 11 times as likely to have Epilepsy/Seizures
- Twice as likely to have Migraines
- Two and a half times more likely to have Autism.
www.vaccineinjury.info/.../resu.../results-illnesses.html

The Pharmaceutical Paradigm is in direct opposition to the continuum of life. For what it's worth I think the concept of vaccination is flawed and ludicrous…it is medieval. The whole focus should be on building a strong immune system and a strong, clean body not pre-infecting the body with disease agents. The body is exposed to disease agents all the time which inform its defensive functions. And now we are being vaccinated from the sky with the most disgusting diseases — Morgellons, Pneumonia and Syphilis (Lyme), aluminum, barium, strontium, mercury, coal ash carbon, bacteria, viruses and mutated fungi. To understand how deeply **eugenics medicine** is now the norm see YouTube: Patrick Jordan ~ *The History of Weaponized Vaccines, Militarized Medicine, & Serum Sickness* . Stay informed at vaccinefraud - YouTube.

Country children who grow up around farm animals and play barefoot in nature for much of their early lives are immune to the infectious diseases of urban dwellers, who are caged within toxic buildings, breathing toxic air and rarely ground their feet on mother earth. A specter of impending disaster haunts our degenerating world. Our children are demineralized and are getting weaker every year since chemical farming began, meanwhile the predatory medical industry's vaccines get more pernicious.

The corporations give us slave labor shoes, disease causing food, harmful EMF devices and then bully us with life threatening disease agents (vaccines) when our bodies are already rotting with candida, tooth decay and chemtrail flu. None of it makes ANY sense, and we should demand proof of concept before we expose any citizen to what is obviously one of the principle strategies of the global genocide. No we should grow up and live true to Nature instead of trying to cheat and rob it with evil life harming potions. The corporate pharmaceutical medical industry needs to be shamed and ridiculed into mending its ways, to stop its criminal charade.

"Vaccines are the backbone of the entire Pharmaceutical Industry... If they can make these children sick from a very early age, they become customers for life. The money isn't really to be made in the vaccine industry. The money is made by Big Pharma with all of the drugs that are given to treat and address all of the illnesses that are subsequent to the side effects of the vaccines." Dr Sherri Tenpenny, D.O.

The principle of immunization is flawed. It is immunization via vaccine that destroys the immune system and causes inflammatory lesions in the brain. There is no point in destroying the immune system in an effort to build disease resistance. The immune system gets enough work, education and training in the course of our daily life. There are no non-toxic vaccines. Vaccines handicap everybody's immune system so you are more likely to get chronic or acute infection. They also brain damage everyone so you can die of frustration from living in a non-sacred (insane) society.

Getting ANY vaccine lowers the immune system's capacity to respond to ALL diseases and triggers a permanent inflammatory cascade and inflammatory brain damage which impairs all functions including the nerve supply to the teeth. When the immune systems in the mouth and gut are compromised, the body basically rots from dysbiosis and fungi. Vaccinations cause permanent autoimmune inflammation and impaired immunity that allows harmful bacteria, fungi, yeast, viruses, and other parasites to basically eat us alive over the course of our lives; and then our rotting teeth contribute to cancer, heart disease, diabetes and all the other degenerative diseases.

Vaccines containing the mercury-based preservative thiomersal contribute to the development of autism and other brain development disorders. Mercury blocks the action of acetylcholine, the neurotransmitter that passes the nerve impulse from the vagus nerve to the heart and other organs including the digestive system. The vagus nerve of the Parasympathetic Nervous System (PNS) uses the neurotransmitter, acetylcholine to regulate breathing, the heart and digestion.

The truth of the obsolescence of the entire foundation of allopathetic medicine is out, and the pharmafia are fighting back trying to hold onto their market share of the disease business. See the GcMAF scandal and why over 100 natural doctors have been killed off. Predatory medicine can only infect itself in our lives if we go along with the Thanatos culture and expose ourselves to the insane agriculture, food and medical system. We have to liberate ourselves from victim mode or the maniacal medical mafia will destroy millions if not billions of lives and become increasingly criminal in its modus operandi. Allopathetic medicine can only thrive if the population is weak, ignorant and ill-informed.

To heal from Autism/GI dysregulation you have to start with juiced and blended raw fruits and vegetables and fermented foods grown on remineralized permaculture farms. Avoid all grains, industrial food and supermarket food in general. Chimps forage from over 360 food sources. Try and count how few food types we eat, and consider how they are all largely devitalized by commercial agriculture. Only intact remineralized permaculture can grow food suitable for en-lightened humans, however, vertical farming and hydroponics is a good alternative during biosphere collapse, Grand Solar Minimum and ice ages.

***Check out the rawfood teachers on youtube David Wolfe, Gabriel Cousens, Dan MacDonald (the Life Regenerator), Markus Rothkranz, Tony Wright, Brian Clement, Vaughn Lawrence, Dr. Mercola, Dr Sebi, Dr. Robert Morse, Jerry Tennant and Dr. Robert Cassar on youtube.

"Vaccination is a ritual based on a cultural myth, while claiming scientific righteousness." Liam Scheff.

ALUMINIUM ADJUVANT TOXICOKINETICS

The Ecotoxicology of Aluminum—Aluminum oxyhydroxide (alum) **adjuvant** used in vaccines is a dangerous, biopersistent, and ultimately brain-damaging toxin! Our body has no ability to rid itself of aluminum adjuvant, because its a man-made substance we have no inherent mechanism to eliminate. Aluminum injected under the skin sets up a life long inflammation response that causes immediate damage to the brain, spinal cord tissue and digestive tract. Aluminum in the body acts as a "thickener," like when alum is us used making in pickles—it "gels" the lymph fluid. When pickling the aluminum helps make the cell walls of fruits and vegetables sturdier, producing a crisp pickle or firm cherry.

Alum and other poorly biodegradable materials taken up at the periphery by phagocytes circulate in the lymphatic and blood circulation and can enter the brain using a *Trojan horse mechanism* similar to that used by infectious particles. This can cause long-lasting biopersistence within immune cells in some individuals, and macrophages transport the aluminum into the brain, leading to CNS dysfunction and reports of chronic fatigue syndrome, cognitive decline, myalgia, dysautonomia and autoimmune/inflammatory conditions linked directly to multiple Al-containing vaccines.

We know that aluminum adjuvant from vaccines goes straight to the brain, we know it triggers the production of a cytokine known as "IL-6" that has been implicated in autism, and we know it also triggers "Microglial Activation," which also triggers autism. We found that the majority of aluminum was actually inside cells, intracellular. Some of it was inside neurons, but actually the majority of it was inside non-neuronal cell populations. So we found that these cells were heavily loaded with aluminum. We also saw evidence that cells in the lymph and in the blood were passing into the brain, so they were carrying with them a cargo of aluminum from the body into the brain.

A study on aluminum in the brain and autism found that it was "low dose" aluminum from vaccines that caused the most damage. This speaks to the dangers of lose dose exposure via breathing chemtrail aerosols and their direct access to the brain via nasal passages and into the bloodstream. *Remarkably, the new study found that it was the lowest dosage aluminum (200 mcg/Kg) that was the most toxic!* The low toxicity of the higher dosages appears to be a consequence inflammation at the injection site. Apparently the high dosages caused such intense inflammation at the injection site that "granulomas" or hard nodules in tissue formed, which "walled off" injured tissue and prevented the spread of vaccine born infection or toxins. While the 200 mcg/Kg dosage did not produce granulomas and so the aluminum become systemic in the body and accumulated in the brain.

The two heavy metals (aluminum and mercury) in vaccines are raising the incidence of neurological disorders such as autism, pervasive developmental disorders or PDDs, ADHD and anxiety disorder. Dr. Stephanie Seneff, research scientist from MIT pointed out an important link between autism and sulfation, concluding that children with impaired sulfation chemistry (among other factors) may be particularly susceptible to the toxic effects of the thimerosal and mercury in flu vaccines. Dr Seneff has also extensively researched the harmful effects of the suppression of Cytochrome P450 detoxification system in the liver by Glyphosate (Roundup). Glyphosate based herbicides impair female fertility, retarding and malforming fetal growth, including abnormally developed limbs, in second-generation offspring. Glyphosate inhibits Vitamin D, causes mineral and nutritional deficiencies, and drives aluminum deeper into the brain.

Healing requires respect, attention, non-violence, non-resistance, non-rebellion, acceptance and unconditional love. Medical capitalism is an anathema and an insult to humane values and humanization. The healing and wholing of the whole HUman requires the nurturing of life, not violence and exploitation against it. It is vaccinated kids that are diseased and immune repressed, not to mention brain damaged. The sicker that unaware people get with the chemtrails, the more they will turn to the predatory medical system for their nasty nostrums.

One of my main concerns is chemtrails causing brain damage to the children who are already handicapped via vaccination, and now we are all being vaccinated (brain damaged) from the skies as well.

It is not just vaccinations that cause autism, the baby in the woman in her womb is being fed nano aluminum through the mother's bloodstream which travels to the baby's brain initiating autism before that child is born. There is a vaccine induced autism epidemic in the States and Australia, while these countries are attempting to mandate compulsory vaccines if kids are going to attend preschool and schools. This is madness. Besides the toxic heavy metals and other chemicals in vaccines…every vaccination causes brain damage via mini ischemic strokes in the brain from the body's inflammatory response. See: Video: Vaccine injuries, **Dr. Andrew Moulden**, 2009

The pharmaceutical companies are in on creating the chemtrail cocktails to make people sick, because they are in the sickness business. The more sickness there is, the more profits for them. I am surprised vaccine pharmaceutical companies still exists in that they are the fifth greatest cause of death in the USA. Vaccines are the main strong point of Rockefeller medicine's strategic business plan of making the population sick and stupid so that they become lifelong users of their cut, burn and poison medicine, and consequently die early painful deaths after spending their life savings. Cut, Burn, Poison...funny way to do medi-sin.

The mission statement of Rockefeller medicine is to keep the patient alive long enough to clear out their bank balance. The point is if you do not want to be eaten by lions, don't walk into the lions den. We have to understand the bottom line of the Borg is profiting from destruction, disease, distress and death.

Dr. Theresa Deisher, a PhD in Molecular and Cellular Physiology from Stanford University, determined that residual human fetal DNA fragments in vaccines may be one of the causes of autism in children through vaccination.

Stay away from Rockefeller death medicine entirely, it is med-evil. See the YouTube Video: "Rockefeller Medicine" - corbettreport.com

Patrick Jordan and **Wil Spencer** on YouTube are exceptional for big picture eugenics bioweaponry and eugenic medicine. Vaccinefraud.com

Listen to YouTube: Patrick Jordan | The History of Weaponized Vaccines, Militarized Medicine, & Serum Sickness

Source: New study: Massive Aluminum levels in Autism brains, is this the smoking gun for vaccines? By JB Handley, Founder of Generation Rescue, https://medium.com

Murder by Injection: The Story of the Medical Conspiracy Against America, by Eustace Clarence Mullins (2016)

Watch the videos: *"Age of Aluminum," "Injecting Aluminum,"* and *"Vaxxed"* online.

VACCINE DETOX AND RECOVERY

Detoxification and Recovery From Vaccines is Multfaceted: Get sunshine and grounding, the body detoxifies 20X faster in the sunlight, and ground for as much of the day or night as possible. Natural immunity necessitates Natural Hygiene principles, Permaculture principles and living true to nature.

Water: Drink 8 cups of filtered or alkaline water daily at least during a detox.

Raw Food Diet, Juices, & Smoothies and sprouts.

Everything that increases GLUTATHIONE as it is an antioxidant that is plentiful in the liver and kidneys, which are the major detoxification pathways: NAC, Propolis, Selenium, Whey protein replenishes glutathione by boosting cysteine.

If the vaccine reaction is severe or "disease" results from vaccination then intravenous glutathione and/or IV Vitamin C maybe advised.

Sulfur rich cruciferous vegetables, Garlic Mustard, garlic and onions; and MSM.

Wheatgrass juice increases levels of glutathione and provides the minerals and chlorophyll needed for detox

Milk thistle seed enhances glutathione. Raw soaked milk thistle porridge is a good way of consuming large quantities of Milk thistle seed.

Alpha lipoic and Vitamin C and E, Alpha lipoic significantly regenerates spent glutathione in the body.

N-Acetyl-Cysteine (NAC), Selenium, garlic and other methylators. Methylation Nutrients (Vitamins B6, B9, B12, and biotin.

Krill Oil Omega 3: Since the brain is made largely from DHA-Omega-3 fats, it makes sense that high doses of them following injury might support your brain's natural healing process.

Omega 3 (along with lecithin) to build up the nerves to rise to a higher order of play and novelty. ***It is best to take Omega 3 from whole food sources due to aldehyde toxin contamination of Omega 3 supplements.

CBD oil can help ease many vaccine injury symptoms by reducing inflammation.

Dandelion root has been used throughout the ages to detoxify, restore and increase the function of the liver.

Blood Cleansing: Burdock Root, Sheep Sorrel, Slippery Elm Bark, Blessed Thistle, Red Clover.

Thuja Occidentalis: Thuja has powerful healing action after vaccine injury.

The common broadleaf weed Plantain helps with vaccine recovery by healing, cleaning the blood and it draws toxins from the body with its astringent nature.

Horsetail, Nettle or Bamboo Leaf Tea for Silica, which has been shown to remove aluminum in the body, a grave concern for vaccines.

Cilantro: 1/3 bunch of cilantro blended with pineapple or orange at least three times per week.

Echinacea strengthens the immune system, fights viral infections in the body, and increases the production of T-lymphocytes and macrophages that destroy pathogens and removes toxins.

Olive leaf is an effective remedy against almost every type of disease-causing microorganisms.

Elderberry's anthocyanins enhance immune function by boosting the production of cytokines, helping to fight coughs, colds, flu, bacterial and viral infections and tonsillitis.

Raw pineapple juice contains the enzyme bromelain which is anti-inflammatory and will reduce coughing. Ginger tea also reduces coughing.

Spices (black cumin seed, cardamom, cinnamon and turmeric).

Fruits: blackberries, blueberries, strawberries, watermelon.

Propolis and Royal jelly helps combat infection, inflammation and the stress on the body caused by vaccines.

Probiotics, prebiotics, and fermented foods with good bacteria will boost your gut health and remove toxins and pathogens. Drink a ton of fresh cabbage juice + probiotics.

Baths: Herbs, Epsom salt, Bentonite clay, Kelp and Essential oil baths can all pull toxins out of the skin, which is the body's largest detoxification organ.

Sweating is another great way to rid the body of toxins. Running, jumping jacks, rebounding or a sauna or infrared sauna.

Massage, dry brushing your skin, and rebounding are three of the best ways to get lymph moving.

Earth: Activated Charcoal, bentonite clay, zeolite, humic acids ionically draw toxins out of the body. Earthing provides anti-inflammatory electrons.

Water: Fresh spring water, or depleted deuterium water will provide the H⁻ ions to quench oxidants and inflammation. Negative ions are richer around falling water.

Over the course of a year, your body absorbs **five pounds** of aluminum, toxins and other junk. To remove this toxicity you need to support the detox organs, clean the liver and colon, then do chelators, binders, fibers, clays, zeolite, org-minerals, juicing, lots of silicon water, colloidal silver, anti-candida, anti-biofilm, enzymes, antiparasite, antiseptic herbs, anti-inflammatories, probiotics. Infrared sauna or sauna, rebounding and lymph massage.

GWASHING: Use charcoal or sulfur soap for washing. Cleaning the pores with alcohol scrub and "Gwashing" a skin cleansing technique promoted by **Dr. Robert Cassar**, is vitally important to allow detoxification through the skin. The skin is the largest detox organ. In total, skin accounts for about 16 percent of a person's total body weight. Most adults' skin weighs in at 20 pounds or more. Gwashing is good to do in combo with sauna and steam rooms, plus alternating hot and cold. See Dr. Robert Cassar's YouTube 2 part video "Getting Started with Skin and Pore Detoxification."

In association with Gwashing and skin brushing other detoxification through the skin includes baths with Epsom Salt, Sea Salt, Baking Soda, Borax and lavender, ozone footbaths, infrared saunas and sunbathing. Clay body packs with activated charcoal. Followed by fresh coconut water or Aloe gel from a live plant on the skin.

Greater detoxification and consequent increased nutrition to the cells means less hunger, cravings and fatigue!

THE PERFECT ARSENAL FOR SOFT KILL

The plausible deniability of slow genocide, makes chemtrailing the perfect method of global eugenics.

The combination of heavy metals, pathogens and low oxygen conditions are the perfect arsenal for the depopulation agenda. From our present global condition it is obvious that modern humanity knows full well how to create disease conditions. To move beyond this pointless suffering we have to use our mystical intuition to get real with the "reality of Nature," beyond the myopia of cultural degeneration.

Reducing the oxygen in the air is one of the main tactics of the depopulationists. Whether it is conscious or not, cutting down the lungs of the planet in the Amazon, and spraying herbicide chemicals from the sky which is killing every tree on earth will rapidly reduce atmospheric oxygen. With the loss of photosynthesizing organisms in the ocean due to acidity, radiation and chemtrails—the planet, like our bodies is entering an oxygen crisis. Healthy cells in the body are aerobic, meaning they require adequate levels of oxygen for cellular respiration. When cells are deprived of oxygen for any reason, decay sets in.

Lower oxygen in the blood creates conditions that feed cancer, fungi and disease in general, which in turn creates acid, hypoxic conditions in the body. When we inhale, oxygen from the air is diffused through tissues and into red blood cells. Enzymes then combine with the oxygen to initiate oxidative processes in the body, which serve many purposes including ridding the body of toxins and other metabolic waste in the body can block the flow of blood and other bodily fluids throughout the body. If the body is well hydrated and the blood is free-flowing, the oxygen-rich blood circulates throughout the body and brings this essential nutrient, i.e., oxygen, to the tissues.

SPIROCHETES AND VIRUSES PRODUCE NAGALASE!

Nagalase is a protein made by all cancer cells and viruses (HIV, hepatitis B, hepatitis C, influenza, herpes, Epstein-Barr virus, and others). Nagalase is an enzyme found in the body and it has a role to play in breaking down the sugar we take in our food into other forms that can be utilized in the body. Nagalase is also an extracellular matrix-degrading enzyme that is secreted by cancer cells in the process of tumor metastasis.

If you have cancer or autism you will have high nagalase, and testing for nagalase levels can detect cancer even when it is at the cellular stage instead of the tumor stage. Any amount of Nagalase in your blood means that there are cancer cells that are multiplying and dividing. Nagalase basically cripples your Immune System so that the macrophages that gobble up and dismantle cancer cells can no longer do their job.

Scientists and holistic doctors have recently discovered Nagalase in many different vaccines, which spurs tumor growth by suppressing the bodies Immune system. It is proposed that pharmaceutical Industry deliberately inserted nagalase in to the vaccines to suppress people's immune system, as nagalase inhibits GcMAF. Thus ensuring increased profits from cancer drugs and infectious disease medications.

The protein called alpha-N-acetylgalactosaminidase or Nagalase has been discovered in many different vaccines, which spurs tumor growth by suppressing the body's immune system. It is proposed that these Nagalase molecules have been deliberately included in vaccines to raise cancer levels and thus increasing the pharmaceutical industry's cancer drugs profits. Nagalase is made by all cancer cells and viruses (HIV, hepatitis B, hepatitis C, influenza, herpes, Epstein-Barr virus, and others). Nagalase blocks production of GcMAF, thus preventing the immune system from doing its job. Dr. Jeff Bradstreet discovered that the levels of nagalase are elevated in children with autism. The result of the immune suppression caused by nagalase is seen in digestive disorders, sensory overload, and numerous types of processing dysfunction in the brain. GcMAF has shown the ability to completely reverse autism and cancer. GcMAF is central to the criminal vaccine psuedo-science...it is the body's natural cancer prevention and cure, and vaccines knock it out.

THE NAGALASE - GCMAF MURDERS

Many of those doctors and naturopaths who met sudden deaths over the past three years (more than 80 deaths) were trying to find an alternative treatment for autism and cancer, diseases linked to exposure to nagalase, a wide spectrum biological toxin. "Macrophages (Greek: big eaters) are cells originating from monocytes, a type of white blood cell found in the body. Macrophages function in both nonspecific defense (innate immunity) as well as help initiate specific defense mechanisms (adaptive immunity) of vertebrate animals."

Starting in June 2015 with Dr. Jeff Bradstreet who helped families whose children were believed to have been damaged by immunizations, over 80 holistic doctors have been killed in just over 2 years, including the great Dr. Nicholas Gonzalez, a holistic anticancer doctor in July 2015 who focused on the benefits of GcMAF. The murder of the truth doctors may have begun several years earlier when the great **Dr. Andrew Moulden** died unexpectedly in November of 2013 at age 49, supposedly by suicide. Suicide would never be an option for such a lucid, honorable and caring individual.

Dr. Moulden had a PhD in Clinical Psychology and Neuropsychology. He also had a master's degree in child development, and was a medical doctor. Dr Moulden hypothesized that vaccines cause blood/oxygen starvation and loss of zeta potential in the brain as a result of **inflammatory loss of blood supply,** causing neurological damage, which can then manifest as autism, facial asymmetry and general loss of brain function. Dr. Moulden was convinced beyond a shadow of a doubt that the mini strokes caused by vaccines produce brain damage, disability, lifelong suffering, and premature death.

Dr. Moulden made it clear that vaccines *"given to mothers"* who are nursing their young children can also lead to autism, seizures and lifelong brain damage in their children. At the time of his murder Dr. Moulden was about to release a body of research and treatments, which could have destroyed the pharmaceutical-vaccine model of disease management. www.drandrewmoulden.com

Jeff Bradstreet, MD, Dr. Nicholas Gonzalez, Dr Sebi and 90^+ holistic doctors died in mysterious circumstances or were murdered around the vaccination/nagalase/GcMAF scandal. The death of the "health" doctors is proof of public subterfuge and endangerment on a grand scale by satanic pharma.

GC-MACROPHAGE-ACTIVATING FACTOR

GcMAF activates the macrophages of the immune system so they can attack cancer cells and pathogens. GcMAF is a macrophage-activating factor , which is produced from Gc-Protein is an immune-stimulatory compound. Nagalase is an endogenous enzyme in sugar metabolism that can prevent the formation of GcMAF from Gc-Protein. One Nagalase molecule can thus destroy a huge quantity of GcMAF precursor molecules. When nagalase levels are elevated, it decimates levels of GcMAF – potentially disrupting the activation of macrophages that protect us from disease.

Nagalase can be produced from tumors retrovirus, herpes viruses, influenza, intestinal bacteria, and Human endogenous retroviruses (HERVs). HERVs are a family of viruses within our genome with similarities to present day exogenous retroviruses. Altered intestinal flora and changes in gut permeability as well as Vitamin D and calcium levels in blood may factor in this clinical picture. Nagalase blocks the Gc protein from attaching itself to vitamin D, thus preventing the immune system from doing its job and therefore causing cancer and other serious diseases. Without an active immune system, cancer and viral infections can spread rapidly.

Autism is a relatively recent condition, as is cancer – and the cause of this emergence is the ingredients of vaccines including the protein nagalase, widely introduced over the past few decades. Nagalase blocks the immune system from adequately functioning! The result of this is massive, full-body inflammation, and because of this, the body that 'attacks' itself in perpetual defense-mode, a factor common in autoimmune diseases. Wear a shungite pendant over the Thymus gland to improve the immune system's intelligence.

Lyme bacteria (and other pathogens) send out Nagalase to sabotage the GcMAF and they also build biofilms that block the Vitamin D receptor. Nagalase works in conjunction with heavy metals to cause lasting damage. While GcMAF has a neuroprotective effect against heavy metal-induced neuronal damage. Meaning GcMAF can be used for autism and chronic fatigue syndrome and for treatment of all disease, including Chemtrail Syndrome.

Increasing oxygen levels and ATP production will help prevent the loss of zeta potential, hypoxia, sludgy blood, high ammonia/acetaldehyde and toxic-acidic conditions that pathogens both produce and love to thrive in. Put more energy, sunlight, water and oxygen into the body to combat the negative EMF frequencies and pathogens that make our environment more entropic. Entropic environments are geometrically toxic to life, causing living things to increasingly fall apart and become chaotic and disorganization. Syntropic or biophillic environments naturally support the complexity, the rhythms and the energy of life.

Humans synthesize GcMAF using Vitamin D3, which binds to the macrophages. Sun exposure is the best type of Vitamin D, whenever you take D3 supplements, you need to take Vitamin K2. Wild mushrooms—notably chanterelles, maitake, and morels—are usually rich in Vitamin D when they get sun exposure. The form of Vitamin D produced in mushrooms is D2, unlike the D3 found in animal foods. The D2 form is just as effective as D3 in boosting the biologically active form of the vitamin in the body. If you put your store bought mushrooms in direct sunlight for 15 minutes this can produce 200 to 800 IU in 3 ounces of mushrooms (the RDA is 600 to 800 IU).

GUT BACTERIA AND MOOD

Probiotic cultures will play a significant role in maintaining health during the chemtrail holocaust, both in strengthening the immune system, thickening epithelial tissue against pathogens, and in regulating mood and social bonding. If you make Bravo GcMAF yogurt the rage disappears along with the frustration. Good to do for a few months at least. You can also make yogurt with Lactobacillus reuteri. Also L. reuteri was also shown to improve levels of the "feel good" hormone oxytocin. Dramatic improvement in skin thickness and health, along with mucosal health was achieved in mice trials consuming a probiotic-containing yogurt.

Those consuming the *l. reuteri probiotic* also displayed the skin glow and exuberant hair growth. Female animals in particular, had especially shiny hair coinciding with an acidic intestinal mucocutaneous pH. The control of inflammation and pH levels due to Cytokine IL-10 and immune competency were found to be important for healthy intestinal lining. L. reuteri served to facilitate immune tolerance and fortify the thickness of the GI mucus lining and repair epithelial barriers, thus making the animal more resilient to environmental challenges and dietary changes.

Consumption of *L. reuteri* up-regulates levels of anti-inflammatory serum protein IL-10 while down-regulating levels of pro-inflammatory IL-17A associated with pathogenic microbial infections. There was significant elevations in plasma oxytocin in those animals drinking probiotics daily, compared with untreated controls. Besides the 'glow of health' in mice, increased social grooming behaviors were observed after consuming purified *L. reuteri* due to the increased levels of the bonding hormone oxytocin.

The good gut bacteria,"*Lactobacillus rhamnosus,*" can dramatically alter GABA may be suitable for mood disorders such as depression or anxiety. The production of L-DOPA and dopamine are enhanced by two bacteria, *Citrobacter freundii* and *Erwinia herbicola*. Escherichia and Enterococcus probiotic species all produce 5HT-Serotonin, while Bacillus species produces Dopamine (DA), and Lactobacillus produces Acetylcholine.

Lactobacillus reuteri produce oxytocin thereby improving mood and sociability. Oxytocin was recently discovered to be integral in microbe-induced immune benefits during the wound healing process by a vagus nerve-mediated pathway. Lactobacillus reuteri can a used to rectify emotional distress, however you will also need to consume raw greens/sprouts/juices and fruit to create healthy intestinal bacteria. These bacteria can be cultured in raw cabbage juice in the fridge.

Consider that indigenous tribes are the picture of health until they come in contact with "Whiteman's World." Western culture breeds sickness, addiction, warmongering, ethnic cleansing and insanity everywhere it goes. We need to change that trajectory by studying intact indigenous tribes who will teach us how to recover our cosmic integrity. This is not regression, this is going back to living knowledge that proved successful, prior to our progressive fall away from cosmic truth.

The Bravo GcMAF yogurt (recipe below) helps reset the intestinal bacteria promoting greater immunity, less aggression, alleviating depression and reducing frustration. While using antiseptics/ anti-pathogen herbs and therapies like colloidal silver, we need to alternate their use with probiotics like GcMAF Yogurt, fermented cabbage, miso, etc…Key allies in healing the chemtrail syndrome include GcMAF yogurt, Philosopher's Water and Oxygen enhancers like green leafy vegetables or Stabilized Liquid Oxygen Drops.

BRAVO GCMAF YOGURT RECIPE

The following Bravo yogurt culture makes Macrophage Activating Enzyme (GcMAF). Macrophages (Greek: big eaters) are a type of white blood cell that engulfs and digests cellular debris, microbes, cancer cells, foreign substances and anything else that does not have the types of proteins specific to healthy body cells on its surface.

Buy one weeks starter kit from www.marsvenus.com/p/gcmaf-bravo-probiotic-yogurt

One Liter Full Cream Milk (Use Organic Milk from cows with no hormones & antibiotics)

1. Heat milk to just before boiling point then put in a glass bowl to cool to lukewarm.

2. Take off the skin if formed on the top of the milk and discard.

3. Mix Bravo Culture, Skim Sachet and Colostrum Sachet in ½ cup of the cooled milk.

4. Whisk the Bravo Culture mixture into the milk.

5. Pour Yogurt Milk into 3 clean glass jars, cover with cotton fabric, fasten with rubber band.

6. Put jars in a flat plastic container that has warm water in it and cover with cotton cloth..

7. Place this in a warm place…boiler room/closet, or in stove with pilot light on.

8. Keep in the warm undisturbed for 24 hours, then a further 8 hours on your kitchen counter. Cover jars with lids, then refrigerate.

To Duplicate: To ½ gallon of Organic Whole Cream Milk (heated and cooled as above) add as your starter 1/2 cup of your Bravo Yogurt to the next batch along with 1 heap Tbsp of Colostrum. Use ½ cup of the cooled down milk to blend these (or shake in one of your yogurt jars) before adding to the bulk of the milk. For those who can afford it, organic New Zealand grass-fed colostrum is the best.

***Besides eating it like normal yogurt, take 1 Vitamin D3 and 1 K2 capsule put 1 tsp GcMAF Yogurt in your mouth and swish several times a day. While consuming Bravo Yogurt, do not consume artificial sweeteners as they kill the friendly gut flora. Do not consume food for at least 1 hour after taking the yogurt.

PROBIO-SLAW: You are more likely to reach for a raw probiotic salad, when you have the slaw base already prepared and in the fridge in serving sized bowls. Just one quarter to one half cup of fermented veggies, eaten with one to three meals per day, can have a dramatically beneficial impact on your health. Typically sauerkraut is fermented for at least three or four days at room temperature. However, here is a method of making a more convenient slaw-salad base without the time and salt, which may not be quite as potent as traditional sauerkraut but it is more convenient. You can juice half a cabbage and mix the juice in with the pulp, then thinly slice or grate the rest of the cabbage and mix this all together. Dissolve the content of 2 probiotic capsules into some of the cabbage juice and add to the mix. Probiotics mixed with celery juice also makes a good starter. Put the probio-slaw in glass storing containers and leave in the fridge for 1 or more days before using as a coleslaw base. When preparing your salad add carrots, beets, radishes, red bell pepper, apples, raisins, dulse, nuts, caraway and other seeds, fenugreek and other sprouts, avocado, cheese, fresh-squeezed pure lemon juice, coconut oil, fresh herbs and garlic etc… *Coconut oil is readily converted to fuel for ATP and doesn't get stored as fat in the body.

BLIS M18: Carotec's Oral Probiotic contains bacteria that produce three potent antibacterial BLIS (Bacteriocin-Like-Inhibitory-Substances) molecules that fight bad bacteria in the mouth. These oral bacteria have unique enzyme producing abilities that allow it to break up dental plaque and neutralize acid that can be harmful to teeth and gums. Research has shown that BLIS M18 produces an enzyme called urease which neutralizes acid in the oral cavity. If you make fermented vegetables like Probiotic Slaw with Carotec's Oral Probiotic then you greatly expand the value of a bottle of these very important bacteria. BLIS oral probiotic would be an ideal culture for cabbage juice kept in the fridge, which swigs can be take throughout the day and swished around the mouth for a minute. A 4-6 ounce serving of the fermented vegetables there were literally ten trillion bacteria. That means 2 ounces of home fermented sauerkraut had more probiotics than a bottle of 100 count probiotic capsules. www.carotec.com

SWANSONS BLIS K12: Oral Probiotics helps to grow *S. salivarius* bacteria that preserve teeth and keeps the bad bacteria away. https://www.swanson-vitamins.com   Oral-Probiotic-Formula.

PROBIOTICS: Probiotics are essential to a radioprotective anti-chemtrail diet. In turn, prebiotics like pectin and inulin (chicory root) are essential to probiotics, as they are food for the beneficial bacteria. As people age, they have a greater proportion of pathogenic microbes to beneficial microbes in their intestinal tracts. This was particularly pronounced in seniors with dementia. The health of your brain is shaped by bacteria in your digestive tract. Bacteria in your gut actually control how your brain cells express specific genes. Other studies report that disturbed gut flora in seniors contributes to accelerated aging, frailty and premature death.

PROBIOTIC FERMENTS: Also make up some coconut milk and coconut kefir to use instead of drinking cow's milk. Probiotics are needed for healthy gut function, which in turn produces healthy brain function and healthy immunity. You can learn how to make your own fermented foods such as cabbage-probiotic cider, kefir, sauerkraut, kombucha and yogurt. Possibly use to ferment cabbage and other vegetables as a component of salads to maintain, support and promote the balance of the total microbiome of good bacteria in the digestive system. I make a grated cabbage mix it with sauerkraut and add probiotics, I keep it in the fridge and make salads with it for a week. Ferment vegetables with probiotics and keep them in the fridge to add to your salads.

CABBAGE THERAPY: Buy (or grow) a ton of red or green cabbages and juice them, put probiotics in the glass bottles and keep them in the fridge, drinking at least 10 oz per day. Cabbage Juice works wonders for digestive problems and aids in digestive health. Sulfur compounds as found in the cabbage family increase the expression of glutathione, which results in both metal detoxification and free radical neutralization. Cabbage Juice contains sulforaphane, which kills off the H. Pylori bacteria that causes stomach ulcers. Cabbage juice also helps reduce acid reflux and gastritis, heals colitis, prevents cancer, and even lowers bad cholesterol. Make red or green cabbage juice with probiotics in it, keep in the fridge and sip throughout the day. This will drop inflammation, improve the immune system and provide sulfur for methylation in the liver. With the cabbage fiber blend it up with water and add probiotics or sourkraut water, put this in a glass container in the fridge for a few days to use to make dehydrated seed crackers.

DEHYDRATED SEED CRACKERS: Any cooked carbs or
processed sugar will create blood sugar swings, promote insulin resistance and the potential for seizures and kundalini kindling. But there is a way to have your cake and eat it too! For us bread addicts, we can change over to sprouted exotic grain Essene breads and seed crackers! Seed crackers and Essene breads are an ideal way to eliminate regular cereal grain breads, which are very disruptive to the GI tract, and feed systemic candida, leaky gut, cancer, inflammation and diabetic conditions. The carbohydrates in raw vegetables, sprouts and low glycemic fruit are perfectly fine however. I also find sprouted or cooked Quinoa to be easy on the body. To satisfy the carb cravings you can make your own dehydrated seed crackers. These provide the Omega Fatty Acids necessary to build strong nerve sheaths, brain fat and cell membranes. Making an effort to balance out your Omega 3 to Omega 6 to 50:50 will go along way to alleviating many chronic mental, physical and emotional health conditions.

These seed crackers can be made with a vege fiber base, or with water. Not that you need to use the cabbage fiber to make seed crackers, you could use veggie juice or water, but it adds a fiber component and flavor to the crackers. You can blend the fiber with 1 cup of water, add probiotics and keep in glass in the fridge a few days, and use this as the liquid-fiber base for making dehydrated seed crackers. After a few days in a large bowl put approximately 1 cup each of ground up sunflower, sesame, flax seed, along with a 1 cup of whole chia and course chopped pumpkin seed. Mix in ground caraway seed, perilla seed, herbs, spices and seasoning and then add the wet cabbage fiber. Form a ball in the bowl, cover with plastic and leave in the bowl to hydrate for several hours or overnight. Chop into quarters and mold each 1/4 into a ball, roll flat on a cutting board with the use of (sesame seeds or poppy seeds) and cut into crackers. Dehydrate till dry and crispy. For freshness store the cooled crackers in an airtight glass container.

6

PREVENTING ALZHEIMER'S AND DEMENTIA

NANO-ALUMINUM VS. SILICON

Aluminum has the remarkable ability to turn the body's own defensive resources against itself...thus manifesting chronic inflammation and autoimmune conditions.

It was the great Viktor Schauberger's understanding that silicon carries the light of life in nature, via its architectural relationship to water. It is the density and perfection of the mineral body that contributes most intensely to the radiant quality of "animal magnetism" and "spiritual magnetism." This is so because the light of life needs a perfectly aligned and coherent liquid crystal body in order to shine with greater force. Genes and personality aside, it is the power inherent in the synchronic wave radiation or sympathetic resonance through the mineral body of the individual, which gives them greater Presence of consciousness and power of heart consciousness. It is this sympathetic resonance or "love" that we are "attracted" to in others."

Those with Alzheimer's disease are more likely to have aluminum deposits in their brain than those without the disease. Aluminum also has xenoestrogenic effects and linked to breast cancer. Aluminum accumulates in long lived cells and tissues like the neurons in the brain, macrophages, bones and heart cells. To eliminate aluminum out of the body, silicon, calcium and magnesium must pull it through the kidneys. Silicon deficiency contributes to Alzheimer's simply because excess aluminum cannot be easily pulled out of the body, and especially out of the brain. The majority of those who live in Western Civilization are silicon deficient duet to chemical agriculture, cooked diet and failing digestive fire. And if you are silicon deficient the body absorbs and stores more aluminum.

If nano-aluminum competes with or counteracts the absorption and use of silicon in plants, animals and other lifeforms we can expect to see the complete collapse of the biosphere on land and in the ocean from chemtrail spraying alone if the omnicidal program continues. Not to mention "mad," or madder humans...rendering vast sections of the population helpless and unable to fend for themselves.

Dr. Chris Exley who has a PhD in Ecotoxicology of Aluminum, University of Stirling has shown that Spritzer water which is high in silica (35 mg/L) improves cognition in people with Alzheimer's. Professor Chris Exley has been researching and thinking about aluminum for over thirty years and has published over 150 scientific papers on the subject. www.keele.ac.uk/aluminium/groupmembers/chrisexley/

His research found that through regular drinking of mineral waters which are rich in silicon (more than 30 ppm silica) the excretion of aluminum in urine is facilitated in such a way that over extended periods of time aluminum is removed from the body. Drinking silicon rich water flushes aluminum from the body and reduces the level of neurotoxin aluminum in the brain. According to Doctor Chris Exley, PhD Spritzer Natural Mineral Water from Perak, Malaysia, and Volvic Natural Spring Water from the Auvergne region of France are high silicon waters that pull Aluminum deposits from the brain and remove it through the urine. Fiji water has approximately 45 mg silicon/liter, however they put fluoride in it, and David Wolfe claimed that Fiji water is not recommended because they don't outgas their plastic bottles for a year before using them.

Silicon-rich mineral water can 'significantly reduce' the levels of neurotoxin aluminum which is linked to dementia. Drinking a liter of silicon rich mineral water every day can prevent memory loss and cognitive decline in Alzheimer's sufferers by removing aluminum from the body. When you drink silicon-rich mineral water aluminum throughout the body is gathered up into the blood and then excreted through the urine.

Organic silicon is found in significant amounts in cartilage, in the walls of blood vessels, and in glands and organs—the thymus, adrenals, liver, spleen, pancreas. Silicon is needed for connective tissue in the body to make it strong and flexible; silica is the glue for ligaments that anchor the brain to the skull. Silicon also provides the structural strength of plants, and their surface protection against the elements and to wall off bacteria, fungi and insects.

Water loving Silicon is the keystone architectural element in the body's collagen structure...which carries the biophoton lightbody...ie: the shining ones. Silicon is the keystone - the architectural element to our carbon (collagen) based structure. Silicon deficiency is one of the main reasons we are losing our water holding capacity and collagen strength as we age.

Our focus should be on silica rather than calcium for building and maintaining strong and healthy bones, and to maintain the shine, elasticity, suppleness and hydration of youth. Silicon also enhances the function of iron, calcium, magnesium, potassium and boron. Horsetail can be mixed 50:50 with yerba mate for tea and is at herbalcom.com under the name "Shavegrass." Biosil is a more expensive supplemental form. umosilica.com Japanese silicon concentrate. Bamboo: Lamberts Healthcare Silica 200 mg.

NATURAL SOURCES OF SILICON

Silicon is more essential in some plants, as silicon deficiency reduces their growth and vice versa, addition of silicon improves growth and guards against attack by pathogens. Silicon (for collagen and hydration)is found in Alfalfa, Bamboo sap, Bamboo leaf, Blue cohosh, Chickweed, Ephedra, Chaparral, Dandelion, Horsetail, Oatstraw, Nettles, Hemp leaves, Eyebright, Cornsilk, Comfrey, Lemongrass, Ginger, Raspberry leaves. Other food sources include the stalks, peels and cores of fruit and vegetables like celery, spinach and broccoli stalks, cucumber peels, Asparagus, Bell peppers, Soybeans, Oats, Brown Rice, Barley , Burdock root, Apples, Oranges, Grapes, Jerusalem artichokes, Radish, Romaine lettuce, Tomato, Nopal cactus, Jungle Peanuts, Almonds, Flax Seeds, Parsley, and Sunflower seeds.

ALUMINUM DETOXIFIERS

At cellular and molecular level, many cell components are implicated in Aluminum toxicity including DNA in nucleus, numerous cytoplasm compounds, mitochondria and the cell membrane. Al can alter the function of cell membrane and mitochondria membrane by interacting with the lipids, thus inducing lipid peroxidation. Al can bind principally to phospholipids within the membrane causing an increase oxidation by highly toxic reactive oxygen free radicals. Moreover due to Al toxicity there is change in the membrane potential that directly correlates with changes in the membrane surface potential i.e., zeta potential causing Al-induced cellular depolarization.

Exposure to higher than normal aluminum levels show a range of adverse effects, including damage to the brain and the nervous system. Alzheimer's sufferers exhibit the accumulation of a toxic protein called beta amyloid in the brain which binds metals including aluminum, copper, zinc and iron. The Nano Aluminum in chemtrails is perhaps the most damaging cause of "Chemtrail Lung" or congestive respiratory conditions. Aluminum clogs the lungs, just as it clogs the root hairs of plants.

Besides having a direct effect of clogging cell membranes, Al also inhibits cell division and causes the restructuring of cell contents by changing the zeta potential, or electrokinetic potential in colloidal dispersions, causing cell protoplasm to coagulate. That is, causing cytoplasm, cell contents, blood plasma and lymph fluids to "gel." **Adjuvants** like aluminum keep pathogens in the body longer so that the body's prolonged inflammatory response creates free radical damage and can present a danger to life. The chemtraitors are essentially spraying us with "live" vaccines from the sky. Dr Christopher Exley on YouTube

Besides preventative measures like moving out of the chemtrailing zones, wearing a mask on heavy trail days, locking up the house and using a hepa air filter, there are various remedial solutions we can take to avoid respiratory problems and dementia. Cleaning out the nostrils and steaming the face with essential oils or herbs after you have been out in the chemtrail soap is probably a good idea considering we really have no idea what they are doing to us, so it is better to be safe than sorry and adopt some new hygiene rituals.

Neurotoxin exposure can include widespread central nervous system damage such as mental retardation, persistent memory impairments, epilepsy, and dementia. Aluminum detoxifiers include cold pressed unrefined organic coconut oil, chia and flaxseed, Milk thistle, Vitamin C (and foods rich in this vitamin), Alpha Lipoic Acid, lemon water, spirulina, chlorella, kelp, Astaxanthin, Magnesium Malate, Malic acid, Apple pectin, L-Theanine a component found in green tea. Saffron is known to remove aluminum from the brain. Saffron has been reported to contain more than 150 carotenoid compounds and is a rich source of B vitamins and riboflavin. B6 supports the elimination of aluminum.

Aluminum is eliminated by foods such as garlic, onion and sulfur rich foods, cilantro, parsley, turmeric, fresh Aloe vera leaf juice, wild blueberries and other berries. Avoid aluminum and alum to prevent and stop the progression of Alzheimer's disease and memory loss and increase your consumption of silicon rich water and foods that aid the excretion of aluminum. All silicon rich sources including diatomaceous earth, cucumbers, bananas, zeolite clay, bamboo resin and horsetail herb. For silicon rich drinking water that removes aluminum see the principle Chemtrail cure that I call **Philosopher's Water**. (*See The Conclusion). The silicon/colloidal silver water helps to with detoxing aluminum out of the brain, reducing inflammation, painful joints, and infectious agents from the population being exterminated via chemtrails.

Silicon rich drinking water is an easy way to raise our vitality up enough to have the presence of mind to look after ourselves in other ways. Hence it is foundational for the movement away from tuning out, to tuning in.

Diatomaceous Earth is approximately 3% magnesium, 33% silicon, 19% calcium, 5% sodium, 2% iron and many other trace minerals such as titanium, boron, manganese, copper and zirconium. A silica drink led to significant excretion of aluminum in the urine, lower the risk of Alzheimer's plaque and dementia and also helps in the prevention of osteoporosis. A glass of water with 2 tsp DE twice-times daily lowers serum concentrations of cholesterol, HDL, LDL, and triglycerides levels, reducing blood pressure and atherosclerosis. Diatomaceous earth has been used for years in the holistic community for gastrointestinal health and its action on microbes including parasites. Other authors have found silica useful in the treatment of aged skin, fragile hair, and brittle nails. Another excellent source of silica is zeolite, as a way to lower the aluminum and heavy metal burden.

Structured water (and shungite water), infrared saunas, steam room/cold shower, ocean swims, mineral baths, and regular exercise. 3-day "water or raw juice fasts." The Scientology drug detox "**Purification Rundown**" system is ideal: ½ hour run, followed by a sauna in which niacin, Vitamin C, Omega-3 (krill) and a ton of water are consumed, then shower and scrub the skin afterwards. Along with chelation amino acids the "Purification Rundown" can actually get rid of lead and other heavy metals, as well as PCBs, Dioxin, pesticides, and petroleum products.

The heavy metals released into the body by chelation therapy can be handled at least partially by Alpha Lipoic Acid. Lipoic acid can be synthesized internally from Caprylic acid (octanoic acid) found naturally in coconuts and breast milk. Following up with colonics may also be helpful for eliminating waste and harmful compounds that have accumulated in the body over time. Aluminum and heavy metal detox is not to be taken lightly, so read up, and get help from professionals in the field.

BIOSILICA BEER: Biologically complexed Silicon has maximum bioavailability. If you have weak digestion it is best to use silicon rich plant material when making herbal beers or some other form of fermentation to make the silicon readily bioavailable. Consumption of moderately high amounts of beer in humans and ortho-silicic acid in animals has shown to reduce aluminum uptake from the digestive tract and slow down the accumulation of this metal in the brain tissue. However horsetail, cucumbers, and diatomaceous earth powder lack the ionic suspension of Orthosilicic (H_4SiO_4) or ionic silicic acid found in the mineral waters and biosilica beers to penetrate the blood-brain and reduce aluminum toxicity in the brain to help ward off Alzheimer's Disease.

To process Horsetail (Shavegrass) you need to split and dry it, then grind it up to a powder. It is poisonous in quantity while it is raw without drying or cooking, or in this case fermenting. Makes good sun tea after processing. Use silicon in conjunction with shungite for a powerful youthifying effect. Since I charge my distilled water with shungite prior to making Philosopher's water, the water has exceptional "drinkability." It is also a lot easier than making tons of horsetail-nettle tea, cucumber-spinach juice, eating expensive bamboo sap and other forms of plant-chelated silicon. Philosopher's water can be used in along with a high silicon plant-based diet for powerful detoxification and exceptional anti-aging. A wine could be made from silicon rich plant material (nettle, hemp, horsetail, bamboo sap) and a fruit such as grapes.

More Herbal Beer ideas in: *Sacred and Herbal Healing Beers: The Secrets of Ancient Fermentation,* Stephen Harrod Buhner

ALZHEIMER'S DISEASE AND DEMENTIA

Alzheimer's disease (AD) is a progressive dementia resulting from altered processing of amyloid precursor protein, the formation of beta-amyloid plaques, hyper-phosphorylated tau protein containing neurofibrillary tangles, and the loss of synapses in the brain. A third of people over 65 have elevated amyloid plaque in the brain, and it is predicted that most people with elevated amyloid will progress to symptomatic Alzheimer's within 10 years. When the aged lose their minds what does that say about the culture at large?

Alzheimer's disease with its full blown dementia and memory loss symptoms, is already the sixth leading cause of death in the United States. By 2025 it is anticipated that 16 million Americans will have the disease, up from 5 million today. By 2050, that number is expected to expand to 88 million or 22 % of the population. The latest figures reveal that dementia, including Alzheimer's disease, has overtaken heart disease as the leading cause of death in England and Wales.

We are on the eve of a crisis of dementia that the world has never before seen. Thus we can anticipate the overwhelm and breakdown of mainstream **allopathetic medicine**. According to research reported at the Alzheimer's Association International Conference 2015 the cost of caring for those with Alzheimer's will consume nearly 25 percent of Medicare spending in 2040. Alzheimer's and chemtrail related dementia will be the #1 cause of death in 20 years.

Dementia is essentially the slow and progressive dying of brain cells, usually resulting from a neurodegenerative disease like Alzheimer's. Brain deterioration and dementia take decades to cause serious and visible harm, eventually, however, dementia is fatal. "Alzheimer's" is now being used incorrectly as a catch-all term for all kinds of dementia. The main cause of dementia is the buildup of toxins, chemicals, and heavy metals in the brain, along with nutritional deficiencies and drugs that block acetylcholine. In the United States more than 28 million baby boomers will develop dementia in the next few years.

As the pandemic of chemtrail cognitive decline and dementia unfolds we can expect to see "mad" or madder humans…rendering vast sections of the population helpless and unable to fend for themselves. From the global chemtrail program we can expect a pandemic of Alzheimer's, accelerated aging and damaged human fetal brain development (cretinism). By 2050 it is expected that 135 million will be rendered with Alzheimer's with costs rising towards a Trillion. One out of every two people over 85 years old will have Alzheimer's by 2050. It is apparent that mindless industrialism and the war against Nature is a failed experiment.

FACTORS CONTRIBUTING TO ALZHEIMER'S

- Aluminum toxicity is mostly due to its enhancement of excitotoxicity by immune system mediators, via crosstalk between cytokine receptors and glutamate receptors.

- Aluminum exposure increases immune cytokines and glutamate in the microglia and astrocytes of the brain generating immunoexcitotoxicity.

- A hyper-excitatory response due to persistently primed microglia leads to dissonance (brain fog), poor brain efficiency, and neurological exhaustion and depression.

- Pesticides interfere with the mechanism that normally switches off the microglia immune activation when the danger has passed, thereby leading to chronic inflammation.

- Glyphosate in Roundup drives aluminum deep into the brain, thus a detox from aluminum is also a detox from Roundup. See Dr Dietrich Klinghardt on YouTube.

- Deficiency of neuro-essential fatty acids, especially Omega-3 DHA, and of monoamine neurotransmitters, which leads to impaired antioxidant capacity and sulfate supply to the brain.

- An ongoing state of secondary neurodegeneration, with the consequent impaired ability to recycle cellular debris and backed up glymphatic drainage. Deficiencies in important minerals such as magnesium and zinc prevent the normal control and protection mechanisms of excitotoxicity.

- Fluoride, at levels added to drinking water, significantly inhibits DNA polymerase, the enzyme that builds and repairs DNA.

- They use industrial waste in chemtrails also, but they mostly seem to dump it over urbanized areas, so depopulation seems to be the raison d'etre.

- The "work around" processes the body initiates in response to brain injury produce undesirable by-products downstream, such as increased β-amyloid plaque (glucose metabolism work around) or encephalopathy (sulfur deficiency).

- EMF-mediated changes in mitochondrial function may affect cognition and even perpetuate development of neurodegenerative diseases such as Alzheimer's and Parkinson's in which mitochondrial dysfunction has been demonstrated.

- Porphyromonas gingivalis, the key bacteria in chronic gum disease been found after death in the brains of people who had Alzheimer's.

Fluoride in municipal drinking water removes copper from copper water pipes, and Alzheimer's sufferers carry higher free copper levels. Copper in the brain inactivates the removal of accumulated toxic β-amyloid sludge that eventually kills neurons. Zinc is copper's natural antagonist that protects against cognitive decline. Zinc deficiency also induces excess free radical production, through allowing inflammatory minerals and metals to impact cells.

Over years, aluminum accumulates in the brain, tissues, and to a lesser amount the bones. It causes BRAIN DEGENERATION, dysfunction and damage due to blocking and reducing blood flow and oxygenation of brain arteries.

Synapse elimination, or "synaptic pruning," is a normal process that occurs during brain development. However in Alzheimer's the mechanisms involved in such pruning might be aberrantly turned back on or hijacked, so to speak, contributing to synapse loss. In the pruning process, microglia eat away at synapses to assist the immune system.

Heparan sulfate, is a linear polysaccharide produced by mast cells, found on the surface of cells (including neurons), where they interact with a plethora of ligands. Heparan sulfate essentially "traps" β-amyloid peptides, causing them to aggregate and form deposits that will eventually lead to amyloid beta peptide plaques and tangles in the brain that trigger inflammation and result in the loss synaptic connections—the effect most strongly associated with cognitive decline, neurodegeneration and dementia.

Dr. Richard Deth found autism and other attention disorders like ADHD, schizophrenia and Alzheimer's disease can be attributed to impaired function of the D4 subtype of dopamine receptor due to high oxidative stress and reduced folate-dependent methylation reactions, including their regulation by dopamine and growth factors, and their inhibition by neurodevelopmental toxins.

Molliver et al. (1989) found a similarity between serotonergic axons damaged by the drug Ecstasy and those seen in Alzheimer's disease. The early vulnerability of aging to the **Locus coeruleus** (Blue Spot), the major noradrenergic nucleus of the brain and to neurodegenerative disease (Parkinson's and Alzheimer's diseases) is of considerable significance.

Loss of the tribe, separation, alienation, rejection, abuse and inattention or lack of care, leads to the production of anaesthetizing chemicals in the brain which numb out emotional pain, leading to memory loss and a general amnesia or suppression of the self. Stress, noxious or anxiety-provoking extremes cause heightened arousal and overactivation of the sympathetic nervous system, which overworks the dopamine and noradrenaline circuits which ages the protective neuromelanin pigmentation and causing nerve cell death. "Connection" is the antidote to stress.

Imagine a time when the majority of people over 40 suffer from dementia - there will be no social services to tend to them.

ALZHEIMER'S RECOMMENDATIONS

- Eliminate all processed sugars
- Eliminate gluten, sugar, meat and processed food from the diet,
- Increase vegetables, fruits, seeds and nuts;
- Reduce stress with yoga and deep breathing, meditation
- Increase sleep 7-8+ hours per night as early to bed before midnight
- Exercise for a minimum of 30 minutes-45 min, 4-6 days per week
- Get earthing/grounding and negative ions in nature.
- Get B-12 methylcobalamin from Nori (seaweed) each day
- Get out in the sunshine each day, sungaze at dawn and dusk
- Take coconut oil, eat soaked walnuts or blackseed oil
- Fast for a minimum of 16 hours between dinner and breakfast.
- Have a minimum of three hours between dinner and bedtime.
- Cultivate warm, stimulating and supportive relationships

Intermittent fasting was actually found to increase basal metabolic rate after both 36 and 60 hours of fasting, likely due to an increase of norepinephrine (caused by lower blood sugar induced by the fast). Fat metabolism also increased (meaning fat was preferentially burned for energy over glycogen, or carbohydrate), likely caused by the increase in norepinephrine levels rather than a decrease in insulin levels. After a 36-hour fast, when you start eating again you continue to burn fat in excess of glycogen (carbohydrate) for energy. Muscle breakdown wasn't seen until the end of the third day of fasting.

Long-term use of Intermittent fasting may, in fact, shift the substrate the body uses for energy preferentially to fat, but also 82 genes that encode proteins involved in energy metabolism, inflammation, immune function, aging, and neurological function. Intermittent fasting doesn't appear to make you hungrier on days you eat. In fact, studies show people actually eat 20% less on eating days. This may be because eating less itself seems to reduce the amount of food that makes you feel full.

Water fasting reduces the chances of getting Alzheimer's and Parkinson's, grows dendrites and revives synapses, renews stem cell growth, enhances mitochondria, repairs DNA and reduces inflammation and histamine. Alzheimer's disease is a loss of memory potentially from an accumulation of plaque in the brain and chronic dehydration. Intermittent fasting, as the name implies, involves reduced calorie restriction (i.e., reducing caloric intake by 20–40 percent) may mitigate some of these risks.

If caloric restriction can slow the body's aging, there is a chance that it could delay age-related diseases such as Alzheimer's. Intermittent fasting needs to be observed to start the process of autophagy to regenerate the tissues of the brain, this will also activate ketosis on a daily basis which removes fat (a contributing factor) and the brain thrives on ketones, not only this but burning fat at this rate will generate **Embryonic Style Stem Cells** and play a role in replacing weak and damaged tissues of the body including brain cells.

Drink one liter of water with a pinch of salt first thing in the morning. Then go for a 45 minute walk out in the sun. If possible include swimming in the ocean or some other water activity. Get interactive with other people, and look for some nutrition to enhance memory. Blueberries, activated walnuts and pecans, different types of fruits all stimulate the brain. High water content fruit like watermelon is especially good for the brain.

 Silicon deficiency contributes to Alzheimer's simply because excess aluminum cannot be pulled out of the body, and especially out of the brain. If nano-aluminum competes with or counteracts the absorption and use of silicon in plant, animal and other lifeforms we can expect to see the complete collapse of the biosphere on land and in the ocean from chemtrail spraying alone if the ecocidal program continues. (***See P. for more on Silicon)

Resveratrol, found in the skin of red grapes, is a powerful antioxidant that helps to protect your cells from the damaging effects of oxidation. It helps the body guard against cancers, cardiovascular disease, and neurodegenerative diseases like Alzheimer's.

Vitamin D could quite possibly be the most important and crucial nutrient for all dementia sufferers. Vitamin D deficiency has been repeatedly linked to brain problems such as poor memory and recall attainability. Researchers believe that vitamin D protects brain cells and may even be able to help damaged neurons regenerate. Vitamin D and K2,sunshine and grounding are vital to fight chemtrail flu and ongoing Lyme-type symptoms.

The Vitamin D binding GcMAF is a universal cure for cancer. It's also believed to be capable of treating and reversing autism, HIV, liver/kidney disease, diabetes, Parkinson's and Alzheimer's disease and rheumatoid arthritis, as well as reduce cancerous breast, prostate and kidney tumors. MAFActive Cream for lesions, molds and skin cancers. It is suggested that GcMAF be taken along with Vitamin D3 and Vitamin K2. https://therivertorecovery.com/gcmaf/

For vitamin E, the best source is without a doubt unprocessed red palm oil. The benefit of red palm oil is not only is it incredibly high in the eight different forms of molecules categorized as vitamin E (including alpha-tocopherol), it's also high in the healthy ketone fats all dementia sufferers need. B group vitamins, in particular, vitamin B6, B12 and folic acid, can help slow the progression of Alzheimer's disease. B vitamins, and especially the Methylcobalamin form of B12 prevents brain shrinkage by reducing homocysteine.

The red algae pigment **Astaxanthin** crosses the blood-brain barrier, allowing its antioxidant properties to protect and feed brain tissue and counteracts the oxidative impact of abnormal proteins in both Alzheimer's and Parkinson's diseases. Take in association with a teaspoon of Lecithin in your smoothie, or other phospholipid rich food like sunflower seeds for better intestinal absorption of supplemental carotenoids. B vitamins, and especially the Methylcobalamin form of B12 prevents brain shrinkage by reducing homocysteine. The best Omega-3 to use is omega-3's Krill Oil because it contains a neuron protective substance called Astaxanthin. Omega-3 regenerates the cones of the eyes.

Chlorella is a powerful detoxifier, with a unique ability to pull heavy metals out of the body but leave the good minerals (essential minerals) alone. Alpha lipoic acid and Vitamin C pulls heavy metals out of the cells.

CANNABIS OIL CURE: Researchers found that cannabinoids permitted a two-fold increase in β-amyloid plaque able to pass through the blood brain barrier (BBB). The nanometals in the chemtrails can easily pass through the BBB, and the infectious agents in the chemtrails can damage the BBB and create meningitis or inflammation of the membranes that surround the brain and spinal cord. In particular Mycoplasma, a type of very small bacteria found in chemtrails are likely to get into the central nervous system. The absence of a conventional cell wall allows mycobacteria to penetrate into the white blood cells of the immune system and once hidden inside the white blood cells they cannot be killed. Mycoplasma can alter the chemical composition of its surface each time the bacterium divides so antibiotics may be useless against it.

Daily curcumin from turmeric lowers plaque deposits in the brain. When fed to aged mice with advanced plaque deposits similar to Alzheimer's disease, the curcumin reduced the amount of plaque. Cannabis oil containing THC can relieve the symptoms of Alzheimer's, and also slow the onset of new cases. THC prohibits the growth of toxic β-amyloid plaques, stopped the inflammatory response from the nerve cells caused by beta amyloid and allowed the nerve cells to survive. Two important components of cannabis are THC and CBD, which have a range of physiological effects relevant to Alzheimer's—If taken regularly they can not only slow the progression of existing Alzheimer's cases, can reduce inflammation, act as antioxidants and neuroprotectants, lower the β-amyloid plaque production, promote the cellular removal of β-amyloid , and even stimulate the growth of new neural tissue. Reduce inflammation through diet, cannabis consumption, and exercise.

THC at low doses also reduced levels of glycogen synthase kinase 3 beta (GSK3ß), an enzyme that is normally involved in energy metabolism and neuronal cell development but is also responsible for the development of neuro-fibrillary tangles in the brains of Alzheimer's patients. If you are investigating cannabis oil, look for a product with a coconut oil base to harness the added benefit of ketones. A 2006 Spanish study found that cannabinoids could even help cure pancreatic cancer – one of the most aggressive forms of cancer.

Consider cannabis as an alternative to anti-spasmodic pharmaceuticals. Mega-dose on fresh cannabis leaf juice – yes this is very healthy and won't get you high.

HERBS FOR ALZHEIMER'S: One of the main therapies for Alzheimer's disease is Ginkgo biloba leaf extract. Insulin and insulin receptors located in the brain are also essential for memory and cognitive functions, and these have been found to be significantly lower in Alzheimer's patients. Sage and Lemon balm have been found to have some effect on the enzyme thought to play a part in the development of Alzheimer's. Turmeric, Ginger, Cinnamon, Black pepper, Chillies (Cayenne pepper), Coriander and Garlic, Reishi and Cordyceps mushrooms, Rosemary, Ginkgo, Ginkgo nuts, Ginseng, Ashwagandha, Chinese Club Moss, Licorice, Cat's Claw. Individuals may also want to add the herb Ginkgo Biloba or Gotu Kola (as tea) to a daily regime as it has shown efficacy in scientific studies.

OLIVE LEAF/OLIVE OIL: Olive Leaf is a natural remedy used to fight Flu, colds, chronic fatigue syndrome, herpes, shingles, diabetes, yeast, fungus, increase energy, and for the Herxheimer reaction. The breakdown in dental health produces severe toxins that lower the voltage in the organs attached to that acupuncture meridian. With low voltage and inhibited protective proteins, the Candida can begin to flourish. Oleic acid in Olive oil and Biotin can prevent the conversion of the yeast form of Candida to its fungal form.

Cancer cell growth is encouraged dental and fungal toxins and are not the cause of the problem but rather the result of the problem. **Dr. Tullio Simoncini** from Rome has shown that the cancer is a RESULT of the fungal growth, which he dealt with baking soda! In recent years, the incidence of skin cancer has been on the increase. The disease is associated with environmental pollution and other factors causing the destruction of the ozone layer, resulting in an increase in ultraviolet radiation reaching the earth.

Certain polyphenols from olives slow down disease processes in the brain, improve mitochondrial dysfunction and, hence offer protection against Alzheimer's disease. A constituent of olives known as Oleuropein was found to inhibit the development of brain cell β-amyloid protein precursor along with β-amyloid metabolism.

Olive leaf is antibacterial, antimycoplasma, anti-inflammatory, antihypertensive, antidiabetic, antifungal, anti-candida, anticancer and antiviral. It appears to inhibit viruses ability to replicate, preventing viral shedding and budding within the cells and cell membrane. Olive leaf (The Tree of Life) is also the best protector of nerve sheaths when going through a kundalini awakening.

Panax ginseng not only protect the brain by reducing inflammation, but also providing the potent ability to promote neurogenesis and thereby regenerate parts of the neuronal network in damaged brains by stimulating the production of a protein, **Brain-Derived Neurotrophic Factor** (BDNF), which is key in creating new neurons. Considered as the poor man's ginseng, Codonopsis (dang shen) is an important Chi tonic of status equal to that of some ancient ones (such as astragalus, ginseng, and jujube). Jiaogulan or Gynostemma pentaphyllum (Southern Ginseng) is an adaptogenic herb known as "immortality tea" and said to be more powerful and less expensive than Ginseng. Jiaogulan is a herb that has been shown to restore homeostasis and increase glutathione production while reducing nitrate levels.

The Alzheimer's brain is "insulin resistant" so cinnamon helps with that and it also helps stop the disintegration and dysfunction of the tau protein. By keeping this protein strong, scientists believe neurofibrillary tangles can be prevented and even reversed. Building up the body's immune system and keeping these microglial cells healthy is absolutely vital for the prevention and reversal of dementia. Add more virgin coconut oil and olive oil to your diet. Eliminate processed sugar intake and avoid transfats in the diet.

DHEA (Dehydroepiandrosterone), and melatonin could be administered along with the herbs initially to obtain more obvious early results from the treatment. DHEA is one of the most abundant circulating steroids endogenous steroid hormone, which is produced in the adrenal glands, the gonads, and the brain.

DMAE (Dimethylaminoethanol) is a choline molecule with one less methyl group, and has the ability to reduce build-up of the age pigmentation known as β-amyloid . Centrophenoxine, an ester of DMAE, is used as a neuroprotectant and for enhancing memory formation. Mixed research supports centropheoxine's ability to attenuate lipofuscin buildup, a cellular wear and tear pigment associated with aging which is thought to reduce the ability of lysosomes to effectively clear cellular waste. You can tell how up lipofuscin (AGEs or glycation) you have in your brain from the extent of age spots you have on the back of your hands. **Centrophenoxine** increases the amount of acetylcholine, a neurotransmitter that resides in the synaptic vesicles. Centrophenoxine has been proven to be effective in treating dementia by showing an increase in skills on cognition testing after several weeks of a 2g daily dose. **Huperzine** has been used for Alzheimer's and senile dementia with positive results.

CHINESE TRADITIONAL MEDICINE FOR ALZHEIMER'S: In Chinese medicine, the brain is said to be an outgrowth of the kidney, therefore, brain deterioration may be prevented or reversed via nourishing the kidneys with tonics and qi tonics, such as rehmannia, ginseng and cistanche; along with kidney essence astringents, such as rose hips and schisandra. A general Chinese formula for Alzheimer's disease and senile dementia would go something like: acorus, polygala, platycodon, ginseng, atractylodes, licorice, cassia cinnamon, astragalus, citrus, pinellia, crataegus, shen-chu, curcuma, gastrodia, salvia, cnidium, red peony, zizyphus, rehmannia, lycium fruit, tang-kuei, cistanche, morinda, aconite, dioscorea, and hoelen (or fu-shen).

Acetylcholine, a neurotransmitter essential for processing memory and learning, is decreased in both concentration and function in patients with Alzheimer's disease. The following Chinese Herbs inhibit the acetylcholinesterase enzyme from breaking down acetylcholine, thereby increasing both the level and duration of action of the neurotransmitter include: Ginkgo biloba, Ginseng, Lycorus radiata, Huperzia serrata, Macleaya cordata, Macleaya cordata, Berberis, Coptis chinenses and Securinega suffruticosa. **Aluminum** inhibits cholinergic functioning and synaptic uptake of dopamine, norepinephrine and 5-HT-serotonin. Avoid anticholinergic drugs!

NEUROTROPIC BOTANICALS considered useful enhancers of brain-derived neurotrophic factor (BDNF) for neuron growth and optimization and central nervous system (CNS) diseases: Bacopa, Coffee Berry, Saffron, Siberian Ginseng, Green Tea, Ginkgo, Olive Oil, Olive Leaf, Rhodiola Rosea, Red Sage (Danshen), Grapeseed, Ashwagandha, Korean Perilla Mint.

FUNGAL ORIGINS OF ALZHEIMER'S

Researchers found "several fungal species" in all of the deceased who died of Alzheimer, but no evidence of fungus in Alzheimer's-free people. A fungal cause would explain the slow progression of the disease and the inflammation caused by Alzheimer's, which is a natural response to fungi. Researchers theorize that the presence of chronic fungal infection in Alzheimer's sufferers, causes the body to produce β-amyloid peptide in an attempt to fight the infection, but the consistent high levels of β-amyloid peptide ultimately leads to the formation of amyloid plaque build-up.

So, amyloid plaque may just be a symptom of the fungus, with the fungus being the actual underlying cause of Alzheimer's disease. Poor diet and hypoxic conditions that feed fungi, combined with low life-energy, poor immunity and separation from Nature's energies are implicated in the progression of the crippling disease. Beta amyloid peptides in Alzheimer's disease trigger the same inflammatory immune response as amyloids created by bacterial biofilm. Immune suppression of the planet since vaccines, antibiotic overuse, chemical agriculture and processed foods is depleting the body's terrain and promoting conditions suited to fungi and other infections predisposes us to Alzheimer's and dementia. Patients with Alzheimer's had signs of fungal infection in their neurons, suggesting that a fungal cause for β-amyloid maybe the actual culprit of the disease. It is hypothesized that Candida albicans may be the gateway fungi to other kinds of fungal brain infections. Besides fungi like Candida species, Alzheimer's is also associated with brain infections of other pathogens including Herpes Simplex virus type 1 (HSV 1), Chlamydia pneumoniae, and several types of spirochaete including Lyme. Also Alzheimer's is thought to be a causal factor in Multiple sclerosis, Asthma, Chronic fatigue, Rheumatoid Arthritis (RA), Fibromyalgia, Interstitial cystitis, and Crohn's disease.

Candida overgrowth is symptomatic of a sick human culture and bad personal lifestyle habits. It is the job of fungi to reduce dead and dying life back to the soil to be recycled into new lifeforms. If the human species is infested with a pandemic of candida, it means that it is the culture, the civilization itself that is anti-life and unsustainable—ie: cosmically unsanctified. Now with the life-toxic EMF technologies and increasing separation from Nature's life-giving energy we can expect vast widespread dementia and increasing numbers of people being recycled back to the soil.

The Candida yeast/fungus and Alzheimer's disease have a common denominator – a certain kind of sticky deposit known as Beta-amyloid plaque! Beta-amyloid forms sticky clumps, or 'plaques', in the brain that are one of the key ways of diagnosing Alzheimer's disease. Candida makes the same amyloid (beta) plaque as found in brains of deceased Alzheimer's patients. The β-amyloid peptide chain of amino acids has a strong antimicrobial activity, especially against Candida albicans (commonly found in "yeast" or thrush infections).

Pathogens can cross the blood–brain barrier via movement through epithelial cells (transcellular), passing through the intercellular space between the cells (paracellularly) and/or via the called Trojan-horse mechanism within infected immune phagocytes. Consequently, pathogens can cause blood–brain barrier (BBB) dysfunction, including loosening tight junctions and increased permeability, which allows heavy metals and toxins greater entry into the brain.

The fungal aspect of chemtrail survival is fundamental, due to the loss of immune strength from heavy metal exposure and the fact that candida and other fungi collect and store heavy metals in their structures, preventing their elimination from the body. The infection of the brain with candida sp. etc... in association with heavy metal and radionuclide sequestration in the beta-amyloid plaque formations and other biofilms makes recovery from chemtrail fallout the most pressing health crisis we face in the world today, especially so since fungi are an intrinsic component in the concoction of the chemtrail formulas.

The most common fungi to cause brain infections include filament-forming fungi like Aspergillus, Mucor and Rhizopus and yeast-type fungi such as Candida and Cryptococcus. To invade the CNS and cause meningitis, Candida albicans must cross the blood brain barrier, and the metals and pathogens in chemtrails undermine epithelial barrier integrity. Meningitis symptoms typically show as fever, headache, eye problems, difficulty concentrating and seizures. The diseased state of the blood vessels found in most patients with AD can also be explained by the presence of fungus.

Chronic candida yeast infection and cancer is created by the impaired function of the stomach and pancreas to operate at full functional capacity and produce sufficient enzymes for their metabolism needs. When enzyme production is impaired, proteins, fats and carbohydrates will become insufficiently broken down to their smallest components, robbing the body's trillions of cells of the fuel they require to generate sufficient energy to supply your needs.

The colon is ideally between pH 5.5 and 7 (slightly acidic to neutral), and our friendly intestinal flora produces lactic and acetic acid to make the gut more acidic, which keeps the candida yeast under control. In addition, poor digestion allows bacteria and yeasts to thrive in an intestinal environment feeding on the partially broken down foods. Without adequate pancreatic enzymes the body cells only create minimal levels of energy (cellular voltage), so your body must now resort to the process of fermenting sugar anaerobically (without oxygen) to make up for this energy loss.

This anaerobic fermentation process increases lactic acid that acidifies the pH of the blood, creating an ideal environment for candida, cancer and other infectious and degenerative diseases. As the pH of the blood goes more acid, fatty acids which are normally electro-magnetically charged on the negative side switch to positive and automatically are attracted to and begin to stick to the walls of arteries which are electro-magnetically charged on the negative side.

ANTIFUNGALS

Both fungi and the heavy metals need to be systematically addressed because fungi, along with fat deposits and biofilms, harbor heavy metals. Calcium deposits and Alzheimer's plaques both harbor heavy metals, while Alzheimer's is associated with fungi. A lifestyle that includes sunshine, grounding, exercise and steaming or sauna on a daily basis. Leaky gut, fungal infections, and oral health problems must be addressed to eliminate systemic inflammation. It is just a matter of changing the terrain to that which nature intended.

Candida, foot/nail fungus and tooth/gum decay needs to be treated systemically via detoxification and diet change off of cooked-industrial food. While we are undergoing our chemtrail detoxification program we must also focus on eliminating ALL chronic infections which are symptomatic of the general degeneration of our body due to the 12 thousand year agricultural civilization.

To conquer MetaboliX and clean up one's terrain in order to build a powerful immune force against whatever high tech demonic pathogen the dark side are going to spray on ustwe need to clean up all our local infections from toenail fungi, to candida and oral issues. Candida has a multitude of underlying causes many of which directly link to potassium deficiency and its role in maintaining candida by aiding in the production of hydrochloric stomach acid and bile excretion. Potassium sorbate stops the fermentation of yeast. Also avoid all sugars and carbohydrates as they feed candida promoting its growth throughout the body. Fasting is advised for all inflammatory conditions and all degenerate and infectious conditions.

The fungal aspect of Alzhiemer's Disease points to a lifestyle and dietary approach including coconut oil, Monolaurin and MCT oil which may be effective at treating and preventing AD. Treatments for fungal infections such as Birch Bracket, Turkey Tail and Red Reishi mushrooms could be used as treatments of Alzheimer's and other amyloid related disease. These mushrooms alter the balance of gut bacteria that create biofilms and resulting amyloids, are anti-fungal, anti-viral, anti-bacterial, anti-inflammatory and anti-aging. Reishi Mushroom is known to digest or block the following pathogens: Aspergillus niger, Bacillus subtilis, Candida albicans, and Escherichia coli.

OTHER ANTIFUNGALS:

Gedunin and nimbidol found in the leaves of neem are powerful antifungal agents that destroy fungi which cause athlete foot, ringworm and nail fungus. To stimulate the immune system we could combine the medical mushrooms with neem leaves, clove, olive leaf, wormwood, black walnut husk, oregano, tea tree, Pau D'Arco, Turmeric, Goldenseal, Barberry, Sea buckthorn, Aloe, Garlic, Lemongrass, Calendula, Lavender, Thyme, Red Sage, Skullcap, frankincense, myrrh and Cassia leaves and bark, black cumin seed. Echinacea provides a "protective shield" by increasing interferon, killer t-cell function and phagocytes (cell-eaters) and has become the herb of choice for such ailments as candida infections. The porous surface of activated charcoal has a negative electric charge that causes positive charged toxins and gas to bond with it. By removing toxins activated charcoal helps eliminate the terrain that supports fungal growth. Colloidal Silver keeps overgrowth of candida albicans under control, thereby reducing leaky gut syndrome, irritable bowel, bloating, itching, headaches and brain fog, etc.

CHITIN CELL WALL OF CANDIDA

Candida albicans grows optimally at pH 4, which is very acid, but it can grow between pH 3–7. You might want to try long baths with Epsom salt and baking soda to raise your pH. Changing the body's terrain to a more alkaline pH with increased oxygen helps reduce candida, along with antifungal and immune support herbs and diet, however to actually get the fungi out of your system you must first dissolve the outer protein layer with proteolytic enzymes, and dissolve the chitin with hemicellulase. The wall of candida is composed of hemicellulose. The enzyme hemicellulase digests hemicellulose.

Candida begins to build this biofilm over itself within 24 hours of initial colonization. The cell wall of candida is composed of the plant polysaccharide fibrin, chitin or cellulose, mannoprotein-1, glucan and mannoprotein-2. Once the biofilm is fully developed, prescription drugs such as Diflucan no longer work because they don't dissolve this film. Once the enzymes get through the biofilm they begin to digest the cell wall that is composed of polysaccharide carbohydrates, proteins and cellulose plant fibers commonly referred to as chitin. Chitinase (cellulase and hemicellulase) enzymes start breaking apart the cell wall, so that the immune system can then see it, and mounts an immune response, inducing macrophage activity against the candida yeast.

Cell wall lysis enzymes that break down cellulose and beta glucans include: serrapeptase, glucanases including beta-glucanase, cellulases and xylanase. It looks like beta-glucanase, xylanase and serrapeptase might be the best combo to start with—in association with papain and bromelain.

- Protease breaks down proteins into amino acids

- Lipase breaks down fats for the proper absorption of lipids

- Amylase breaks down carbohydrates

- Cellulase breaks down fiber/cellulose

Vitamin C with bioflavonoids are needed to reduce oxidative damage to tissues during the cleansing crisis. Obviously fibrous sweepers including clay, psyllium, ricebran, yucca etc... should also be used in conjunction, but taken at a different time of day than the enzymatic agent itself, so that the enzymes don't simply dissolve the fiber broom instead of the fungi.

Candida eradication needs a multi-pronged approach of stopping alcohol, sugar and cereals. Bread feeds candida, and the candida demands bread. Basically you need to strip the outer cell membranes off the fungi with an enzyme blend, while using antifungal herbs. Start researching YouTubes on the ketogenic diet. It is a good idea to starve the fungi by cutting out most carbs and all sugars. Dr. Thomas Seyfried, a leading cancer researcher and professor at Boston College says that the low-carb, high-fat ketogenic diet can replace chemotherapy and radiation for even the deadliest of cancers. Ketogenic metabolism is anti-cancer because it is anti-inflammatory and raises energy production by creating more mitochondrias in the cells.

The Ketogenic diet involves eating those vegetables that grow *above* ground, all fruits that end in "berry," meat/fish, fat (olives, nuts, seeds, avocado, butter, olive oil, coconut oil) and grass fed dairy (mostly cheese and yogurt), pasture fed eggs, along with probiotic fermented cabbage, or sauerkraut. After the 3rd day your metabolism will change over to ketosis and you will lose appetite for sugars/carbs. This is a short-term (from days to a few weeks) detoxification reaction in the body. As the body detoxifies, it is not uncommon to experience flu-like symptoms including headache, joint and muscle pain, body aches, sore throat, general malaise, sweating, chills, nausea or other symptoms. (You may get a Herxheimer Reaction as the fungi dies off. ***See P.)

The carbohydrate addicted master-slave culture is hitting the wall with escalating Metabolic X, insulin resistance, depression, dementia and insanity. Therefore the failsafe way out of the mental sludge of the control Matrix is a series of water fasts for 3 or more days, so that the brain goes into fat burning or ketosis rather than glucose burning. As we burn up our fat stores we eliminate cell receptor resistance and can undergo deep detoxification from heavy metals, pesticides, chemtrails, pharmaceuticals and all manner of consciousness impairing agents that cause so much "noise" in our system that we fail to enter into sympathetic resonance with our soul and cosmic consciousness.

If the wage-slave class is addicted to substances that feed candida, are the predator class also? It is mostly the slaves resort to junk food, alcohol, tobacco and other life harming, numbing substances, because they have to abdicate their self-determinancy in order to remain a slave. It is a Catch 22 that by suppressing themselves with their escapist tools, they are forever locked into slave mode.

SUBSTANCES FOR FIGHTING CANDIDA

• **Baking Soda**—Dr. Simoncini says that the substance that works better than anything else to kill fungus is sodium bicarbonate (baking soda). His patient's tumors were seen to melt away as the fungi were killed with the solution of baking soda. The fungus cannot grow if the voltage in the tissue is normal, and bicarbonate works as an electron donor to raise the voltage. The alkaline effect of Baking Soda stops fungi growth. Alkaline puts 10 times the oxygen in tissues and fungus cannot survive alkaline nor oxygen rich tissues. Baking soda binds with uranium, and can remove up to 92% of uranium from contaminated soils. Baking soda, clay and Epsom salt baths are used for radiation sickness. It is also used intravenously to protect patients from the hazardous toxicity of chemotherapy.

• **Bitter melon juice** induced apoptosis or programmed cell death along several different pathways, and also activated a pathway, which shows that it knocks out the cancer cells' metabolism of glucose. Thus starves them of the sugar they need to survive. Yeast (a fungus) also carries out fermentation in anaerobic conditions, thus their primary mechanism of ATP production is glycolysis.

• **Bitters:** Candida hates bitter herbs like Gentian, Swedish bitters, Andrographis and bitter melon and lemons.

• **Eat raw salads** like watercress, spinach and turnip greens. Essential fatty acids like Omega-3 combat inflammation and retard fungal growth while mending mucus membranes and cell membrane destroyed by candida.

• **Ginger root**, turnips, cabbage family, barley and barley sprouts, rice and oat bran, wheat germ and wheat grass, chlorophyll, flaxseed, psyllium husks, guar gum and apple pectin, olive oil, a little papaya or pineapple with meals to improve digestion.

• **Garlic** and onions are antifungal. Whenever your anus itches take 3-4 Kyolic Garlic pills with a glass of water.

• **Shatavari** is a potent anti-candida herb. Candida has been shown to decrease thyroid function. Ashwagandha may increase thyroxine levels and treat hypothyroidism.

• **Nystatin** is a harmless prescription drug used for Candida.

• Anything that strengthens the immune system will help fight Candida; cut well back on the cooked food in your diet and concentrate on eating plenty of fresh green salads. Parasites are a terrain problem...make sure you are plugged into the earth and sky by going barefoot and sungazing.

• **H2O:** Remember to drink plenty of water to flush out the toxins that the yeast produces.

• **SUPPLEMENTS:** Take a stress multivitamin and a chelated mineral supplement daily. Plus vitamin C 1000mg, vitamin B6 200–600 mg, vitamin E 800iu, Propolis 500 mg 3 times per day, take Kyolic Garlic pills or fresh, and Primrose, Borage or Linseed oil. Use digestive enzymes or raw food with every meal. Candida impairs the liver's ability to store vitamin B12.

• Take one teaspoon per day of Bentonite clay, zeolite and diatomaceous earth in a glass of water and use it topically to allay symptoms such as athlete's foot and eczema.

• **Marine Collagen** derived from fish scales has a high concentration of glycine, hydroxyproline and proline. Fish collagen peptides have the best absorption and bioavailability due to their smaller particle sizes compared to other animal collagens. This allows the collagen to be absorbed at a higher level through the intestinal barrier into the bloodstream and carried throughout the body. The collagen rich parts of the fish, mainly skin and scales, can be made into homemade fish stock.

• **Collagen** has an important structural role in animals contributing to the architecture and resilience of bone and connective tissue. Fungi and other pathogens break down collagen, while silicon is a structural molecule of collagen with antifungal properties, due to its inherent inertness to bacteria, mold and fungi. Collagen provides the cushion for your bones and joints and it is strengthened by silicon, glycine, hydroxyproline and proline.

• **Hyaluronic Acid:** The stronger our collagen the more resistant the body is against microbe attack and proliferation. The polymer Hyaluronic Acid found in human skin assists in retaining moisture, providing cushioning, helping to repair damaged tissue, maintaining the collagen and elastin matrix and creating a protective barrier against microorganisms.

• **Silicon:** To "cure" candida the body needs to be made more mineral dense, and lifestyle and diet changed to be more immune supportive. Bamboo silicon, horsetail and nettle are good sources of the "youth" element. In plants silicon alleviates abiotic and biotic stresses, activates the plant's defense mechanisms and increases the resistance of plants to pathogenic fungi.

• **Garlic:** Kyolic Candida Cleanse & Digestion Formula 102 features a unique combination of aged garlic extract, ginger, and the enzyme (glucanase, lipase and protease) to support internal cleaning, healthy intestinal function and digestive balance. Combine this with the enzyme Serrapetase.

• **Knockout Tincture:** Broadspectrum knockout tincture with chaparral, olive leaf, pau d'arco, wormwood, clove, galangal and St John's Wort.

121

BETA GLUCANS: The walls of plants and fungi contain numerous sugar homopolymers (cellulose, chitin, and beta glucans). Beta Glucans compose up to 60% of fungal cell walls of candida, along with mannoproteins (mannose-containing glycoproteins) and a chitin layer (polymer consisting mainly of unbranched chains of N-acetyl-D-glucosamine). The polysaccharide Beta 1, 3D Glucan is a biological response modulator that stimulates immune response thus used against high cholesterol, diabetes, cancer, and HIV/AIDS. Maitake mushroom contain unique beta-glucan polysaccharides, known as grifolan and D-fraction, it is especially helpful for stimulating immune functions, raising Natural Killer Cells and offering antitumor effects. **Beta glucans** are found in barley and oat bran, nutritional yeast, marmite.

BIRCH BRACKET MUSHROOM: *Piptoporus Betulinus* or Birch Bracket Mushroom is anti-candida, antibiotic, anti-fungal, anti nano-bacteria, anti-inflammatory, anti-cancer, kills worms and is laxative. The birch polypore was among two mushrooms that were found in the bag belonging to **Iceman Ötzi**. Ötzi who lived 5,300 years ago, likely suffered from arthritic joint pain, *Lyme disease* and tooth decay, and atherosclerosis. This mushroom is also known in Chinese traditional medicine where it is used for the treatment of various diseases including oral ulcers, gastroenteric disorders, cirrhosis of the liver, inflammation, and various cancers. Birch Bracket contains (1-3)-α-d-glucan in its cell wall which increases enzymes that degrade biofilms, therefore is ideal to use in removing heavy metals and protecting against the infectious agents in chemtrails.

ANTICANDIDA HERBS: Birch Bracket Mushroom, Pau d'Arco, Black Walnut, Clove, Shatavari, Echinacea, Goldenseal, Suma, Chaparral, Siberian Ginseng, Aloe, Ginger and Garlic. Baikal skullcap roots, Senna, Houttuynia cordata (Chameleon), Prunus pendula (Weeping cherry tree), Paeonia suffruticosa, Cortex pseudolaricis, Alpinia officinarum, Gold thread, Cloves, Cinnamon and Olive leaf. Cinnamon oil.

Euphorbia Extracts from *Euphorbia hirta* and related species contain diterpenes that significantly inhibit Candida growth by changing the fungi's efflux pumps, which they use to become resistant to antifungals.

Hopseed Bush or *Dodonaea Viscosa* blocks candida growth by 85% by preventing the ability of Candida to expand its germ tube.

New Zealand Pharmacopeia: New Zealand Red Leaf Horopito, Kawakawa, Kiwifruit seed, Manuka seed pods, Willow bark and Gorse flowers for pain.

Olive oil (Oleic acid) and Biotin can prevent the conversion of the yeast form of Candida to its fungal form.

Neem has antifungal properties that help athlete's foot, ringworm, candida and thrush. It has been most helpful in treating a variety of skin problems and diseases including acne, psoriasis, eczema and other persistent conditions.

Oregano essential oil is known to be one of the most profound antifungals, and also has antibacterial, antiviral, and anti-protozoa properties, as well as being sedative and calms down hyper-sensitivity.

Horsetail (Shavegrass) has a high silica which normalizes bowel function and is active in clearing the intestinal tract naturally, the mineral silica is necessary in the reconstruction of damaged and inflamed intestinal walls.

ANTIFUNGAL HERBS: African Bird Peppers, Astragalus, Barberry, Black cumin seed, Black Sesame Seed, Black walnut, Burdock Root, Cat's Claw, Chamomile, Chaparral, Chanca Piedra, Chinese Wolfbane, Cardamom, Cayenne, Clove, Cinnamon, Echinacea, Fennel seeds, Fenugreek seeds, Garlic, Gentian, Gold thread, Grapefruit seed, Grapeseed extract, Graviola, Ginger, Goldenseal, Gymnema sylvestre, Rhubarb (da huang), Dahurian angelica, Huang Bai, Di Fu Zi, Olive leaf Extract, Oregano, Mountain Ash, Orrowan Berry fruit, Mullein, Nettle Papaya (leaf, pulp, peel, root, seeds), Pau D'Arco, Parsley, Pinebark- Pycnogenol, Pumpkin Seed, Pokeroot, Quassia Bark, Suma, Turmeric, Siberian ginseng, Aloe, Shield Fern, Spanish Black Radish, Self All, Skullcap roots, Seneca snakeroot, Senna, Wormwood, Plum Seed Powder, Reishi, Turkey Rhubarb Root, Turmeric, Wild Indigo Root.

ANTIFUNGAL SUPPLEMENTS: Calcium-magnesium, Magnesium oxide, Monolaurin or Caprylic acid complex from coconut is a potent antifungal that kills Candida cells, 10-Undecenoic Acid by Thorne Research (derived from castor bean oil), sorbic acid, Probiotics, Biotin, Colloidal Silver, Vitamin D. Take a stress multivitamin and a chelated mineral supplement daily. Plus vitamin C, vitamin B6, D3, D-Mannose, Vitamin E, and Propolis 3 times per day; take Kyolic Garlic pills or fresh garlic, and Primrose, Borage or Linseed oil. Candida overgrowth is sometimes a reflection of a lack of digestive enzymes, so use papaya or pineapple enzymes, or raw food with every meal. Take at least one teaspoon per day of Bentonite clay or the PM Cleanser in a glass of water to eliminate toxins from pathogen die-off.

BARK TEAS: Because the barks of trees contain antifungal agents to protect the tree from attack, barks are useful anti-candida remedies. Slow simmered tea from barks are anti-inflammatory, antioxidant, anti-viral, anti-parasitic, anti-septic, anti-cough, anti-asthmatic, expectorant, cardiotonic, aphrodisiac, hypotensive, laxative, stomachic (beneficial to digestion), lymphatic and Spleen tonic. Barks contain natural fungicides to protect the plants from infection. You can make your own bark tea infusion or capsules using the inner bark from a variety of local and foreign edible plants such as Pau d'Arco, Anamu, Bellaco-caspi tree, Black walnut, Babul bark (Acacia nilotica), Birch, Beech, Brazilian peppertree, Buckthorn, Graviola (soursop), Wild cherry, Peach, Pine, Slippery elm, Cinnamon sticks, Eucommia bark (Du Zhong), Jatoba, Matico, Fedegoso, Guaco, Mangosteen and Apple tree bark, Piri-piri, Ubos. Bark infusions are used topically for bacterial and fungal infections. Pau d'arco is a very common bark used as a potent antifungal agent.

Pau D'arco and H202—Cat's claw and pau d'arco—in which you put a couple of drops of hydrogen peroxide...to oxidize the pathogens.

TOENAIL FUNGUS: The solvent DMSO improves the penetration of antifungals when treating stubborn toenail fungus. DMSO is rich in sulfur, which has antifungal, antibacterial, and keratolytic activity. Apply 50:50 DMSO and 20% Salicylic acid treatment via dropper bottle on base and cleft of toenails once a day and the nail will grow out fungus free. This acid mixture speeds senescence of inferior tissue and speeds cell regrowth, so frequently clean and scrub your nails. Eliminate toenail fungus you might try various topical treatments such as propolis tincture, Colloidal Silver, Lugol's, hydrogen peroxide or essential oils (oregano, savory, hyssop and clove oil).

Before bed rub Castor oil on the feet and cover with socks. After your shower rub feet with Baking Soda and Borax Powder. Spray feet several times a day with organic apple cider vinegar and essential oil (either oregano, savory, thyme or sage). Make your spray bottle at the ratio of 1 tsp essential oil to 1 cup of vinegar. You can really get on top of excess bad bacteria and fungi by rubbing Baking Soda on your feet and toes before putting your socks on at least once a day. If you keep a dish (large enough for both feet) of baking soda with some borax in it in the bathroom, you can step into it and rub your feet in the stuff after you have dried off from the shower. Sulfur ointment rubbed daily into the feet gets rid of athlete's foot, chapped feet and fungi growing in the soles of the feet. Lugol's between the toes eliminates athletes foot. Helichrysum oil rubbed between toes is a powerful antifungal, and silicon water strengthens nails against fungal infection. After one year drinking Philosopher's water both toenail fungus and ingrown toenails will disappear and nails will become youthful and strong.

DETOX FOOT BATHS: Detoxing the brain through the feet ~
Overnight is an ideal time to detox through the feet. Before bed…first scrub the feet with a strong bristle brush and clean the nails. Make a strong concoction of herb tea with wild crafted local plants or dried herbs (you can also add organic lemon skins or other fruit skins).

Foot baths are a great way of giving a systemic antifungal treatment to the whole body due to the absorbent nature of the bottom of the feet. Hence you can make concoctions with boiled coffee grounds, the grounds from chaga/chicory coffee, baking soda, Borax, Epsom salt, Sodium Thiosulfate, MSM, kelp, clay, humates, antifungal herbs like Pau d'arco and silicon rich herbs like horsetail and nettle, and medical mushrooms.

The dechlorinator, **Sodium thiosulfate** is said to be a powerful detoxing agent to remove mercury and other heavy metals from the body. It is also a topical antifungal such as can be used for ringworm and cancer treatment. Soak feet for 30 minutes. Then cover them with a clay masque with activated charcoal in it…allow this to dry, while watching a movie or reading a book. Put natural fiber socks on your feet and go to bed. In the morning wash and scrub your feet thoroughly. Reuse your footbaths in a bath, then use the water for your garden with the addition of EM-1 Microbial Inoculant from Teragenx.

DETOX BATH: Borax, Epsom salt, Sea Salt and Baking soda baths and
foot baths help to remove heavy metals from the body, including the brain and nervous system. Make your detox baths as hot as possible and for around 30 minutes. As an anti-inflammatory agent, borax effectively treats arthritis, gout, swollen gums and other inflammatory diseases. It also is an antiseptic and helps stop the growth of nanofibers, nano-bacteria, mycoplasma and fungi. Skin brushing followed by a **Miracle 11 Detox Bath** is a great combo.

Additionally, the substance eliminates infection such as bladder infection, urinary tract infection and others. Research online for how Borax is used in treating Morgellons. Kelp and clay baths are also recommended for chemtrail and radiation detox. You can use ½ cup of kelp heated on the stove with some water and put into a bath, then after a long bath, let the bath cool and use the water for the garden and houseplants—they love it!

"Existentialism means that no one else can take a bath for you." Delmore Schwartz

THE BRAIN'S GLYMPHATIC SYSTEM

The brain actually has its own unique waste disposal system, dubbed the glymphatic system, which is similar to the lymphatic system, that "piggybacks" on the blood vessels in the brain. The glymphatic vessels could act as a pipeline between the brain and the immune system. The "g" in glymphatic points to the "glial cells" of that manage this detoxification system. Keeping the glymphatic system open and flowing ensures heightened brain power and the avoidance of Alzheimer's disease and dementia.

Molecular lesions have been detected in Alzheimer's disease, but the overarching theme to emerge is that of an accumulation of misfolded proteins in the aging brain resulting in oxidative and inflammatory damage, which in turn leads to energy failure and synaptic dysfunction. An imbalance between the production and the clearing, and aggregation of peptides causes B-amyloid peptides to accumulate.

Fenugreek Seed Powder nullified aluminum chloride-induced tau pathology, oxidative stress, and inflammation in a rat model of Alzheimer's Disease. Fenugreek seed extract could be able to inhibit the activity of acetylcholinesterase (AChE), a key enzyme involved in the pathogenesis of AD, and further shown to have anti-Parkinson's effect. Fenugreek seed sprouts contain lecithin, an emulsifying substance which works to cleanse the lymph nodes and entire lymphatic system, and are exceptional for maintaining healthy breast tissue. Fenugreek seed sprouts and extract may be an important ally to aid the removal of aluminum from the brain via the **glymphatic system**.

The cerebral spinal fluid (CSF) pumped into brain tissue flushes away waste through the glymphatic system, including the proteins beta amyloid and tau that are associated with Alzheimer's disease and other forms of dementia. The glymphatic system is more active while we sleep, it can be damaged by stroke and trauma, and improves with exercise. Any lymphatic assistance—raw diet, living-hydration, exercise, vibe machine, cervical and lymph massage, vibratory massage for the spine and neck, spinal shower etc...will help to clean and clear the central Mohawk of the brain allowing us to become more self-initiatory, executive and sovereign.

Apparently self-reflexive awareness (and witnessing) is a phenomena of the central line of the brain. A Mohawk over the top of the head. The glymphatic system of lymph vessels associated with microglia in the brain drains off 3 lbs of toxic lymph and plaque per year. Therefore if we are sedentary, poorly hydrated, inflamed or otherwise metabolically "clogged up" our center for "Selfhood" and self-reflexivity is impaired. As is evidenced by the sense of a dull, numb crown... ie: a numbskull. Rubbing your hand or a magnet over the central (Mohawk) region of the head helps to wipe stale energy and emotions from our field.

Glymphatic Clearing: Some ways to keep the glymphatic system of the brain clear include: hanging from the hips over a bar, or aerial yoga, while rubbing the skull and massage the back of the neck and the shoulders. Massage the jaw and down the front of the neck; continuing under the collar bones, the breasts and into the stomach to assist the lymphatic system. Put your thumbs in your ears with fingers at the temples, take a deep breath and blow your cheeks up like a balloon. Pinch the top of the nose and sniff-breathe; and tap fingers around the eye sockets and down the side of the nose and around the jaw. Bend over forwards and massage the scalp with essential oils (rosemary, thyme, sage etc...) mixed with jojoba oil. Put your hands on your hips with your thumbs at the back and arch your spine backwards toning AHHH. Toning HUUU or any sound you like is great for detoxing the brain, so make sure you sing, hum or tone every day. Toning while in the bath is an added bonus.

Rebounding is the ultimate lymphatic drainage practice, with running a close second. Soaking in hot mineral springs water alkalizes the body allowing for the decontraction of tissues and more efficient elimination of wastes. Transcranial Electromagnetic Stimulation, Scenar Devices and Accupens may also be effective. The Accupen stimulates muscles hence moves lymph and promotes healing with eliminating pain. You put it directly on the skin—starting out with #3-#4 until you are used to it. Excellent for injuries, shoulders, joint inflammation pain and facial toning. (Only $12 from China).

The enzyme Serrapeptase dissolves only dead tissues such as the old fibrous layers that clog the lining of our arteries and dangerously restrict the flow of blood and oxygen to the brain. It is recommended for anti-aging, because much of aging has to do with the accumulation of scar tissue, inflammation, and dis-regulation. Juicing and cucumbers and watermelon etc... provides the structured living water necessary for good hydration. Electric massagers, infrared wands, heat pads, Castor oil packs, Magnesium chloride spray and rosemary oil massage on the face, head, jaw and neck helps with all issues to do with the head, brain and sense organs.

Early to bed early to rise! During sleep the brain's glymphatic system becomes 10 times more active than during the waking state, thus insomnia is unhealthy for a "clean" brain. When we sleep, our brains are pumped with cerebrospinal fluid. This fluid washes away waste proteins (such as beta amyloids) that build during the time we spend awake. The glymphatic transport was by far the most efficient in lateral sleepers, that is sleeping on one's side. Research shows that the immune system needs 8-9 hours of sleep in total darkness to recharge completely. A weak immune system cannot keep your body clean inside, and the resulting congestion threatens cellular life.

Lack of circadian obedience to nature's rhythms contributes to Alzheimer's. Quality sleep is crucial for a healthy brain because sleep is when your body clears toxins from your brain, repairs damaged cells, grows new ones and organizes your memories. Getting plenty of outdoor sun exposure every morning helps to fortify your circadian rhythm, which is important to getting the quality sleep necessary to reduce the risk of Alzheimer's. It is also important to avoid blue light in the evening such as that from the television, computers and cell phones as it prevents melatonin production and increases insulin resistance.

Establishing a relaxing bedtime ritual, and exercising daily also make it easier to get your full 7-8 hours quality sleep. Avoid eating late at night so the brain can cleanse itself fully while you sleep. The earlier you eat your last meal in the afternoon, the greater the glymphatic system can work to detoxify the brain overnight. Melatonin has antioxidant potential that is five times greater than Vitamin C and two times greater than Vitamin E, stimulating antioxidant enzymes, enhancing the activities of other antioxidants or protecting other antioxidant enzymes from oxidative damage. melatonin reduces chronic and acute inflammation, preventing neurodegenerative disorders and brain oxidative damage.

Avoid fluoride as it undermines the pineal gland's capacity to produce melatonin.

CLEARING THE ATTIC

The glymphatic system must be clear and flowing for the feeding of the brain with new blood and energy. This is especially important as it relates to the crown and our connection to the cosmos. The glymphatic system (crown chakra) becomes dull giving us a sense of cosmic separation when we eat late at night, fail to get enough fresh air and exercise or when we endure ongoing psychological abuse from authority figures who have no idea (nor potential for conception) of who and what we are.

One way to open the **glymphatic Mohawk** is to roll the crown of cranium on the ground...similar to both when praying to Mecca and the Rabbit's Pose in yoga. However, the hands are out in front Sphinx–like, and you carefully roll the top of your head over the carpet, without hyperextending the back of the neck, while sniffing to clear the sinuses. Hanging from the hips and moving the spine around also helps to open the brain's glymphatic highway. Most importantly though, is to become so ALIVE, that the social psychosis and competitive, exploitative power wars do not gravitate in our direction and clog up our cerebral hardwares.

Narcissism is simply the material human fallen from the cosmic soul connection. Once opened and released, "connected" and communicating our brain can naturally work to spontaneously create the best of possible lives. Whatever the situation, self-realization gives us the expansive safe space we need to heal and grow. The way to free ourselves from the arrested development of the hive-mind of the Borg is to open up and expand our own higher HUman capacities.

Advanced Human Character Traits Include: Honesty, Fairness, Tolerance, Fortitude, beyond Ego-defensiveness, Joy, Peace, Generosity, Magnanimity, seeks to Further All Life, Faith-Trust, Patience, Universal Compassion and motivated by Kindness, Self-discipline, Chastity, and speaking Truth to Power. Along with these traits are psychic abilities such as Precognition and Visions, Expansive Dream Life, Creative Genius, Telepathy, Reading Minds, Medical Intuition, Ability to Heal, Ubiquitous Desire to Assist All Beings, Fair Witness or Universal Judicial Capacity; plus a Visceral Understanding Of Nature, the Tao and the Fibonacci Nature of Cosmic Design, and invariably inflamed with a Inspired Soul Vocation.

> *"By merely restraining his passions a man can never arrive at peace, can never actualize his ideal; he must purify those passions. True strength and power and usefulness are born of self-purification, for the lower animal forces are not lost, but are transmuted into intellectual and spiritual energy."* By James Allen, Dignity and Self-Discipline www.renegadetribune.com/

The paradigm of destruction that is presently killing the planet is governed by narcissism. Narcissism makes us malleable and vulnerable to the directives of the empire's mind control. Goodness explodes beyond the boundaries of "the control system." Goodness arises from a clear glymphatic system in the brain, that "clears out our attic," and allows for an expanded EMF egg of the body, which connects us to the wider cosmos beyond both the personal and collective sphere. Narcissism, materialism, war-capitalism, empire and all aspects of Borgism are propagated by a "**dirty attic**," aborting our HUmanity and cutting us off from cosmic design and sacred Destiny.

It is recommended you put a soft plush carpet near your bed, so you can roll your cranium on it before you sleep, and when you first get out of bed in the morning. This is an easy habit to program, and it makes for far deeper sleep and more soul orientation and navigation during your day. Clearing the Attic allows us to disengage from material enslavement and the commodified world, which gives us access to free will, and the discipline to improve spiritually rather than mindlessly following the flock.

Basically I am saying that clogging up your glymphatic system by eating late at night, when coupled with experiencing the stress of social pathology acts to "cut us off from God," unless we undertake lymphatic detox practices. When we run from social toxicity, predators, parasites or power-plays in general we may stagnate our lymphatic system in order to go unconscious so that we numb ourselves out against emotional pain. However by doing so we fail to develop more advanced social adaptive skills and merely prolong "victim energy," which sets us up for further abuse in the future. Clearing the Attic is a simple daily exercise we can do to maintain mindfulness around the need to keep our glymphatic system open and flowing.

Sovereignty and self-determinancy is the only way to arrive at a transcendent destiny.

SLEEP PERCHANCE TO DREAM OF THE NEW

Over-excitation of specific cortical and limbic neurons due to the failure of inhibition of certain excitatory pathways within the brain, causes innervation and degeneration of these excitatory pathways. This provides a rational explanation for the pattern of degeneration seen in Alzheimer's disease.

The importance of deep restful sleep, the earlier from midnight as possible cannot be overstated. When we sleep our brain cells are reduced in size by about 60 percent to create more space between the cells, giving the cerebrospinal fluid room to flush out the debris. Restful sleep is therefore important to allow your brain to clear out toxins, including harmful Amyloid-beta proteins linked to brain disorders such as Alzheimer's.

Interestingly, Alzheimer's disease is associated with both reduced REM sleep and the calcification of the pineal gland which messes with melatonin production. Sleep disorders are also linked to autism as well as other neurological diseases, including depression, schizophrenia, Lou Gehrig's disease (ALS), Parkinson's disease, multiple sclerosis and others.

Chemtrail nanoparticulates calcify your pineal gland, necessity for intuitive thinking, spiritual gnosis and is the pleasure and satiety center (satiated, enough food). When the pineal gland's ability to make sulfate is impaired, this, in turn, reduces production of melatonin necessary for adequate and healthy sleep. It may come as no surprise, then, that melatonin impairment has been implicated in autism. Autism is essentially the loss of "self" via being totally self-focused due to turning the body's own defensive resources against itself!

Avoid fluoride as it undermines the pineal gland's capacity to produce melatonin.

SLEEP AND ALZHEIMER'S

Since WW2 the widespread fluoridation of the water supply has lead to the calcification of the pineal gland, and a systemic arthritic-sclerotic degenerative process in the biochemistry of Western Culture. Jennifer Luke's Ph.D. hypothesizes that one of the four enzymes needed to convert the amino acid tryptophan (from the diet) into melatonin is being inhibited by fluoride. Besides providing restful sleep, melatonin is also one of the body's main antioxidants and protects against cancer, as well as being the essential link in the chain of biochemistry leading up to the spirit molecule DMT. Thus our entire body, mind and spirit is being downgraded and undermined by fluoride in the water supply and fluoride falling down on us from the chemtrails.

Good sleep and an efficient lymphatic system are essential to provide adequate glymphatic drainage of the brain at night. Disrupting just one night of sleep in healthy, middle-aged adults causes an increase in amyloid beta protein, a brain protein associated with Alzheimer's disease. And a week of tossing and turning leads to an increase in another brain protein, tau, which has been linked to brain damage in Alzheimer's and other neurological diseases. The brains of people with Alzheimer's are dotted with plaques of amyloid beta plaque and tangles of tau protein, which together cause brain tissue to atrophy and die. Black Seed Oil cuts inflammation in the brain allowing deeper sleep. Avoid eating food late at night as this the capacity of the glymphatic system of the brain to drain at night.

INSOMNIA HERBS: Herbs for calming nerves, insomnia, neuralgia, pain, shock, Die-off and depression of the down cycles, for tea, baths or capsulation: Syrian rue oil; Coptis Root, Horsemint or Bee Balm, Reishi, Catuaba bark, Bala, Borage, Burdock leaves, Chamomile, Catnip, Chinese Arborvitae, Chinese date seed, Gorse flowers, California poppy flowers, Comfrey, Cowslip, Evening primrose, Ginger root, Goldenrod, Green Tea, Hop flowers, Juniper berries, Kava kava, Lemon balm, Linden flowers, Lobelia, Lotus seed, Passion Flower, Peppermint, Magnolia bark, Meadowsweet, Mimosa root bark, Motherwort, Mullein, Nettle, Oatstraw, Passion flower, Polygonum Vine Stem, Red clover flowers, Red sage root, Rosemary leaf, Skullcap, St John's Wort, Sweetflag Rhizome, Valerian, White Peony Root, Yarrow, Yellow dock. White willow and Wood Betony can be used as an anti-inflammatory for nerve pain and headaches.

SLEEP AID: An oil made from marijuana in a base of black cumin seed oil or olive oil can be used on the temples, wrists and on the neck under the ears to produce a deep restful night's sleep. Grind up some buds, put them in a dark glass jar, cover the powder with oil and shake the jar once a day. The oil will be ready to use in less than 1 month. Sieve and put the oil in an attractive bottle for the bedside table. Cannabis is being legalized to reduce public aggression and as a soporific to put dissenters to sleep.

DETOXERCISE: The lymphatic system circulates through the movement of the skeletal muscles, therefore it is even more important to exercise while cleansing than ever. If due to your fast or the release of toxins you feel too tired to exercise then drink some water and either take a sauna, spa, or enema to help eliminate your immediate toxic load then do some gentle stretches or yoga.

A walk along a beach or in trees while deep breathing in through the nose will also help restore your energy level. Remember the Thyroid regulates your metabolic rate i.e.: energy level and this gland responds to the amount of airflow through the pharynx, so breathe deep into the back of your throat through your nose in order to energize your Self. We need plenty of energy to deal effectively with the toxins as they are released and escorted out of the body.

Stagnation at this point could lead to autointoxication damage and leaves one vulnerable to colds, flus and infections. Moderate aerobic exercise such as walking for one hour a day would be OK, with some additional stretching or "rolling around on the floor." The body will want to move at this time to help deposits move to the eliminative organs. This is why the American Indians incorporate dancing into their cleansing rituals. Acidosis creates depression but any exercise or deep breathing will help oxygenate the blood and thus reduce acidity.

HERBS FOR CIRCULATION: Improving circulation is essential in order for the blood system to do the field work of picking up heavy metals and carting them out of the body. Cayenne is a circulation booster par excellence. Slowly build up to 2-3 tsp of cayenne per day for a therapeutic dose…put into vegetable juice, Master Cleanser, Tom Yum soup and other cooking. Other circulation assistants include Ginkgo biloba, Ginger, Galangal, Garlic, Willow bark, Bilberry, Butcher's broom, Green Tea, Chinese moss, Triphala, Guggulu, Arjuna bark, Bala, Hawthorn berry, Ashwagandha, Nettle, Chickweed, Lime leaves, Maral root, Maca, Horseradish, Black radish.

Seaweed helps maintain lower levels of triglycerides and cholesterol, smooth circulation in the blood vessels, and prevents fatal conditions like heart failure, atherosclerosis, and peripheral artery ailments. The hand held infrared wands are great for pain relief, increasing circulation and detoxing. In Chinese medicine, Dragon's Blood resin is commonly prescribed to invigorate blood circulation for the treatment of traumatic injuries, blood stasis and pain. It can reduce the formation of blood clots and has been shown to promote blood circulation, alleviate inflammation, stop bleeding and may be beneficial for arterial and vascular diseases.

BLOOD BUILDING: Include iron, vitamin B-12 and folic acid-rich foods in your diet. Some vegan foods that are good sources of iron include: lentils, kidney beans, prunes, green vegetables, molasses, and dried apricots. Beetroot is a good source of iron and folate, and can help lower blood pressure, boost exercise performance and prevent dementia. The blood's pH is naturally 7.365 but our acid-forming cooked diets can cause the balance to shift slightly in favor of acidity, which scours the arterial walls resulting in plaque buildup. Fruit and vegetables are packed with nutrients and phytonutrients that build blood and reduce arterial plaque, making them allies in building blood and cardiovascular health.

Vitamin A (retinol) and Sida acuta (the common wireweed, a member of the mallow family), also supports red blood cell production. Foods rich in vitamin A include: Chlorophyll rich dark, leafy green vegetables, spirulina, carrots and red peppers, watermelon, grapefruit, and cantaloupe. Aloe vera juice is a natural blood booster that cleans arteries and is anti-inflammatory. Dandelion root has been shown to improve liver conditions by purifying the blood. Copper intake doesn't directly result in red blood cell production, but it can help your red blood cells access the iron they need to replicate.

ADRENAL FATIGUE AND DARK CIRCLES

Dark circles under the eyes are a primary indicator of adrenal/kidney overload. Zinc from pumpkin seeds, poppy seeds and celery help to rectify this. Overdosing on bananas causes an excess of potassium and the depletion of salts which can contribute to dark circle syndrome. Also dark circles under the eyes indicate that your immune system has become overactive, that autoimmune processes are taking place in your body. When your intestinal flora is not fully populated with healthy bacteria it compromises the mucus membrane on the gut wall leading to the progression of Leaky Gut Syndrome.

In Leaky Gut Syndrome, the epithelium on the villi of the small intestine becomes inflamed and irritated, which allows metabolic and microbial toxins of the small intestines to flood into the bloodstream. This event compromises the liver, the lymphatic system, and the immune response including the endocrine system leading to the inflammation and autoimmune condition underlying all diseases and those dark under-eye circles. Gelatin (containing proline and glycine) protects against leaky gut, regulates insulin and boosts metabolism.

Prolonged stress exhausts the adrenal glands and other glands and organ systems resulting in Hypoadrenia. Hypothyroidism, reactive hypoglycemia and depressed immunity are often associated with this condition as well. The adrenals are the site of the highest concentration of Vitamin C in the body. To build up your adrenals to recover from fatigue take 1000 mg buffered vitamin C four times per day with plenty of water between meals. Nutrients like pantethine (vitamin B5) have been shown to support your adrenal glands and mood, while directly metabolizing stuck fat out of your liver. Nutrients like phosphatidylserine have been shown to recalibrate cortisol response in your brain, helping to prevent exaggerated cortisol in response to stress in the adrenals. Pantothenic acid or B5, vitamin B1 and vitamin B6 work synergistically to nourish and strengthen the adrenals.

REDUCING STRESS HORMONES: The adrenal cortical hormones suppress inflammatory processes, healing processes and the immune system. They also convert glycogen stores into glucose and elevate blood sugar levels--to counteract this catabolism chromium and Corosolic acid from Banaba leaf improves glucose entry into cells. Consume raw-complex/low glycemic carbohydrates and high quality protein to potentially deflect the ill effects of elevated cortisol. Acetyl-L-carnitine and phosphatidylserine are used to reduce cortisol production and repair receptor sensitivity in the hypothalamus. Adaptogens are herbs help coping with stress by restoring hypothalamic cortisol receptor sensitivity.

ADRENAL HERBS: Ashwagandha, Astragalus, Chaparral, Siberian ginseng, Licorice, Ma huang, Rhodiola rosea, Sea-buckthorn, Maca, Moringa leaf, Borage, Skullcap, Dandelion and Suma. Licorice root slows down the deactivation of cortisol, and aldosterone - essential for salt conservation in the kidney, salivary glands, sweat glands and colon. Sauerkraut and sea vegetables (seaweeds) support adrenal health, as do phytonutrient rich antiinflammatory herbs like ginger, turmeric, rosemary, thyme, basil and oregano. Proteins are necessary for stress hormones, good blood sugar balance and anti-inflammatory enzymes: hemp seed, chia, quinoa, sprouts and spirulina..

ADAPTOGENIC HERBS: Ashwagandha root, Basil, California poppy, Echinopanax elatum, Devil's claw, Dong quai, Codonopsis, Goldenseal, Gotu kola, Green tea, Hawthorn extract, Hops Flowers, Kava kava, Licorice, Magnolia bark, Manchurian Thorn Tree extract, Rhodiola rosea, Schizandra, Suma, Valerian. Perhaps the most well known adaptogen is ginseng of which there are three types: Asian (Panax ginseng), which produces the strongest stimulation, American (Panax quinquefolium), which soothes and Siberian (Eleutherococcus senticosus) for stamina. The Aralia family includes Ginseng, Echinopanax, Aralia, and Eleutherococcus. One of the best ways to control elevated cortisol levels is to keep well hydrated for dehydration causes cortisol levels to increase.

Only intact nature's energy can revive our dis-eased energy and metabolism. Spirit is a river flowing back to its oceanic self, pretty much everything humans do prevents this full cycle of return. The more we turn to Nature to heal and whole us, the closer we come to Goodness, Godliness and Holiness

LECTINS

The Fall of Homo sapiens was greatly exacerbated by agriculture, and grain production in particular. Principally because of the **lectins** in grains interferes with our metabolism by imposing upon the body's main metabolic hormone **leptin,** which is predominantly made by fat cells and governs energy expenditure. Lectins are a protein that can cause irritation that can result in symptoms such as diarrhea and vomiting, and damage the gut wall and reduce nutrient absorption. Lectins are form of natural defense in plants, essentially as a toxin that deters animals from eating the plants. Plant lectin proteins are involved in the defense mechanisms of the plant against viruses, bacteria, fungi and herbivorous invertebrates and vertebrates. Knowledge of how lectins and gluten affect the GI tract and metabolism is especially important to those who are autistic, vaccine damaged, have mercury amalgams or are otherwise exposed to heavy metals.

Like gluten, Lectins can attach to the intestinal wall, and break the tight junctions in the gut lining creating leaky gut. Simply put, the lining can become more permeable, allowing food particles such as lectins to slip into the bloodstream, which can trigger an inflammatory response and/or the production of antibodies to lectin. Lectins are harmful and cause inflammation and autoimmune diseases, including celiac disease, diabetes, and rheumatoid arthritis. Lectin toxicity produces weight grain, brain fog, loss of energy, loss of motivation etc...from the endotoxin reticulation due to Leaky Gut.

"The Leptin Diet," by Byron J. Richards explains how to unleash the power of hormones to resolve fatigue, food cravings, thyroid problems, and body weight issues. Leptin is the principle metabolic hormone that controls thyroid, adrenals, sleep, energy, and metabolism. A low carbohydrate diet increases the sensitivity of leptin receptors in the hypothalamus. Omega 3 increases sensitivity to insulin and leptin. By preventing spikes in blood sugar, eating a low carb diet and increasing the Omega-3:Omega-6 ratio, leptin and insulin sensitivity can improve. ***It is best to take Omega 3 from whole food sources due to aldehyde toxin contamination of Omega 3 supplements.

Obese people have high levels of leptin which produces insulin resistance and belly fat. Lower leptin and increase leptin sensitivity lowers appetite. Refined sugar boosts leptin, which stimulates cell migration and cancer metastasis. Since the ketogenic diet is so low on carbohydrates the usual blood sugar spiking that initiates excessive levels of insulin and leptin and associated down-regulation of receptors is avoided.

Dr. Steven Gundry popularized the **lectin-free diet**. According to Dr. Gundry, people should limit the following foods when trying to avoid lectins: legumes such as beans, peas, lentils, and peanuts, squash, nightshade vegetables, such as eggplant, peppers, potatoes, and tomatoes, fruit - although in-season fruit is allowed in moderation, grains, corn and meat or milk from corn-fed animals. Lectins in raw or undercooked kidney beans can cause symptoms that mimic food poisoning, such as vomiting and diarrhea.

Food preparation ways to decrease the lectins in foods include: boiling, fermentation, sprouting, peeling, deseeding, pressure cooking. The sprouting process – for grains, beans, legumes and seeds – releases enzymes that lowers the levels of lectins in food. Besides avoiding lectins in the diet Dr. Steven Gundry recommends supplementing with L-Glutamine, Licorice, Marshmallow, Clove, Mushroom extract, Pine bark Extract, Zinc, N-Acetyl Glucosamine and other GI lining restoring agents.

See: "The Plant Paradox: The Hidden Dangers in "Healthy" Foods That Cause Disease and Weight Gain, by Dr. Steven R Gundry M.D., 2017

"We will use soft metals, aging accelerators and sedatives in food and water, also in the air.

They will be blanketed in poison everywhere they turn.

The soft metals will cause them to lose their minds. We will promise to find a cure from our many fronts, yet we will feed them more poison.

The poisons will be absorbed through their skin and mouths. They will destroy their minds and reproductive systems.

From all this, their children will be born dead, and we will conceal this information.

The poisons will be hidden in everything that surrounds them; in what they drink, eat, breathe, and wear.

We must be ingenious in dispensing the poisons for they can see far. "

~The Illuminati Covenant

7

HEAVY METALS AND RADIONUCLIDES

HEAVY METAL AND ALUMINUM POISONING

Heavy metal used to be rock music our parents didn't like us to listen to, now we are besieged by a scourge heavy metals raining down on us from the skies. The chemtrails slowly degrade the living environments wherever chemtrails are sprayed, breaking apart organisms and their tight knit relationships. Meanwhile The National Institute of Health, National Center for Biotechnology (NCBI) has officially declared atmospheric aerosols and their particulates, chemicals, metal oxides are of severe detriment to human health and the entire biosphere. A USDA biologist Francis Mangel tested and found elevated levels of aluminum in water and soil samples of 4,610 parts per million which is 25,000 times the safe guidelines of the World Health Organization in California's Mt. Shasta region.

There are no safe levels for heavy metals! Heavy metals are naturally occurring elements that have a high atomic weight and a density at least 5 times greater than that of water. Even at lower levels of exposure, these metallic elements are considered systemic toxicants that are known to induce multiple organ damage. Their toxicity depends on several factors including the dose, route of exposure, and chemical species, as well as the age, gender, genetics, and nutritional status of exposed individuals. [*In this book, for convenience I include aluminum under the term "Heavy Metal"].

Toxic metals have an imposter effect in the body, replacing the biological slots meant for the correct metals, and thus creating havoc with our form and function, and the continuum of life.
   * Strontium Mimics ⇨ Calcium.
   * Cesium and Barium Mimics ⇨ Potassium.
   * Plutonium Mimics ⇨ Iron.
   * Fluorine, Chlorine and Bromine Mimics ⇨ Iodine.
   * Cadmium Mimics ⇨ Iron and Copper.
   * Lithium Mimics ⇨ Sodium.

Because of their high degree of toxicity - arsenic, cadmium, chromium, lead, and mercury rank among the priority metals that are of public health significance. Mercury in particular is the second most toxic metal known to man, second only to plutonium. Because heavy metals compromise the immune system allowing opportunistic infections to occur, people with heavy metal toxicity often also manifest an overgrowth of candida, or parasitic (worm) infestation. To get rid of worm infestation eat 2 cups of raw pumpkin seeds per day for a week. Take a weeks break and repeat the process for another week.

Any chemtrail survival protocol is focused on detoxifying the body and keeping it as clean as possible so that internal resources can be rallied to deal with whatever environmental hazards come out way. The human body is designed to eliminate toxins, but can only do so if the detox organs are strong and the body resources are available to do the job. The cleaner the blood, the lymph, the tissues and organs, the less likely pathogenic micro-organisms will take up residence. Resilience against pathogens is achieved via a pure body uncontaminated by chemicals, toxins, pollutants, poisons, insecticides, fungicides, herbicides, chemical fertilizers, heavy metals, food additives, stimulants, etc.

Heavy metals set up conditions that lead to inflammation in arterial walls, joints and tissues, causing more calcium to be drawn to the area as a buffer. Heavy metals set up conditions that lead to inflammation in arterial walls, joints and tissues, causing more calcium to be drawn to the area as a buffer. Leaky gut and leaky blood brain barrier allow heavy metals to enter and accumulate making us more vulnerable to electrosensitivity. EMF pollution in turn actually promotes leaky gut and a leaky blood brain barrier.

Heavy metal poisoning, glutathione deficiency and methylation insufficiency are contributing factors to candida, dysbiosis, leaky gut and all digestive disease, changing the gut flora to those species less conducive to health and "happy" neurochemistry. Body, mind, soul and earth are inseparable. Like leaky gut, leaky brain is associated with inflammation and infection. You need to heal a leaky gut in order to heal a leaky blood-brain barrier and vice versa. Gelatin (containing proline and glycine) protects against leaky gut, regulates insulin and boosts metabolism.

> *"As human suffering is caused by separation from our inner life, the only path to enjoying a healthy and joyful life is to achieve a oneness between our body-mind-spirit. Such is a universal law, which is called "Changes" or "Oneness.""*~ Hu Li Za Zhi. 2008

ACCUMULATION AND BIO-CONCENTRATION

Nano-particles accumulate in biological systems and persist for a long time, which makes such nano-particles a very real threat to life, equivalent to that of nuclear radiation.

Radiation and nano-particles accumulate and bio-concentrate up the food chain from the smallest algae up the food chain to the largest carnivore. It is important to consider that toxins in the body have an accumulative, synergistic negative effect thus, it is vital to cleanse the system of heavy metals along with radionuclides. Thus it is vital to protect our own life from their disruptive and carcinogenic effects, as well as protecting our genetic lineage from the genotoxic effects. The health-weakening effects of eating non-organic foods contaminated with nano-particles and radiation increases with every generation as more and more of these biohazards accumulate in the environment.

The bioaccumulation of all these elements in different body tissues is influenced by the pH of the body. With the accumulation of heavy metals an overall body (tissue) acidification and inflammation takes place. In an acid environment, all metabolic and digestive and detoxification processes are slowed down, liver and kidney function are diminished, and all enzyme activity is also decreased. Heavy metals eventually bind to body proteins, then the immune system recognizes these proteins as a foreign and attacks them, leading to so-called autoimmune disorders or chronic inflammation. In an acid environment is the perfect terrain for chronic inflammation, a major source of free radical production. Sulfur compounds as found in the cabbage family increase the expression of glutathione, which results in both metal detoxification and free radical neutralization.

Children and infants are up to 500 - 2,000 times more sensitive to the same exposure of low dose of radiation or nano-particles. Women and girls are 50% more sensitive to radiation compared to men and boys, and we can expect nano-particles as well to be highly toxic to an egg, sperm, fetus and small children. Damage to form and function of our human bodies and our food supply is inherited by subsequent generations in a geometrically degenerative fashion. Strong immunity and healthy bio-terrain is paramount to withstanding the effects of chemtrails, until the world's 7 billion people can make THEM stop the slow genocide by the accumulative boiling frog effect.

HEAVY METAL TOXICITY SYMPTOMS

Heavy metal exposure precipitates and aggravates all degenerative diseases and poor health conditions. Heavy Metals can directly or indirectly cause, contribute to, or make worse, nearly every disease or illness known to man: Chronic pain, Chronic fatigue, Cancer, Parkinson's, Hormone disruption, Low libido, PMS, Impotence, Prostate problems, Alzheimer's, Multiple sclerosis, Amyotrophic lateral sclerosis (ALS), Autistic spectrum disorder, Parkinson's, depression, Weight gain, Cardiovascular disease, Crohn's disease, kidney disease, Liver disorder, Lupus, Reproductive disorders, Diabetes.

Chronic pain, chronic malaise, fatigue, brain fog, chronic infections such as candida, gastrointestinal complaints, such as diarrhea, constipation, bloating, gas, heartburn, and indigestion, mood swings, depression, and/or anxiety, nervous system malfunctions – burning extremities, numbness, tingling, ringing in the ears, paralysis or electrical sensations, dizziness, nausea, migraines or headaches, visual disturbances, joint and muscle pain, loss of cognition and memory, dementia, immune system damage, hormonal disturbances, infertility.

ALUMINUM POISONING

Aluminum, while it is the most abundant metal and third most abundant element of the Earth's crust - has no known biological function and is a recognized environmental toxin.

We are being sprayed/poisoned with nano particles which are one-billionth of a meter in size. Thousands of these particles are flooding each individual blood cell in our bodies, interfering with metabolism and breaking us down. Normally, aluminum is poorly absorbed from the GI tract, but nano aluminum is absorbed in much higher amounts. However, the nano sized particles are infinitely more reactive and induce intense inflammation, hence the arthritic conditions most of us are being plagued with in the last 5 years.

Nano-particles, can have the same dimensions as biological molecules such as proteins and easily cross cell membranes and interfere on a mechanical level with the form and function of cells. Nano aluminum from chemtrail aerosols goes directly into the brain through the nasal passages, bypassing the blood brain barrier, causing immuno-inflammatory-excitotoxicity, a significant increase of lipid peroxidation and glutathione depletion in the brain.

In the last ten years, respiratory disease in the US has moved from 8th to 3rd highest cause of death. Aluminum in the lungs and brain shows significant accumulation with age. It is thought that aluminum decreases spontaneous nervous discharge, thereby reducing nerve activity. Aluminum (Al^{3+}) is a light metal, however for purposes of convenience the mention of "heavy metals" in this book automatically includes aluminum. Today, nearly 93% of those people tested for metal toxicity reveal excessively high aluminum levels in their hair. Sources of aluminum poisoning include vaccinations, cookware, baking powder, antacids, beverage containers, foil, cigarette smoke, cosmetics, antiperspirants, sunscreen, and "chemtrails."

Aluminum along with other heavy metal toxicity is commonly the cause of chronic inflammation, chronic fatigue, chronic adrenal fatigue and chronic pain. Aluminum also can alter the replication and reassociation of DNA. Aluminum induces DNA damage through triggering the oxidative burst, resulting in genotoxic stress, leading to mutation, genomic instability or cell death (apoptosis). The synergistic effect of aluminum combined with barium and strontium is many times more toxic than aluminum alone. Barium and other heavy metals are well known to reduce immune function, setting up conditions for a global pandemic of infectious and degenerative disease of epic proportions. Plus, the solar dimming effect of daylight chemtrailing reduces our Vitamin D levels, making us more vulnerable to the disease-causing metals and biological warfare agents in the chemtrail cocktail itself.

Aluminum is a desiccant - it sucks moisture from the air, soil, man-made structures, trees and other plant life — and our bodies. Perhaps you have noticed the drying out, depreciation and oxidation of your city or property from the chemtrail spraying. Aluminum strips the body of the boron needed for strong bones and metabolizing phosphorus and magnesium. In plants, aluminum produces chlorosis, a condition where there is insufficient chlorophyll for photosynthesis.

Aluminum accrues to toxic levels over time in slow apoptotic cell turnover tissues, such as bone matter, the heart and the brain. The brain and its associated nervous system is where diseases such as Alzheimer's, Parkinson's, MS, chronic fatigue and other neurological or autoimmune diseases manifest, including the complete autistic spectrum, from learning disorders to full blown autism.

The energy dependent exchange of cytoplasmic Na+ for extracellular K+ in mammalian cells is due to a plasma membrane bound enzyme system, the Na,K-ATPase. Aluminum has also been shown to inhibit Na-K-ATPase, and since the brain uses 20% of the body's energy, when energy generation is impaired that is when we start getting depression, poor cognitive function, dementia and fatigue. If you're tired, then consider using Succinic Acid, NADH 20mg Sublingual + CoQ10 + Adrenal Cortex + liposomal glutathione with liposomal vitamin C to boost energy and mental alertness.

Aluminum inhibits cholinergic functioning and synaptic uptake of dopamine, norepinephrine and 5-HT- serotonin. Aluminum and EMF electro-smog are poisonous to the very phase conjugate nature of consciousness. Aluminum activates Monoamine oxidase (MAO) which may contribute to lowered levels of monoamines in the brain and pineal gland. Aluminum also causes the significant reduction of Glutathione (GSH) the body's most important antioxidant.

The effect of overstimulation of immune cell activity is as harmful as immunosuppression (inhibition of functional activity), inevitably increasing the susceptibility to invading pathogens, setting the perfect terrain for the overgrowth of yeast and fungus (candida). Heavy metals - are highly toxic, and very effective at killing the friendly bacteria in our gut. A compromised, leaky GI tract opens the door to all kind of toxins and allergens, which, in turn overburdens the immune-system and leads finally to all kind of allergies. Chronic-inflammatory reactions, cancer development, hypersensitivity, allergic and autoimmune diseases are known consequences of persisting overstimulation related to heavy metal exposure.

ALUMINUM AND VACCINE ILLNESS

The nano-aluminum from chemtrails is a major causal factor in the dramatic rise of Alzheimer's, as it directly enters the brain via the nasal passages. Aluminum nano-particles accumulate in particular in the bone marrow, lymph nodes and cell membranes. Barium deposits in the muscles, lung and bone and strips immune protecting selenium from the body. Barium, Aluminum and other chemtrail aerosols can cause difficulty breathing, stomach and chest pains, increased blood pressure, heart arrhythmia and damage to the heart, kidneys and liver. Aluminum is excreted principally through the urine. Adequate kidney function is therefore essential for detoxification. Any therapies that stimulate the activity of the liver, kidneys, bowel and skin can be helpful.

Depending on where they occur in the brain the mini seizures and lesions caused from vaccines damage the function of various organs...eyes, teeth, heart, lungs, GI tract etc.... These damages are permanent without serious rehabilitation such as hyperbaric oxygen, but may not express noticeably till much later in life. We don't know who we would be, or how our life would have unfolded if we were not damaged as children with the eugenic poisons fluoride, chlorine, vaccines and mercury fillings. Plus most of us were brought up on deficient cooked industrial food which has neither the content nor spiritual energy necessary to create genuine HUmans. Remineralized organic food contains higher life-energy, and a coherent, ordered template conveying essential information to build the liquid crystal structures of living creatures.

Aluminum is also a known carcinogen and has neurotoxic effects. The long term genetic integrity of United Dire States is of particular concern considering the widespread industrial-chemical agriculture, Fukushima radiation and daily chemtrailing with nano-particles. Broadly speaking, long-term exposure to toxic heavy metals can have carcinogenic, central and peripheral nervous system and circulatory effects. High level of exposure to heavy metals during pregnancy is directly associated with autism in children. Heavy metals are not filtered by placenta from mother to child and are directly deposited in growing fetal tissue. Prenatal exposure to mercury, lead and aluminum poses a permanent health threat particularly to the developing brain.

The ischemia, hypoxia and lesions in the brain caused by vaccines not only distorts the symmetry of the facial features, but it also damages the affluent nerves feeding the mouth. This damage is relatively permanent if not suspended and repaired through treatments like hyperbaric oxygen. Having lost nerve supply the mouth's immune system is compromised and is subsequently filled with mercury to cover up the potholes of decay. The mercury exhausts the body's main antioxidant glutathione and causes permanent digestive problems, dysbiosis and disease.

The perpetrators of mass lobotomization via inflammatory ischemia to the brain due to vaccines need to be stopped immediately. This travesty is a medical war against the people of the earth. Willful compliance with the agenda to chemically lobotomize Homo sapiens in order to keep the masses as dumb commercial slaves is immoral. To submit one's children to brain destroying vaccines is murder...it is a crime against life. Just as the chemtrails are a crime against the planet and all life. The pharmaceutical model of "healthcare" system is a surefire way to ensure the progressive degeneration of the population. There is no point damaging the nervous system, immune system and GI system with life harming drugs and vaccines in the name of preventing disease. That is, you cannot prevent disease by causing it. The grand deception of the vaccine regime for clipping the spiritual wings of the population is up!

- See the YouTube videos of the great scientist and doctor Andrew Moulden PhD. explaining this compound crime of epic proportions!

- For how aluminum from vaccines etc... affects genetic and epigenetic expression and how to reverse the negative effects see the work of **Dr. Ben Lynch,** *Dirty Genes: A Breakthrough Program to Treat the Root Cause of Illness and Optimize Your Health* www.drbenlynch.com/vaccinesdirtygene/

- Check out this YouTube video on the autoimmune crisis created by vaccines: *The Exploding Autoimmune Epidemic* - Dr. Tent - It's Not Autoimmune, you have Viruses.

BEHAVIORAL SYMPTOMS OF AL POISONING:

Oppositional defiance, frustration, anger, inappropriate verbal responses, name-calling or false accusations toward others, slander, continuous talking, or telling stories to strangers, forgetting words, difficulty speaking (fragmented sentences, etc.), forgetfulness (short-term memory loss), difficulty naming ordinary objects (keys, lamp, etc.), difficulty managing time and meeting deadlines, diminished capacity to plan ahead, inability to organize, difficulty learning new concepts and skills and following instructions or directions, vagueness, confusion, disorientation, dizziness, inability to focus, strategize or sort through problems; difficulty listening to others, difficulty performing simple tasks and the activities of daily living, poor personal hygiene, wearing inappropriate clothing; difficulty establishing or maintaining relationships, difficulty in showing affection or overly affectionate, weepy and groveling, feelings of inadequacy and dependency, codependent on others who are abusive or demoralizing, decreased impulse control, obsessive, compulsive behavior, addictiveness, divulging personal/private information to strangers, loss of boundaries, inappropriate interest in others' belongings/activities, delusional beliefs not based on facts, poor judgment, weak navigation of moral dilemmas, decreased capacity to be self-reliant and handle personal finances, lacking foresight, vision and preparedness, irresponsible, loss of awareness of surroundings and not eco-conscious.

DETOXING HEAVY METALS AND RADIONUCLIDES

CHELATION THERAPY

Chelation is the chemical bonding that works to build biochemical substances or, in this case, bond to the atoms of pollutants and radioactive isotopes so as to transported out of the body to be eliminated rather than incorporated into tissues where they can do very considerable damage. Medical chelation is done to reduce calcium plaques on arterial walls using a synthetic amino acid EDTA (ethylene diamine tetraacetic acid) and numerous natural chelating agents. EDTA is said to work in vascular conditions either by removing calcium found in fatty plaques either directly via chelation effect or alternately by stimulating release of hormones that in turn cause calcium removal or lower cholesterol levels. Research suggests that EDTA therapy may reduce the oxidative stress injury and inflammation in blood vessel walls as well by eliminating inflammatory chemicals.

Chelation also removes the calcium deposits from the body which are complexed with stored heavy metals, so eliminative organs must be highly active and supported by antioxidants. By removing heavy metals chelation therapy simultaneously helps to dissolve and remove calcium plaques…which are complex accretions of nano-bacteria, their biofilm, calcium deposits and heavy metals. I dissolved the calcium scale in my distiller with lemon juice in less than one minute, I was amazed—so lemon squeezed into distilled water may be great to deplaque the body and removing heavy metals, arthritic deposits and candida. Apple cider vinegar, magnesium and Chanca piedra (stone breaker) can assist breaking down deposits, reduce inflammation and relieve pain.

There are no safe levels for heavy metals. Mercury in particular is the second most toxic metal known to man, second only to plutonium. So don't start an applied chelation regime without first removing the mercury amalgam fillings from your mouth, because the chelators will mobilize the oral mercury load and liberate it into circulation. Inflammation that occurs in the gut as a result of mercury poisoning from amalgams etc... changes the flora in our gut and shuts down the body's glutathione antioxidant system. Mercury lowers T-Cell count thus contributing to cancer, autoimmune diseases, allergies, Candida overgrowth, and multiple sclerosis.

Glutathione may have complexed the mercury and toxins, but if the exit doors out of the body are closed by inflammation, dysbiosis, impaired GI immune system, and poor functioning GI, liver and kidneys, the heavy metals and toxins cannot get out of the body through the kidneys and GI tract. Mercury when combined with endotoxins from leaky gut, dysbiosis and candida yeast is 8 times more toxic!

Because heavy metals compromise the immune system allowing these other opportunistic infections to occur people with heavy metal toxicity often also manifest an overgrowth of candida, or a parasite (worms) infestation. Any chemtrail survival protocol is focused on detoxifying the body and keeping it as clean as possible so that internal resources can be rallied to deal with

140

whatever environmental hazards come out way. The cleaner the blood, the lymph, the tissues and organs, the less likely pathogenic micro-organisms will take up residence. Resilience against pathogens is achieved via a pure body uncontaminated by chemicals, toxins, pollutants, poisons, insecticides, fungicides, herbicides, chemical fertilizers, heavy metals, food additives, stimulants, etc.

When the body cannot eliminate toxins it will naturally attempt to lock them away out of circulation to try and protect vital organ systems such as the brain. Both the biofilms of pathogens, mucoid deposits and calcification (deposits of calcium phosphate) in joints, tissues, blood vessels, or organs contain stored heavy metals. To eliminate the "bad bugs" you have to breakdown their protective biofilms associated with your pathogen load in order to release the heavy metals during a specially designed cleanse.

As we attack the biofilms and plaques, Kyolic garlic and enzymes taken throughout the day will help clean up and eliminate the pathogen load, while using chelators like EDTA. Plenty of antiseptic and antifungal herbs, along with silicon rich herb teas (Oatstraw, Pineneedle, Horsetail, Nettle, Hemp Leaf), plus medical mushrooms such as Chaga Tea and Reishi will give the body the resources it needs to remove pathogens, toxins and heavy metals safely. Also nettles, red clover, catnip and ginseng are chelating agents. These remedies should be taken daily as infusions, tinctures or vinegars for this purpose.

Some of the best natural chelating agents are black and green tea catechins, burdock root (Arctium lappa), and brown seaweeds which bind strontium to create sodium alginate which is then excreted. Sodium alginate removes strontium, barium, radium and other radioactive isotopes. It is present in most sea vegetables, wild garlic or onions, watercress, artichokes, pears, citrus fruits, pineapples, egg. An important assisting agent is the amino acid Taurine, which can protect against radiation as well as chelate heavy metals, and brewers yeast helps build and regenerate cells damaged by radiation.

MINERAL ANTAGONISTS

Detoxifying Heavy Metals Is A Specialist Job — Regular detoxification techniques like fasting, the liver flush, kidney zinc and colonics do not work with heavy metals. First mineral antagonism is necessary to dislodge the toxic metals from the tissues, (brain, liver, kidneys, muscles etc.). Detoxifying heavy metals involves balancing mineral antagonists that dislodge the competing metals from the tissues into the blood, along with chelating agents that bind the metals in the blood and prevent them from being re-deposited somewhere else so the kidneys can excrete them.

This is done by flooding the body with nutritional minerals like zinc, selenium, potassium and magnesium that compete for the same deposit sites and dislodge the heavy metals and radioactive elements. Algaes, Seaweeds, Green juices, vege juicing and smoothies are a great auxiliary to a heavy metal/radiation cleanse. Check online for a full list of Mineral Antagonists.

To eliminate aluminum out of the body, silica, calcium and magnesium must pull it through the kidneys. Magnesium citrate has low molecular weight so it easily crosses the blood-brain barrier, and helps increase the number of synapses in the Hippocampus and help improve cognition and memory. Magnesium is also needed for the production of the body's energy molecule ATP. Epsom salt foot baths and baths, and putting the remaining water on the garden is also an integral use of magnesium.

Aluminum can be eliminated to some extent by the skin, so saunas, mineral pools, spinal showers, and hot baths with Epsom salts may be beneficial. Due to the substantially toxic levels of aluminum poisoning in the general public it is recommended to wear flip flops in a public sauna to prevent being exposed to the aluminum coming out of people as they sweat.

ESSENTIAL MINERALS FOR DETOX

Selenium boosts glutathione and is a potent detoxifier of mercury. Selenium binds with mercury and deposits it in the liver in an insoluble form, as well as aiding the manufacture of glutathione which is the main mercury detox pathway. Selenium has a protective effect against aluminum, cadmium and reduces the toxicity and oxidative damages caused by mercury. (See YouTubes by Dr. Christopher Shade, a mercury and glutathione expert). Zinc supplementation at 330mg/day restores normal intestinal permeability in Crohn's patients. Zinc reduces the toxicity of aluminum and the cell damage that comes with it. Can remove also lead. The presence of cadmium often causes a lack of zinc.

AGED GARLIC: It is believed that there is a benefit in combining EDTA with other chelators, because EDTA acts slowly and could potentially lead to redeposition of metals. Kyolic Garlic Extract is an effective enhancer of EDTA and other chelators. Garlic will chelate lead, cadmium, and mercury.

Garlic should be crushed, sliced, or chewed (prior to cooking) in order to ensure maximum allicin production, since allicin is responsible for its labile chelating ability. Allicin chelates heavy metals such as Cadmium, Gold, Lead and Mercury, and acts as a detoxifier. The alliums – garlic especially but also onions, ramps, chives, shallots are also excellent antioxidant sources which protect red blood cells from radiation damage. Aged Garlic extract (2g/day) resulted an 8-fold increase in T-cells relative to control and has shown antiproliferative effect and it has been shown to lower LDL. Aging your own garlic will take 20 months. You can also employ powered, minced flake and granulated garlic, or dehydrate your own.

STANDARD CHELATOR MIX: Chelating agents are substances that have a strong ability to grab onto toxic metals such as mercury, arsenic, copper, iron, aluminum and others. Medical chelation is done to remove heavy metals and calcium plaques on arterial walls using a synthetic amino acid EDTA (zinc acid). In a glass of distilled or reverse osmosis water add 1/2 tsp EDTA, 1 tsp MSM, ¼ tsp Magnesium Citrate, 1 tsp buffered Vitamin C, ½ tsp Potassium Bicarbonate, drink immediately on an empty stomach. This taken every 3 hours around the clock, for 72 hours. Along with a regular daily dose of Alpha lipoic acid, Taurine, Zinc and Selenium, plus Vitamins A, K2, D and E, N-acetyl cysteine (NAC)), which are important in combination with oral chelation.

ALPHA LIPOIC ACID: Alpha lipoic acid is a chelating agent that is especially important to eliminate heavy metals from the brain and other nervous tissue. Being a very small water and fat soluble molecule, Alpha lipoic acid has access to almost any tissue in the body and work within cells too. It increases the intracellular level of glutathione, the important cerebral antioxidant. Alpha Lipoic Acid (ALA) is a mercury-chelating antioxidant that mitigates heavy metal toxicity when used in association with Vitamin C. Taking ALA with like EDTA and DMSA made chelation much easier. ALA is able to cross the blood-brain barrier and can remove mercury from the brain. However Alpha Lipoic Acid should not be used alone, as it only mobilizes mercury with a weak bond. Vitamin C, alpha-lipoic acid, and CoQ10 regenerate glutathione.

EDTA *(Disodium Ethylene-Diamine-Tetra-Acetate)*

The synthetic amino acid EDTA is a weak acid closely related to vinegar, or acetic acid. If you put an eggshell in vinegar, it'll dissolve. In the same way, EDTA will take calcium off your arteries. EDTA treatment has been shown to improve circulation resulting in better memory function, reversal of diabetic gangrene, peripheral ischemia, decreased macular degeneration and improved vision in people with diabetic neuropathy, reduced cramping pain, and improved heart function, helps dissolve kidney stones, and reduces osteoporosis. EDTA actually stimulates bone growth through a complex action of the parathyroid gland. Chelation therapy helps to correct, reverse, or eliminate a vast array of serious and prevalent health conditions, ranging from senility to cancer. EDTA chelation tends to INCREASE skeletal integrity.

Oral chelation works best through the synergistic effect of combining EDTA with numerous natural chelating agents. For the most part, oral chelation products with EDTA are designed to remove cholesterol and calcium deposits in the arteries. The removal of toxic heavy metals and aluminum is a secondary function through their association with the calcium plaques and nano-bacteria.

Oral EDTA is a safe and effective blood thinner and anti-clotting agent. Oral EDTA is slower acting than intraveinous, because only about 3% to 8% of an oral dose gets absorbed (compared with 100% of an intraveinous dose). Oral chelation is also an option, although it's considered less effective. 1 to 2 months of oral EDTA is chelation equivalent to a single session of intraveinous therapy. Someone taking 800 mg of EDTA per day is generally absorbing only around 40 mg, or about 1200 mg per month.

Recommendations: Take EDTA at least 2 hours apart, in doses comprising 1-2 grams of oral EDTA daily adding a multi-vitamin and mineral supplement, in cycles, 6 weeks on then 2 weeks off. Magnesium Di-Potassium EDTA is more expensive than the calcium and sodium EDTA, and Suppositories are supposed to work better than oral. Magnesium Di-Potassium EDTA can have a very powerful calming effect on the nervous system by both blocking the stress response as well as stimulating the relaxation response. Removing heavy metals from the body will promote a deep sense of calm because heavy metals create havoc, incoherence and discord in the body. Magnesium di-potassium EDTA suppositories can help the body eliminate a variety of toxins in a safe and gentle way. EDTA chelation suppository captures heavy metals, the route of excretion is the bowel. Chelation with EDTA is more effective if taken along with Kyolic Aged Garlic Extract.

IMPORTANT TIP: While undergoing the chelating of heavy metals it is important to remineralize with kelp, greens (wheatgrass juice), humic acids (fulvic acid/shilajit/leonardite) and blue-green algae! EDTA also binds with essential minerals zinc, copper, and magnesium, for this reason, it is recommended that people using EDTA make sure they are also taking a good mineral supplement to make up for what they might be losing. Chelators bind zinc, necessary for immune system function and inhibit free radical scavenging enzymes requiring Zn, Mn or Cu for activity (i.e. SODs). So when undergoing chelation you need to increase your high quality mineral foods and supplements like kelp so that the immune system and enzymes are still supported.

DIMERCAPTOSUCCINIC ACID: Dimercaptosuccinic acid (DMSA), (also called Succinic Acid/Butanedioic/Amber Acid) is used to remove toxic heavy metals such as lead and mercury. DMSA is a non-toxic, water-soluble treatment for heavy metal toxicity, especially for mercury (vaccines/amalgams). Succinic acid is a powerful antioxidant that helps fight toxic free radicals, will reduce hot flashes, increase weight loss, regulate cardiac rhythm. Succinic acid had been shown to stimulate the neural system recovery and strengthens the immune system, and can also help compensate for energy drain in the body and brain, boosting awareness, concentration and reflexes, and reduce stress. 17th Century aristocrats would brew tea in special amber containers knowing that the amber vessel it is brewed in would release its special properties into the tea that would cure them of their ills. Take 1-2 tablets/day, your body will only use what it needs and you will eliminate any excess. www.therussianstore.com/

TRANSDERMAL DMSA: DMSA is safe and quick treatment for lead or arsenic poisoning symptoms. DMSA is used transdermally to treat autism through removing mercury and other toxins from the brain. A topical heavy metal detoxification cream will increase the overall detoxification of heavy metals. Besides oral chelation we may consider making an antifungal/chelation cream for feet, Chemtrail Bug lesions and Morgellons, eczema and other skin conditions. Sulfur cream on the feet before putting on socks does a wonderful job of eliminating fungi in the skin of the feet. To this we may add a form of selenium and DMSA or succinic acid, as well as Zinc Oxide Cream.

Warning: DMPS (sodium 2,3-dimercaptopropane-l-sulfonate) is a sulfuric acid salt which is extremely effective in removing heavy metals when an intravenous shot of DMPS was given, 90 percent of heavy metals were excreted through the kidneys after 24 hours. However DMSA and DMPS carry risks of harm, and should only be used under medical supervision. Owing to redistribution of mercury with DMSA treatment so without additional chelators present, such as EDTA, DMPS or glutathione and metallothionein, the mercury may just redistribute elsewhere in the body instead of being removed.

SELENIUM: Selenium sulfide 1% and 2.5% strengths are used on the scalp to help control the symptoms of dandruff and seborrheic dermatitis. Scalp psoriasis topical medicated shampoos and conditioners often contain pyrithione zinc, salicylic acid, ketoconazole or selenium sulfide. Topical L-selenomethionine combined with vitamin E can prevent UVB-induced skin cancer when applied continuously before, during, and after radiation exposure.

PERFECT HYDRATION

During the chemtrail cleanse you want the GI tract to be loose and open so the released heavy metals are not re up-taken into the kidneys. Perfect hydration, eliminative herbs, fiber brooms, clays and zeolite along with colonics allow for the exit of moribund matter without it recirculating back into our system. Hydration is super important during chelation regimes. Add a pinch of Himalayan salt to compensate for the loss of urinary salt. Salt, along with water, addresses the common symptoms of lightheadedness and fatigue. Water with a squeeze of lemon is particularly effective at stripping biofilms and mineral plaques.

While detoxing from heavy metals avoid bread and other grain foods as these are connected to edema and candida. Avoid all inflammatory, mucus producing foods in general. One of the main benefits of fasting is the dissolving of excess proteins and mucus. Fenugreek seed sprouts and extract help move lymph and may be an important ally to aid the removal of aluminum from the brain via the glymphatic system. Structured water in raw fruits and vegetables and shungite water are superior waters for moving and removing unwanted elements and toxins from the cells. The best thing I found so far to help boost cell growth and counter genetic decay is octagonal structured water made using Tesla technology and frequencies etc...

I dissolved the scale in my distiller with white vinegar in less than 1 minute. Thus apple cider vinegar or lemon juice in distilled water may be an ideal way to deplaque the body when removing calcium deposits, heavy metals, arthritic deposits, arteriosclerosis, candida and cancer tumors.

CHELATION FOODS AND SUPPLEMENTS

Ashitaba, Green tea, Cilantro, Parsley, Nettle, Ginkgo biloba, Red ginseng extract, Green tea extract, Aloe gel, Olive leaf, Water melon juice, Banana tree stem juice, whole pumpkin juice, Hawthorn berry, Cayenne, Grape seed extract and Grape skin extract. Vitamin E and D, Pycnogenol, Quercetin, CoQ10, Vitamin C, Beta-carotene and all antioxidants. Magnesium, Sodium alginate, Selenium, Silicon and Zinc gluconate. Vitamin B's such as folic acid, inositol, choline and niacinamide, about 400-500 mg of each daily. Folate is a B vitamin naturally occurring in leafy greens and fermented foods. Benfotiamine- a lipid soluble B vitamin also reduces glycation, and helps get glucose into the cells, therefore can lessen brain fog and depression and stimulate increased energy.

Unfortunately, our symbiotic ecosystem can be broken down by a number of influences including antibiotics, stress, sugar and chemicals. By consuming probiotic containing foods like sauerkraut and kimchi and supplementing with probiotics we can continue to support the delicate microbiome balance which influences our brain chemistry, mood and skin, not just our digestion. The GI tract contains 80 percent of our immune system; our microbiota (gut flora) is responsible for the secretion of regulatory T cells, IgG and IgA and the production of butyrate, vitamin K2 and vitamin B12.

AMINO ACIDS: Many heavy metal binding proteins contain sulfur and sulfur is also important for liver detoxification. Sulfur makes cell membranes more pliable allowing for improved oxygen transport to the cell and improved waste transport from the cell. Sulfur helps lessen glycation—the process by which sugar cross links with collagen protein to armor plate our cells with AGES. The sulfur-containing amino acids—methionine and cysteine, N-acetylcysteine, S-adenosylmethionine, Alpha-lipoic acid, and the tripeptide glutathione (GSH) all contribute to the chelation and excretion of metals from the human body. L-lysine is an amino acid involved in the structural repair of damaged blood vessels, that has a beneficial effect on lead toxicity and high blood pressure.

SULFUR AMINOS: Heavy metals like cadmium, lead, aluminum and mercury depletes the body's main antioxidant GLUTATHIONE, along with Vitamin C, and inhibits thiamine (B1) and pyridoxine (B6). It is important to repeat that NAC increases glutathione levels.

When there is a **glutathione deficiency** in the digestive system, heavy metal detoxification cannot occur! Hence the role of glutathione, N-Acetyl cysteine (NAC) and alpha-lipoic acid in the treatment of mercury toxicity. N-Acetyl cysteine or cysteine is a sulfur containing amino acid that will assist mercury to cross the blood brain barrier to be removed by the body.

The heavy metals, cadmium, arsenic and mercury bind with sulfur to create sulfides and thus become soluble to be excreted from the body. So you need plenty of sulfur containing amino acids cysteine, methionine, taurine and glutathione in diet both for anti-aging and thriving in the chemtrail holocaust.

Adequate levels of the amino acids cysteine, glutamine and lysine and supplements as Vitamin B12 and Vitamin D are necessary to counteract a heavy metal burden. L-Cysteine and Vitamin B6, Methionine, Taurine, Thiamine and Acetyl CoA. Niacin, NAC and Vitamin C are a useful combo to take prior to drinking alcohol to prevent its conversion to acetylaldehyde.

PROBIOTIC HEAVY METAL DETOX: Specific probiotic bacteria may have properties that enable them to bind heavy metals and other toxins from food and water. The cabbage and probiotics 'good bacteria' help to detoxify chemicals within our body such as Bisphenol A, sodium nitrate, perchlorate an ingredient in jet fuel and fireworks, Heterocyclic aromatic amines (HCA) are mutagenic compounds formed when meat is cooked at high temperatures of 150-300 degrees C, and Toxic Foods. Kimchi degrades a variety of organophosphorous pesticides. The fungal melanins in Chaga mushroom improve its metal binding properties. Drinking Chaga-Chickory root coffee in the morning will assist your heavy metal detox. A quarter of a cup of grated ginger made into 6 cups of ginger tea per day will settle your digestive system. You can keep this tea hot and ready in the glass carafe of a coffee maker.

METALLOTHIONEIN: Metallothionein is one of the most powerful antioxidants that the human body produces. The only way to expulse heavy metals and control their level in cells is to immobilize the heavy metal atoms by linking them to biological molecules, such as proteins like metallothionein. Metallothionein (MT) is a cysteine-rich protein with a low molecular weight that has the capacity to bind to certain minerals and heavy metals. The main functions of MTs are related to metal metabolism, acting in the detoxification and storage of heavy metals and in the regulation of cellular copper and zinc metabolism in response to physiological and environmental changes.

It is found in the membrane of the Golgi apparatus which are the central organelle modifying protein and transporting lipids within the cell. One of the most important functions of metallothionein is the protection against heavy metals. For this reason high concentrations of this protein are present in the mucous membrane of the intestine where it serves as a binding agent for heavy metals by exchanging zinc for mercury, lead, platinum, aluminium etc. Not only is it present in the intestines, but metallothionein is also found in the liver, pancreas, mouth, stomach and the brain.

Metallothionein and Autism: Metallothionein is the first line of defense against heavy metals passing through the blood-brain barrier unhindered! Research of **Dr. William J. Walsh**, PhD., author of the book *"Nutrient Power: Heal Your Biochemistry and Heal Your Brain,"* suggests all problems of autists, both immunological, brain and intestinal, can be explained by poorly functioning metallothionein. Children with a dormant metallothionein deficiency syndrome are in danger of acquiring developmental arrest (autism) when their metallothionein system is overloaded by a vaccine, a bacterial or viral infection, antibiotics, or amalgam fillings of the mother during pregnancy etc.

Several other diseases and behavioural disorders are likely associated with malfunctioning metallothionein such as like ADHD, fibromyalgia, fibrosis, ME and CFS (chronic fatigue syndrome), and it could possibly be a factor in cancer Metallothionein also plays an important role in several other processes in the body: It is indispensable in the development of nerve cells (neurons) in the brain together with the Omega-3 fatty acids.

It has a regulating influence on hippocampal behaviour and is involved in the emotional development and socialization (amygdala). Metallothionein regulates the concentration of zinc and copper in the blood. It is essential in the development and functioning of our immune system. It prevents intestinal infections and protects against excessive yeast growth in the intestines. It is involved in gastric acid production and influences taste and texture sensation of food in the mouth.

Isolated Metallothionein could be used by rich people who are accidentally vaccinated or otherwise exposed to heavy metals or arsenic etc... for the rest of us NAC, Alpha Lipoic Acid and Milk Thistle seed, and the cabbage/mustard family vegetables will suffice. To ensure that our body is protected from heavy metal accumulation we must look to incorporating food sources that support metallothionein on a daily basis.

FOOD SOURCES THAT SUPPORT METALLOTHIONEIN: Hops, pomegranate, watercress, cruciferous vegetables, quercetin, Cordyceps mushroom, zinc. B6 is required by the liver to produce detoxification binding proteins such as cysteine, glutathione, and metallothionein. NAC and cysteine foods improve metallothionein metabolism. All polyphenols appear to enhance the expression of metallothionein, however only tannic acid and quercetin stimulated the uptake of zinc. Blueberry juice can augment the antioxidative capability of the liver presumably via stimulating Metallothionein expression and superoxide dismutase (SOD) activity, which decreases extracellular matrix collagen accumulation in the liver, and thereby alleviating hepatic fibrosis.

POLYPHENOLS: Depending on their level and persistence, excessive free radicals, or Reactive oxygen species (ROS), can cause diverse pathological conditions, such as oxidative damage to DNA, proteins, and lipids, that may contribute to cell degeneration and tumor genesis. Reactive oxygen species can perturb the mitochondrial permeability transition pore and disrupt electron transfer of the cell's energy generating center triggering apoptosis and necrosis. There is a direct relation between total phenol content of the plant with its free-radical scavenging potential. Thus the antioxidant properties of plants are correlated with defense against oxidative stress, degenerative disease and the aging process. Polyphenols are efficient in scavenging ROS, plus they reduce the catalytic activity of enzymes involved in ROS generation and thereby prevent various ROS-mediated human diseases. In Ayurvedic medicine the poly-herbal formulation called Vayasthapana Rasayana is used for quenching free-radical and promoting longevity.

Foods Highest in Polyphenols: Cloves, peppermint, star anise, cacao, oregano, celery seed, sage, rosemary, flaxseed, chestnut, chokeberry, elderberry, blueberry, blackcurrant, aronia, acai, goji berry, maqui berries. Rose hip polyphenols include catechin, anthocyanin, quercetin, taxifolin and eriodictyol.

BINDERS

An hour or two after the chelators use binders to help mop up the debris. The quicker and more efficiently chemical toxins are removed by the body's detoxification pathways, the less likely they will cause damage. Russian black radish, MSM, the cabbage family, garlic, and garlic mustard are sources of sulfur, which binds with copper and other heavy metals so they can be eliminated, and many heavy metal binding proteins contain sulfur. Organic sulfur binds with aluminum, mercury, copper and other heavy metals so they can be safely removed from the body. Sulfur is also important for methylation and liver detoxification. **Cilantro with Chlorella:** To eliminate heavy metals the combination of cilantro and chlorella is helpful to detox. The algaes, spirulina or chlorella are needed to bind up the liberated heavy metals to carry them out of the body. Seaweed, Kelp and chlorella contains the powerful chelating agents mannitol and polysaccharide alginates.

Other binders include chitosan, citrus or apple pectin, a special bicarbonate formula, organic germanium, and others. The skin of fruits and vegetables are high, not only in pectin, but also in a wide range of antioxidants and other phytonutrients. The pith of the citrus contains about 30% pectin. Apple Pectin reduces Cesium-137 load by over 62% in one month and pectin is also a chelator of other positively charged heavy metals. Potassium - reduces uptake of cesium-137. Rice bran chelates reactive iron.

BROOM CLEANSERS

Every cell of your body is affected by self-poisoning making you feel irritable and depressed as these toxins accumulate in your tissues and nervous system. When you rid the colon of toxins and its buildup of waste, you will feel lighter than air, loaded with energy, and filled with good health.

Never fast or drink solely liquids when doing heavy metal detox, as you need the fiber to absorb some of the toxins and metals in order to protect your body. Also for broom action in the GI tract to speed elimination of heavy metals use flaxseed, chia seed, rice bran and psyllium powder. When you add enzymes to rice bran this releases the β-glucan and protein from the rice bran.

PM CLEANSER recipe includes equal parts Psyllium powder, Bentonite Clay, Yucca root powder, Magnesium citrate powder, and papain/or bromelain enzyme powers. Mix this together and put in a jar in the fridge. Take 1 heaped teaspoon in a 10 oz glass of water before bed. Or if cleansing or fasting take 3 times a day alternating with cleansing herbs every 3 hours or so. Vitamin C is also a great addition. Ingredients can be bought by the pound at herbalcom.com

SOOTHERS: To Prevent GI Irritation — Aloe, rose hips, slippery elm, mullein, mallow, yucca root, flaxseed, chia seed, chamomile, horsetail and ginger will help to reduce inflammation in the GI tract. Eat flaxseed and flaxseed oil to help detox the body. This superfood is full of fiber and Omega 3s, both important substances for detoxification.

SOOTHING TEA: Licorice, Chamomile, Mullein, Marshmallow, Flax, Chia, Ginger, Galangal, Cinnamon, Fennel. Drink this energizing tea by the gallon during your cleanse to support elimination and fortify the adrenal glands. It is great made in a French Press.

STIMULATE AND SUPPORT DETOX ORGANS

Approximately 60% of the toxins are excreted through the urine and 40% through fecal matter. The happy, relaxed body will stop holding on to what is harming it so establish enjoyable routines during your most intense fasts and cleanses. Exercise, yoga, sweating, grounding on the earth and sunlight are also essential to detoxifying the body.

Before taking chelators to remove heavy metals we must first undertake a colon cleanse to remove the black tar biofilm so that toxins can freely "leave" the body. Also we must raise our Chi (ATP) or cell voltage and support the liver and kidneys, as well as establishing advanced hydration practices. To increase liver detoxification add Milk thistle, Dandelion root, Schisandra and 6000 mg of vitamin C per day along with bioflavonoids and Alpha Lipoic Acid to promote liver activity.

Seaweed/Kelp contains a powerful chelating agent called Mannitol. The algaes - spirulina or chlorella are needed to bind up the liberated heavy metals to carry them out of the body. Rice bran chelates reactive iron. To increase liver detoxification add Milk thistle, Dandelion root, Schisandra and 6000 mg of vitamin C per day along with bioflavonoids and Alpha Lipoic Acid to promote liver activity. Schisandra berries are helpful when used with milk thistle seed and turmeric root for preventing or treating liver damage.

Quick Liquid Detox Recipe: 1 cup pure water, 1 tsp zeolite powder, 1tsp chlorella, 1 Tbsp Aloe Vera Gel. Other ingredients like apple pectin, charcoal, fulvic minerals, magnesium and aloe vera to aid in the detoxification process. Plant-based enzymes (bromelain, lipase, catalase) can be added to ensure optimal utilization of all of the above nutrients and assist in the breakdown and removal of plaques.

A cilantro pesto of soaked raw pumpkin seeds and cilantro is a standard in the chelation diet, as are all colorful fruits and vegetables, raw juices and sprouts.

Probiotics are essential to a chemo and radioprotective diet so you may like to make probiotic cabbage juice and coleslaw. In turn, prebiotics like pectin and inulin (chicory root) are essential as probiotics, as they are food for the beneficial bacteria.

PREVENT RETICULATION

Similar anticancer/anti candida terrain is needed to counteract the effects of the heavy metals and nanobots from chemtrails.

While doing a Heavy Metal Detox the GI tract needs to be open (clean) in order for the toxins to not be reticulated into the Kidneys. A gentle laxative combo is Triphala, Shatavari Root, Hyssop and Bala Root …these increase peristalsis and revive GI function without the negative side effects of other laxative herbs. You will need to increase your water intake because transit time in the colon is reduced. It is the chlorophyll and living protoplasm of raw greens grown in remineralized soil that will protect the body from the heavy metals being released and help them exit safely from the body. Wheatgrass juice and other greens are a powerful detoxifier that neutralizes toxins with enzymes and cleanses the body of heavy metals and other toxic substances stored in tissues and organs.

SAFFRON: Saffron (*Crocus sativus*), the most expensive spice of the world is grown mostly in Iran. Saffron was found to significantly reverse harmful aluminum-induced symptoms, reduce lipid peroxidation and is anti-mutagenic. The use of saffron and honey minimized the toxic effect of aluminum in the liver by alleviating its disruptive effect on the biochemical and molecular levels.

ACTIVATED CLAYS: Most chemical and metal toxins have a positive charge, whereas the clay has a negative charge. Thus, the toxins cannot resist being drawn towards the clay. Bentonite clay has a great capacity for absorbing many times its own weight in toxins. Heavy Metal Cations are positively charged ions or groups of atoms, that are attracted to negatively charged items, such as clinoptilolite zeolite particles. Fulvic acid activates zeolite, bentonite clay, green clays. Clay has an electrical charge opposite from the heavy metals that it helps pull out. You can mix leonardite or humalite into clays to provide the catalyst of fulvic acid, which gets molecules inside and outside the cell membrane.

ZEOLITE: Micronized Clinoptilolite Zeolite is a naturally occurring, negatively charged product of sea water and hot magma. Zeolite is a unique volcanic mineral with a 4-sided honeycomb structure and a negative magnetic charge. This distinctive structure allows zeolite to have a strong osmotic gradient to capture positively charged heavy metals, environmental toxins, and free radicals. Its unique porous, cage-like structure works to absorb unwanted positively charged ions and molecules and trap them. This structure has the ability to loosely hold molecules such as calcium, sodium, magnesium and potassium and exchange them when absorbing the undesirable molecules such as ammonia and heavy metals and bad odors.

Once zeolite captures toxins it then holds them with its magnetic energy until they are excreted out of the body through normal digestion. Zeolites also trap microbes such as pathogenic bacteria, viruses, and yeasts into their matrix where they are eliminated through the bowels and urine. It also grabs hold of xenoestrogenic molecules from plastics, pesticides, and herbicides; and is a hangover cure! Take 1 tsp in a 8oz glass of water on an empty stomach, 1-2 hours away from food, minerals, supplements or prescription drugs.

Topical application of clinoptilolite zeolite to skin cancers effectively reduced tumor formation and growth. Zeolite powder and shungite can be added to drinking water filtration devices to detoxify the body of harmful toxins like mercury, lead, aluminum, arsenic, plastic residues in addition to radioactive isotopes like plutonium and uranium.

Micronized Zeolite is 85% opaline silica that is widely used as a soil amendment for its ability to increase water retention allowing plants to more easily access it. Unbelievably, it can hold up to 55% of its weight in water and slowly releases it to the plant as needed. Micronized Zeolite (Clinoptilolite) www.greenclays.com/

Let us perfect the means; the end will take care of itself.

SULFUR AND METHYLATION

The Methionine/Glutathione Transsulfuration Pathway uses sulfur-bearing molecules to remove toxins through binding the toxins to methyl groups and excreting them from the body — a process called methylation. A methyl group is one carbon atom bonded to three hydrogen atoms (CH3).

Aluminum, Mercury and other heavy metals interfere with the body's natural ability to detoxify itself, through the processes of methylation and sulfation. When methylation is compromised it's like having sticky, sludgy spark plugs. Everything slows down, energy is compromised, and metabolism is impaired and repair is halted.

Methylation or the passing on of methyl groups protects DNA, RNA, neurotransmitters, protein and creatine from free radicals, radiation, UV, EMFs and heavy metals. Epigenetics uses methylation to turn genes on or off—with regards to our relationship to our changing environment epigenetics is more important than genetics in crafting who we become. Epigenetics modifies gene expression rather than altering the genetic code itself.

Stress, poor diet and dehydration represent a challenge to adequate methylation. The alcohol and acetaldehyde produced by yeast/fungi in the GI tract represents a burden on the methylation system, exhausting the liver's resources and interfering with "pro life-growth" epigenetics. Both alcohol and acetaldehyde lowers glutathione levels! Glutathione is one of the body's most important antioxidant molecules for detoxification, quenching inflammation and protecting against heavy metals.

Glutathione is used to remove toxins from the body and is reconverted into Methionine, during methylation process, and the Methionine/Glutathione Transsulfuration pathway cycle is repeated. If this transsulfuration pathway is disrupted, oxidative stress can result and lead to various health problems.

A substance is oxidized when electrons are removed, and reduced when electrons are added. The mitochondria in your cells generate energy by combining oxygen with glucose to gradually oxidize food and store it as ATP. This oxidation of glucose releases energy, but it can also let free electrons escape. Anywhere from 2 to 5% of your total oxygen intake during both rest and exercise can form these highly damaging oxygen-based free radicals (ROS). Because we are an oxygen-based life form, oxygen both provides life and but at the same time can be harmful to cells (in the form of oxidative stress).

151

To maintain health, our body must not only use oxygen but produce antioxidants to prevent the oxygen from damaging tissues within the body. Insufficient antioxidants can result in damage to mitochondria to the DNA, cell membranes, and oxidize fats and proteins. The results of excessive oxidation can include genes being expressed abnormally which can lead to abnormal paths of development, to cells not transmitting information well due to impaired cellular membranes (including neurons in the brain), and to cellular die-off due to toxicity.

Glutathione, most important antioxidant, is synthesized by most cells in the body, particularly those in the liver. The body makes N-acetyl-L-cysteine (NAC) into cysteine and then into glutathione, a powerful antioxidant. N-acetyl cysteine (NAC) can neutralize toxins in the liver because of its ability to boost glutathione and is an unbelievably effective asthma remedy.

The main component of connective tissue is collagen. It is structured as three protein strands arranged in a triple helix, and is the most abundant protein in the body. Sulfur plays a role in the formation of muscle, skin, hair and nails and is a major building block of collagen, the connective tissue that makes up cartilage. Dietary sulfur significantly affects the production of collagen in our skin, and it's also an antioxidant that helps protect your collagen once it forms.

SUPPORT METHYLATION

Micronutrients supportive of methylaton and methionine synthesis include: Zinc, Folinic Acid, Choline, Betaine (trimethylglycine, Methyl-B12 and SAMe.

The micronutrients and precursors to support glutathione synthesis: Glutathione methyl ester, N-acetylcysteine (NAC), B6, Selenium, Glutamine and the antioxidants: Vitamin E, vitamin C, lipoic acid; along with garlic, turmeric and black pepper, ginger and leafy greens. The sulfur containing cabbage family provides sulfur which is important for methylation in the liver.

By supplementing with high doses of buffered vitamin C, MSM, DMSO and niacinamide (vitamin B3), reduces or eliminates fatigue and pain in fibromyalgia, arthritis and chronic fatigue. MSM (Methylsulfonylmethane) is an organic sulfur compound that primarily works extracellularly. As a source of sulfur it helps eliminate heavy metals, just like the sulfur containing amino acids, by chelating the heavy metals and making them soluble.

Topical DMSO Treatment — When rubbed on the skin DMSO and magnesium chloride sol is quickly absorbed into the deeper tissues and is a potent anti-inflammatory helping to relieve any kind of joint or muscle pain. This mixture can be put in a spray bottle to spray on the back of the neck (for hangovers and migraine), or sore muscles or joints.

See YouTubes of Dr Ben Lynch on methylation; and Glutathione/Methylation Depletion Theory of ME/CFS by Rich Van Konynenburg.

 www.tracemin.com/ —To check yourself for heavy metals, and mineral deficiencies you can send hair to this lab.

FAT BURNING TO REMOVE HEAVY METALS

Metal toxicity is a source of an individual's inability to lose weight.

Heavy metals are sequestered in the biofilms of pathogens and in body fat deposits, so we need to clear out all morbid storage areas in order to have a clean machine. By stimulating fat burning through raising Resting Metabolic Rate (RMR) we burn more calories every day and raising ketogenic metabolism by water fasting we can break down fat deposits and eliminate stored heavy metals and toxins. To remove stubborn fat deposits you need to become more active and eat fewer calories than you burn.

Increasing fat burning metabolism through reducing carbohydrates, calorie restriction, fasting and the keto diet reduces the propensity to get Alzheimer's and dementia. The enzyme Lipase helps your body in digestion, fat distribution and fat burning for energy. Lipase breaks down and dissolves fat throughout the body. Without lipase, fat stagnates and accumulates. Since Protease helps break down proteins and eliminate toxins, it is crucial to have plenty of protease during fat burning.

We can reduce the propensity to get Alzheimer's and dementia by increasing fat burning metabolism through reducing carbohydrates, calorie restriction, fasting and the keto diet. Lipase is one of our most vital digestive enzymes that catalyzes the breakdown of dietary fats. The enzyme "Lipase" helps your body in digestion, fat distribution, as well as fat burning for energy. Lipase breaks down and dissolves fat throughout the body. Without lipase, fat stagnates and accumulates.

Low levels of enzymes are found in diabetes, heart disease and most every degenerative disease, due to the lack of live digestive enzymes in the cooked diet. To really improve digestion, and clean up the blood, an enzyme formulation must have a generous amount of protease, amylase and lipase with high activity and high potency. Since Protease helps break down proteins and eliminate toxins, it is crucial to have plenty of protease during fat burning. When your food is poorly digested, you absorb nutrients that aren't fully broken down or usable, which stimulates the immune system to attack and defend your body against partially digested foods that get into the bloodstream.

Garlic has ideal anti-obesity properties that help in the reduction of fat cells. Fatty acids present in coconut oil boost up the metabolism and help reduce the abdominal fat. Another trick to burn fat is have a glass of celery juice before your meal. Chia Seed, perrilla and flax seeds are rich in omega 3 fatty acids and can added to your breakfast in cereal, salads, and soups or in yogurt. This helps reduce abdominal fat in particular and the fat in your thighs as well. Green tea or Matcha is very effective for eliminating fat since it increases fat burning metabolism.

L-CARNITINE: L-Carnitine isn't technically an amino acid, it is considered a vitamin-like compound that is related to the B vitamins. L-carnitine is formed in the liver and kidneys from the amino acids lysine and methionine. L-carnitine helps to transport fat, particularly long-chain fatty acids, into the mitochondria of cells, where they can be oxidized — that is used as fuel to generate adenosine triphosphate (ATP). Without adequate L-carnitine, most dietary fats can't get into the mitochondria and be burned for fuel.

Supplementing L-Carnitine at just 1-2g per day significantly reduces muscle damage and soreness from strenuous exercise, and improved recovery to exercise. The increase in endurance and reduction in fatigue was likely because they burned more fat while preserving muscle glycogen, in addition to having lower levels of lactic acid and higher levels of creatine phosphate. L-carnitine increases nitric oxide blood levels, and reduces oxidative damage from nitric oxide, which not only enhances energy during workouts, but also muscle recovery following workouts. L-carnitine also increases the number of testosterone or androgen receptors, inside muscle cells, stimulating weight loss, muscle growth and strength gains. You can get some L-carnitine from plant products like avocado and soybeans, but red meat is the best source.

CREATINE: Creatine may be key to turning the body toward anabolic building metabolism for it increases protein synthesis, especially within muscle fibers, it is mostly found in meats, fish and chicken. Creatine plays a very powerful role in energy metabolism, for ATP is replenished from creatine phosphate (CP). Our bodies make Creatine from the amino acids glycine, arginine and methionine. Creatine plays a vital role in the release of energy in the muscles of humans and other animals. Creatine also plays an important role in nerve cell function, and also buffers lactic acid production, thereby reducing muscle fatigue.

APPLE CIDER VINEGAR: Bitter flavors also increase digestive enzyme secretion, which improves signaling of fullness cues. Apple Cider Vinegar helps in spot reduction of abdominal fat, as it breaks down fat cells and aids digestion as well. The combination of Garcinia taken with Apple Cider Vinegar makes the body go from a fat-gain to fat-loss state while resting. Garcinia taken with Apple Cider Vinegar in water: increases resting metabolism more than 130%, flushes out harmful toxins, boosts energy levels and increase mood, blocks excess fat production, improves lean body mass, lowers insulin levels and makes it easier for your body to use glucose.

LEMON DETOX DRINK: Add juice from one whole lemon to a glass of lukewarm water and drink this on an empty stomach as soon as you wake up in the morning. Alternatively chop a whole lemon skin, pith and all and make into a hot tea with ½ tsp of unpasteurized honey.

FLAT TUMMY WATER: Take 2 liters of water and add 2 sliced lemons and 1/2 a sliced cucumber, 1 Tbsp grated ginger, crushed mint or basil leaves and a pinch of Himalayan salt. Keep this for overnight, next day at regular intervals drink a glass of this water.

FAT BURNING HERBS INCLUDE: Cardamom, Cumin, Fennel, Dill and Coriander seeds make a perfect detox drink. Fresh Ginseng root, Gymnema, Yerba mate, Guarana berries, Garcinia, Commiphora Mukul, Rhodiola rosea, Basil, Dragonwort, Galangal, cayenne pepper, black pepper, cinnamon, turmeric, mustard seed. Taken before a fat-containing meal Galangal will block up to 38% of dietary fat. Rich in phytonutrients, cardamom helps increase fat metabolism and brain function.

Cardamom can also prevent abdominal fat, lower bad cholesterol and triglycerides, and improve glucose tolerance, lowering the risk of metabolic syndrome. It can also balance the gut flora and boost digestion. Cardamom is thermogenic (meaning it increases your body heat and speeds up your metabolism), has anti-inflammatory properties, and acts as an antioxidant, cleaning up rogue molecules called free radicals and resisting cellular aging.

Basil also helps reduce fat buildup in your liver while detoxifying your body. The piperine in black pepper battles fat by blocking the formation of new fat cells. Cumin is a great fat burner that also aids in digestion. One teaspoon can help you burn up to three times more body fat! The allyl isothiocyanates in mustard seed can boost your metabolism by up to 25% for several hours after eating. The curcumin in turmeric contributes to lower body fat, weight loss, plus is also an anti-inflammatory agent and lowers insulin resistance.

GARCINIA: Garcinia cambogia, a tropical fruit also known as the Malabar tamarind, is a popular weight-loss supplement. It blocks your body's ability to make fat and it puts the brakes on your appetite. It could help keep blood sugar and cholesterol levels in check, too. The active ingredient in the fruit's rind, hydroxycitric acid, or HCA, has boosted fat-burning and cut back appetite in studies. It appears to block an enzyme called citrate lyase, which your body uses to make fat and raises levels of serotonin, thereby curbing appetite.

GREEN COFFEE BEAN: Besides maintaining aerobic respiration Green coffee bean is also highly prized for weight loss. The chlorogenic acid and caffeic acid in green coffee stays intact when the beans are unroasted. The caffeic acid helps with removing fatty acids that are stored in your body while chlorogenic acid helps the liver process those fatty acids. While the chlorogenic acid is a metabolism boosting, thermogenic agent that helps the body to burn its fuel more efficiently, leading to weight loss. Chlorogenic acids hinder the absorption of dietary fat and is also believed to reduce the generation of new fat cells due to its superior antioxidant effects, as well as enhancing fat burning in the liver.

The reason for the powerful effect of Chlorogenic acid on glucose metabolism is that it inhibits glycogenolysis,otherwise known as anaerobic respiration. Glycogenolysis is the breakdown of glycogen to glucose (blood sugar), or the production of glucose from fat and protein in the liver and muscle. Aerobic respiration may utilize glucose or fat to produce ATP. Anaerobic respiration also results in a smaller production of ATP, but does not require oxygen. Creatine phosphate and glucose are the primary fuels of anaerobic respiration. Because these molecules are stored directly in the muscle, they are readily available emergency stores for short, powerful exertion.

Green coffee bean extract has strong polyphenol antioxidant and anti-inflammatory properties, similar to other natural antioxidants like green tea and grape seed extract. Through its ability to help fuel efficiency and increase metabolism thereby lowering insulin resistance, blood sugar and pathogen growth Green coffee bean extract may be one of the most powerful aids to overcoming Borg Metabolic X and the degenerative disease complex.

Cancer is the inevitable result of cooked food, demineralization, lack of enzymes, excess carbos-cereals-sugars, hypoxia, loss of zeta-potential, acid blood, animal protein diet, transfats and altered non-living fats, loss of aerobic ATP energy production and poor cellular detoxification etc… Shifting to aerobic ATP production is the key to fighting cancer so all efforts must be made to tuning the biochemistry towards aerobic respiration. Green coffee in supplements and enemas may be a significant ally in the fight against the cancer and the mutagenic terrain in general. Cancer and candida occur in anaerobic, hypoxic conditions.

FAT BURNING OILS: Savory, Thyme and Sage essential oil cut with blackseed oil or castor oil, and rubbed onto the fatty tissue belly, breasts and inner arms and inner thighs stimulates the burning of fat. While removing heavy metals and infectious agents from chemtrails it is important to raise metabolism and burn excess fat stores. Essential oils encourage the regeneration of cells, support greater immune defense, sustain energy production, and clarify the mind.

INCREASE METABOLIC RATE: As land is becoming infertile and toxic, as food quality falls our bodies fail to get the nutrition for high energy and detoxification. Raise your metabolic fat burning rate with Oolong green tea, sex hormone and adaptogen herbs like Damiana, Dong quai, Green Tea, Ginseng, Catuaba, Chuchuhuasi, Gordonii hoodia, Guarana, Pau d'Arco, Maca, Maral root, Mucuna, Muira puama, Suma, Yerba mate, Tongkat ali. Eat protein with every meal, eat spicy foods, drink more cold water, do a high-intensity workout, lift heavy things, walk more, and get a good night's sleep. Caffeine's ability to speed up the central nervous system makes it a powerful metabolism booster. The healthy bacteria found in yogurt, pickles, and other fermented foods like sauerkraut, may help you lose weight. Stretching every hour wakes up metabolism, as does laughing. Eat fish as fish oil reduce the levels of fat-storage enzymes in the body. Seaweed and seafood contains iodine that revs up the thyroid thus raising metabolism. Megadosing on Vitamin C provides both energy, detoxification and overcomes the adrenal fatigue that tends to lower metabolism. Eat organic food to avoid endocrine disruptors.

FAT AND MUSCLE BURNING RECOVERY: Since fat and protein burning (gluconeogenesis) goes up during the massive energy demand of kundalini glutamine and aspartate might eventually become deficient. Glutamine protects muscle mass by providing an alternative fuel source and has a stimulatory effect on gluconeogenesis. Aspartate is non-essential in mammals, and might serve as an excitatory neurotransmitter in the brain. It is also a metabolite in the urea cycle, and participates in gluconeogenesis. L-Carnitine feeds the heart oxygen and energy and protects the body from ketosis, thus reduces muscle soreness after exercise. Ketosis is the toxic waste products from fat mobilization, which raises blood acidity and causes the body to lose vital alkaline minerals such as potassium, calcium and magnesium. Kelp and wheatgrass juice are good ways of remineralizing.

NADH: Nicotinamide adenine dinucleotide, otherwise known as Coenzyme 1, is a high-energy hydrogen that occurs naturally in all our cells. NAD+: Nicotinamide adenine dinucleotide (NAD) is one of two main metabolically active forms of vitamin B-3. Nicotinamide adenine dinucleotide (NAD), a coenzyme found in all living cells, is needed for energy creation, circadian rhythm and cognitive function. NAD+ enhances cognitive health during aging, controls aging through the regulation of genes, boosts physical and mental energy, enhances efficiency of mitochondria, optimizes a healthier metabolism, improves blood sugar regulation and promotes insulin sensitivity (overcoming insulin resistance). The coenzyme is, therefore, found in two forms in cells: NAD$^+$ is an oxidizing agent – it accepts electrons from other molecules and becomes reduced. This reaction forms NADH, which can then be used as a reducing agent to donate electrons. These electron transfer reactions are the main function of NAD.

NADH is used for improving mental clarity, alertness, concentration, and memory; as well as for treating Alzheimer's disease. Because of its role in energy production, NADH is also used for improving athletic endurance and treating chronic-fatigue syndrome. NADH is the body's most powerful antioxidant, and it can regenerate other important antioxidants. The energy producing organelles of the cell (mitochondria) produce NADH, which in turn produces cellular energy ATP. Free radicals interfere with cellular energy production by destroying enzymes and mitochondria, resulting in fatigue and loss of motivation.

As we get older, our NAD+ levels naturally decrease, however it may be possible to reverse mitochondrial decline with NAD, and promote *Sirtuin Gene Activation* - the same longevity genes shown to become active during caloric restriction and life-extension. NAD fuels the activity of sirtuins, including SIRT1— inducing the growth of new mitochondria. SIRT1 helps insure the communication signals get through from the cell's nuclei to the mitochondria to keep mitochondria running smoothly. NAD boosters might work synergistically with supplements like resveratrol and pterostilbene to help reinvigorate mitochondria and ward off degenerative diseases and aging. Pterostilbene (found in blueberries and grapes) is more potent than resveratrol when it comes to improving brain function, warding off various kinds of cancer and preventing heart disease.

Human digestive enzymes have evolved to act upon right-handed sugar molecules, that is those prefixed with a "D." **Niacin** requires adequate **D-ribose** to form Nicotinamide riboside (NR) and thus NAD+. Take about 1 tsp (5 grams) of D-ribose a couple of times a day along with 1/2 a Niacin tablet because it potentially improves niacin's conversion to NR. Nicotinamide Riboside (NR/ Niagen) 1,000mg of NIAGEN is effective in raising NAD+ levels. A cheaper version is to use Niacin (50mg) to ½ tsp of D-Ribose in a glass of water. If you buy flushing 100mg Niacin "tablets" you can break them in half. Using Niacin and D-Ribose raises cellular energy, especially when reinstating circadian atunement, along with sungazing/grounding. NADH can also be made from the amino acid L-Tryptophan using 60mg tryptophan for 1mg B3. Tryptophan being the precursor to serotonin.

ENDURANCE ERGOGENICS: Humans consume ergogenics to enhance their long-term endurance, performance, stamina, and recovery Caffeine has consistently shown ergogenic effects for both endurance and short-term exercise. Non-coffee herbal sources of caffeine commonly found in dietary supplement products include guarana, kola nut, green tea, and Yerba maté. Ginseng, herbal sources of caffeine and ephedrine and other ergogenic plants such as Chia seed, Tribulus Terrestris, Ginkgo biloba, and Rhodiola Rosea.have also been studied repeatedly for their effects on human physical performance.

ANABOLIC TISSUE BUILDERS: Fulvic acid, chromium picolinate, Arginine, Ornithine, Creatine, Gumar, Ginseng, Maca, Maral root, Bala, Rose hips, yerba mate, Sarsaparilla, Rhodiola Rosea, Fenugreek, wild oats (Avena sativa), Stinging nettle root, Sea buckthorn (Rhamnus frangula), Vitamin C, Siberian ginseng, Aralia, Rhaponticum, Rhodiola, Schisandra berry, Shilajit, Ashwagandha, Eleutherococcus.

EMFS AND METAL DETOX

Mineral metabolism in the body requires both exercise, sunlight and grounding.

EDTA, DMPS & DMSA is all very good, but without the "correct" electromagnetic grounding and negative ions that only pristine nature provides it is harder to detox the heavy metals and poisons completely out of the body. Your body needs electrons in order to recharge, so any lying, walking or sitting outside with flesh in contact with the ground will help. It takes 40 minutes of lying on the ground for red blood cells to recharge their fields so they can unclump and oxygenate the body properly. A foot bowl of magnetite sand to put your feet in while watching videos or on the computer will help make up for the lack of grounding due to the toxic/radioactive earth.

If we think that hiding inside to get away from the chemtrail spraying is the answer, then our detoxification will be diminished from the lack of sunlight and grounding. Thus we need the discipline to set up our detox and enlivening routines and carry them out effectively. In order to get the heavy metals out of the brain the body must be charged and earthed and energized by the magnetic earth. Detoxing while barefoot in Hawaii would be ideal, (except for the fact that Hawaii is now badly radiated from Fukushima).

Most chemical and metal toxins have a positive charge, whereas the clay has a negative charge. Thus, the toxins cannot resist being drawn towards the clay. Bentonite clay has a great capacity for absorbing many times its own weight in toxins. The stronger human energy EMF or "Qi" field the greater the connectivity in the field, and the greater the repulsion and elimination of adverse energies that we are exposed to.

Dr. Dean Bonlie DDS -Magnetism Dr. Dean Bonlie discusses the use of magnets in the detoxification of heavy metals including Mercury. Magnetico Sleep Pad, a revolutionary solution that promotes health by mimicking the full strength of Earth's geomagnetic field. Dr. Bonlie went on to develop a high strength clinical treatment magnet called the Magnetic Molecular Energizer (MME), which is currently awaiting FDA approval. http://magneticosleep.

The basis of Dr. Dean Bonlie's theory is that our only source of magnetism is from the Earth, but now that this source is so drastically depleted, it appears to have a distinct impact on our health. Because the Earth's magnetic field is reducing due to Grand Solar Minimum, your body does not achieve the magnetic resonance necessary to restore and rejuvenate your organs and tissues. Most cell division occurs during your first two hours of sleep, as this is when the brain produces the most amount of human growth hormone. The valence electrons (the critical ones) of the atoms of these new cells will orient their direction of orbit depending on the direction of magnetic field in which they divide.

Initially, his research led to the design and production of the Magnetico Sleep Pad as a form of magnetic supplementation. A supplemental unidirectional field (like the Earth's) is needed to give extra zing to your electrons at the right time and in the right direction. The reduction of the Earth's field is the most likely explanation for why the human body responds so well to magnetism, we are in a deficiency state! Magnetico's patented Sleep Pad is the best way to provide your body with the magnetic environment it needs to restore and rejuvenate itself. Magnetic resonance is essential to health, growth, and longevity.

RADIOPROTECTION

Against Cancer and Oxidation/Free radicals

Nuclear (ionizing) radiation and EMF radation are both defended against by the same health progams. The intense radiation from dozens of RF/microwave antennas surrounding has the same effect on human health as ionizing gamma wave radiation from nuclear reactions. The foundations of an anti-radiation protocol is to megadose on Vitamin C and other antioxidants. Stock up on C, Alpha Lipoic and Glutathione. (Apparently Vitamin C lasts longer in the freezer.) Maximize Vitamin C fruits: Goji berries, blueberries, Amla powder, acerola cherry, camu camu, rose hips, kiwi fruit, black currants, strawberries, elderberry, acai, maqui, raspberries, plums, lemon, lime, oranges, red grapes, cherries.

Also Radiation Protection: Sea-buckthorn berry, aronia, pomegranate, goji and mangosteen. Astaxanthin, Ashitaba, Aloe Vera, Chamomile, Chaparral, Echinacea, Garlic Mustard, Olive leaf, Neem, Ginkgo, Uva Ursi, Yucca Root, Noni Fruit & Seed, Jojoba, Juniper, Turmeric, Graviola, Frankincense, Myrrh, Reishi Mushroom, Niacin, Cysteine, Bentonite clay, Zeolites, Fulvic Acid, Pyrophyllite clay, Activated charcoal. Bladderwrack, Irish Sea Moss, Kelp, chlorella, algae, spirulina, dulse and nori as well as Miso broth.

Adopt a mineral rich diet (natural iodine Lugol's solution, iron, B-12, ginseng, selenium, boron, & zinc). MSM and the cabbage contain sulfur which binds to heavy metals during methylation/detoxification: garlic mustard kale, watercress, Brussel sprouts, antioxidant rich kale, red capsicum, parsley, broccoli, cabbage, turnips, cauliflower, arugula, mustard greens, bok choy, onions, green beans, garlic, spinach, eggplant, Potatoes baked with skin for Potassium. Coconuts and coconut water are very high in potassium and magnesium. Potassium reduces uptake of cesium-137.

Stop all refined sugar/grain consumption and focus on sprouts, green and living foods and living water. Increase beta carotene: papaya, goji, spinach, kale, carrots, chard, swiss chard, yams, squash, carrots, pumpkin, beets, and collards. Purple vegetables (potatoes, yams, onions, beets, purple chard and cabbage).

One of the most powerful antioxidants Megahydrate (*hydrogenated silicon*) invented by Patrick Flanagan sops up free radicals and drives off radiation, take 3-6 capsules/day in combo with your Omega-3s.

Niacin (B3) from food as well as a diet high in whole grains may protect against radiation-induced cumulative DNA damage. Niacin-containing enzymes that are involved in energy metabolism, NAD and NADP, work by quenching free radicals thus protect against excessive tissue damage.

Probiotics are essential to a radioprotective diet. In turn, prebiotics like pectin and inulin (chicory root) are essential to probiotics, as they are food for the beneficial bacteria. Incorporate high fiber for broom action in the GI tract to speed elimination of heavy metals use flaxseed, chia seed, rice bran and psyllium powder. The skin of fruits and vegetables are high, not only in pectin, but also in a wide range of antioxidant flavonoids and other phytonutrients. The pith of the citrus contains about 30% pectin. Apple Pectin reduces Cesium-137 load by over 62% in one month and pectin is also a chelator of other positively charged heavy metals.

Baths with Epsom salts, sea salt, clay, baking soda and borax helps pull out the radiation from your body.

Living-water from raw-plant protoplasm, or structured water via vortexing, and Schauberger tech would be good if one has no access to deep spring water or Glacial water. www.balancedenergystructuredwater.com. Incorporate cysteine (thiol) … amino acid antioxidants. Shilajit or Humalite contains at least 85 minerals as well as Humic/Fulvic acids that are major chelators of heavy metals and radioisotopes. Humalite might assist radionucleotides out of the body.

MELANIN: The biological role of melanin in the human body may extend far beyond simply protecting us against UV radiation, melanin may actually both protect us against ionizing radiation and even transform some of it into metabolically useful energy. Melanin has a diverse range of ecological and biochemical functions including display, evasion, photoprotection, detoxification, and metal scavenging. This protective capacity of melanin to scavenge and sequester [heavy] metals may be a factor in neurological diseases like Parkinson's, which are largely a pathology of the melanin pigment-rich areas of the brain.

www.greenmedinfo.com/pharmacological-action/radioprotective.

POTASSIUM: To counteract the effects of radioactive Cesium-137 from Fukushima increase your potassium from non-contaminated sources. Potassium Sources: High potassium foods from natural food sources like beans, dark leafy greens, spinach, potatoes, sweet potato, squash, yogurt, fish, avocados, mushrooms, and bananas. The RDA for potassium is 3.5 grams. NOW Potassium Citrate is a good inexpensive supplement.

ANTIRAD CONDIMENT: Potassium citrate and Potassium chloride (salts), mixed with spices (turmeric, ginger, garlic, cumin, mustard, caraway seed), herbs (basil, oregano, thyme, rosemary), pepper, papaya enzyme and kelp powder, as a condiment in a salt shaker sprinkled on food to reduce Cesium 137 from Fukushima.

FLUORIDE AND NUMBING-DUMBING

Herodotus (484-425) pointed out a grievous source of frustration at being human when he said: *"The worst pain a man can suffer is to have insight into much and power over nothing.*

Humanity is losing its physical, cognitive and spiritual powers as the earth loses her vitality due to anthropocentric mismanagement. Plus it is obvious that the ruling ĒLite are making us dumber, subdued and compliant through mass poisoning on every conceivable front. The fact that generations from the 1950's on were impacted by the decline of minerals in the soils, by chemical farming and by fluoride in the water, has negatively impacted the sanity of well-being of the majority of Western populations since then.

Fluoride, at levels added to drinking water, significantly inhibits DNA polymerase, the enzyme that builds and repairs DNA. Fluoride disrupts the intestinal microbiome, weakens tooth enamel and interferes with the protein tunneling in enzymes. Fluoride at a mere 1 ppm obstructs an enzyme critical for protein synthesis, glutamine synthetase, by 100%. Plus glutamate is an essential precursor for the synthesis of glutathione, the body's principle antioxidant, thereby lowering cellular defense systems. Plus glutathione is one of the main agents that removes heavy metals and other toxins out of the brain and body. Lowered immunity is known to be connected with autistic behavior and increases social reticence. Thus with the digestive, endocrine and the immune systems compromised in the majority of citizens, this acts to tear the fabric of society apart and disintegrate common weal and collective abundance.

Fluoride also interferes with the Krebs Cycle, that is energy production in the cell. Despite it being a neurotoxin that causes cancer fluoride is still added to approximately 60% of the United States' water supply. When aluminum comes into contact with fluoride, it hitches a ride into the brain as aluminum-fluoride which can bypass this barrier. This just so happens to be the same aluminum compound found in the brains of Alzheimer's patients. Neurological damage from the fluoride-aluminum combo may explain the crisis of moral consciousness we are facing in the political arena today.

Aluminum binds with fluoride and greatly increases fluoride toxicity. Aluminum binds with fluoride in the body and it is fluoride that carries the aluminum across the blood brain barrier. When the body is deficient in iodine fluoride is uptaken and since fulvic acid goes through the blood brain barrier an Lugol's -Fulvic mix will protect the brain from fluoride. Fluoride comes from the phosphate fertilizer industry where aluminum is mined, so fluoride comes from the breakdown of aluminum. Aluminum is very reactive chemically and Water fluoridation to a public water supply "enhances the bioavailability of aluminum," allowing it to cross the blood-brain barrier easier, thereby making it even more toxic.

Normally, aluminum is poorly absorbed from the GI tract, but nano aluminum is absorbed in far higher amounts. This absorbed aluminum has been shown to be distributed to a number of organs and tissues including the brain and spinal cord. Fluoride binds with iodine receptors in the thyroid, displacing iodine. So when we are iodine deficient and when there isn't adequate iodine available, the thyroid can't synthesize thyroid hormones. A daily dose of 120 ppm Fluoride results in highly significant increases in spontaneous lipid peroxidation (rancidity) as well as neurodegenerative changes in neuron cell bodies of selected hippocampal regions.

Once fluoride crosses the blood-brain barrier, it causes degeneration to specific parts of the brain — the hippocampus, the neocortex, and the cerebellum. The hippocampus is considered the seat of memory and is critical for learning, emotional regulation, emotional intelligence and the ability to shut off the stress response. The neocortex is considered the most evolved area of the brain where sensory perception, conscious thought and language skills largely take place. The cerebellum is responsible for movement, kinesthetic sense, coordination and balance. The damage from fluoride doesn't stop at your brain — it continues on to your spinal cord, sciatic nerve and peripheral nervous system.

Sodium fluoride is classified as a neurotoxin – in the same category as arsenic, lead, and mercury, but it's still prevalent in the United States' water supply. Environment toxins such as fluoride disrupt and diminish key enzyme systems making us susceptible to disease. There is a causal link between fluoride and cancer, genetic damage, neurological impairment and bone and dental pathology. Fluoride reduces the activity and the thyroid gland, slowing metabolism and promoting weight gain. A mere 1 part per million fluoride inhibits DNA repair by 50%, plus also inhibits 61% of the enzyme that breaks down acetylcholine at the synapse so that the next impulse can be transmitted across the synaptic cleft.

Fluoride plays a key role in acute Magnesium deficiency! Symptoms of Magnesium deficiency include: fatigue, weakness, depression, anxiety, confusion, mental-emotional disorders, behavioral disturbances, headaches, psychosis, irritability, muscle cramps, seizures and irregular heart rhythms are among the classic signs and symptoms of low magnesium. Green vegetables are good sources of magnesium because the center of the chlorophyll molecule contains magnesium.

Fluoride in municipal drinking water removes copper from copper water pipes, and Alzheimer's sufferers carry higher free copper levels. Copper in the brain inactivates the removal of accumulated toxic beta amyloid sludge that eventually kills neurons. Zinc is copper's natural antagonist that protects against cognitive decline. Zinc deficiency also induces excess free radical production, through allowing inflammatory minerals and metals to impact cells. Fluoride is a category 6 carcinogenic, the same as arsenic and snake venom.

"Fluoride causes mental health issues, it is added in the water supply here in Ireland, the people all have no option but to shower and bathe in it, and skin is your biggest absorber of chemicals, this is why medicine is now coming in patches, and why creams work. So the people of Ireland, buy bottled water to drink, but even this does not help does it, even if they drink spring water, all their clothes and their skin are washed in it every day, there is no escape. It's time to wake up, grow up, take responsibility for our collective actions and their effects on the whole, of planet, and nature and people and animals, its gone too far to be allowing profit and money to be more valuable than clean air and water, good food and happy healthy humans and animals. We have our priorities wrong, and our basis of existence is based on a worldwide failing system built on war and greed, rather than to feed and nurture all beings born here." Julie Kilbride

Aluminum is very chemically reactive. Fluoride increases the uptake the aluminum in your body through increasing the assimilation of aluminum. The combination of nano-aluminum and fluoride further enhances the bioavailability of aluminum, allowing it to cross the blood-brain barrier easier, thus making it many times more toxic. Excess levels of aluminum mobilizes calcium and heavy metals to move from bones to the central neural tissue leading to metal-induced inflammation issues like fibromyalgia and arthritis, chronic fatigue and all manner of mental, emotional dis-eases. Constant exposure to fluoride causes a buildup of calcium phosphate crystals, which contribute to cardiovascular blockages and arthritic inflammation amongst other conditions.

Fluoride accumulates in the pineal gland more than any other part of the body. The British scientist Jennifer Luke discovered that fluoride accumulates to strikingly high levels in the pineal gland, because it is exposed to a high volume of blood flow. Calcification of the pineal gland can cause early puberty in young girls, and reduces the body's ability to regulate melatonin, a hormone that plays a central role in the regulation of circadian rhythm and dimethyltryptamine (DMT), a neurotransmitter implicated in causing dreaming and "spiritual" levels of consciousness. Fluoride is contributing to a worldwide "pandemic of developmental neurotoxicity" that results in "significantly lower' IQ scores and disabilities such as attention-deficit hyperactivity disorder, dyslexia, and other cognitive impairments. Fluoride causes calcification of the pineal gland... undermining the melatonin-serotonin cascade that ultimately results in the spirit molecule DMT. The best way to spiritually castrate a population and reduce them to wage slaves is to put fluoride in the drinking water.

Dr. Russell Blaylock, in his book "*Health and Nutrition Secrets,*" gives extensive evidence of the dangers of fluoride and the colossal social crime of duping the population into believing it helps prevent tooth decay. He also shared what the nano aluminum does to the brain and how it affects diseases like Alzheimer's, Crohn's, Lou Gehrigs, and similar diseases. He includes remedies to counteract the effects of this aluminum that we are breathing due to the massive amount of stratospheric aerosol geoengineering evidenced around the world.

We can find our way back to The Garden of Nature's sanity and sanctity, and we must if we wish to Thrive.

HOW TO REMOVE FLUORIDE FROM THE BODY

• **Avoid Poisoning**—Protect yourself from city water: Never drink chlorinated water unless it is an emergency. A distiller is ideal for drinking water, but always keep such water in glass containers, and add natural salt or ionic minerals. Ideally a chlorine filter shower head is recommended. If you take baths you could use of a dechlorinator such as sodium thiosulfate, which reduces chlorine species to "chloride," which is less harmful. You could also use coconut oil or shea butter on your skin to build up a barrier to harmful chemicals in general.

• **Remove Fluoride from** drinking water. Water with low fluoride values may still become toxic when the silicon content of water or diet is high, as silicon transports fluoride around the body.

• **Lemon juice or Apple cider vinegar**—Drink a glass of water with lemon juice or apple cider vinegar upon rising and eat liver-friendly foods, such as garlic, turmeric, lemons, limes, and avocado, and your body will have an easier time removing heavy metals and toxins.

• A **high quality protein diet**, adequate vitamin C and calcium could prevent the appearance of symptoms of fluorosis.

• **Remineralize**—Eat foods grown in remineralized/high organic matter soils for when minerals are missing, the body substitutes metals such as cadmium for zinc, lead for calcium, and aluminum for many other needed minerals.

• **Chelation Therapy** should remove fluoride as well as heavy metals from the body. Cilantro is best used in conjunction with chlorella for mobilizing and removal . New research has revealed that fluoride in drinking water makes the aluminum that we ingest more bio-available. The combination of aluminum and fluoride causes the same pathological changes in brain tissue found in Alzheimer's patients.

163

• **Iodine** pushes the fluoride from your body via urine, so use Lugol's or nascent iodine and incorporate seaweeds (kelp, nori, dulse, wakame, etc…) in your diet.

• **Boron** is helps flush fluoride from your body so add 1 cup of borax and 1 cup of Epsom salt and maybe ginger tea to a bath. Mix 1/8 of a teaspoon (up to ¼ teaspoon) Borax into a liter of distilled water and sip it throughout the day. Boron-rich foods include most nuts, dates, prunes, honey, broccoli, bananas, and avocado.

• **Tamarind** can be used in a tincture or tea to cleanse the body of fluoride.

• **Turmeric** offers protection against fluoride. Curcumin attenuates neurotoxicity induced by fluoride, preventing and even reversing damage.

• **Tulsi** (Holy basil) is a potent anxiety and stress relieving herb, and is a powerful 3rd eye, pineal gland activator. Put leaves in drinking water to counter Fluoride.

• **Magnesium** helps attract fluoride away from bones and teeth, allowing the body to eliminate it. It also inhibits the absorption of fluoride into your cells.

• **Liver Detox**—Doing liver cleanses, especially through coffee enemas, are a great way to get rid of fluoride as well as other toxins and heavy metals in the body.

• **Raw Cabbage Juice**, freshly prepared is particularly good for your liver and digestive system.

• **Lymphatic Exercise** like rebounding, as well saunas are great for ridding your body of toxins, as they inspire the body to sweat them out. Just be sure to keep hydrating—with distilled water—and to protect your kidneys with chickweed tea.

• **Grounding and Sunlight**—Electrons from the ground and Photons from the sun are essential for the calcium flux in mitochondria and to prevent calcium plaques including those in the pineal gland. Fluoride increases the calcification of the pineal gland, while grounding and sunlight—circadian compliance reverse this.

• **Shilajit**—In its raw form, Shilajit is a black/brown tar–like liquid, composed almost entirely of trace minerals, humic and fulvic acid. Fulvic acid is a transporter molecule. Fulvic acid is one of the most powerful antioxidants - free radical quencher known to man and will remove toxins like fluoride at a cellular level. Fulvic acid enters the Blood Brain Barrier so mineral and herbal preparations can be produced in a Fulvic acid base…with shilajit and antifungal herbs. Humic acids like humate or leonardite help remove fluoride from the body. Shungite and kelp will also help remove fluoride from the body.

• **Fluoride Shield Fluoride Shield**™ eliminates "toxic forms of fluoride and other dangerous compounds like mercury, chlorine, and bromine" from the body! The ingredients include tamarind, zeolites, organic fulvic acid, shilajit, cilantro and nascent iodine. Shungite and kelp will also help remove fluoride from the body. Increasing iodine by taking kelp or Lugol's will help "out compete" the other harmful bromides.

8

GASTRO-EMOTIONAL HEALTH

The gastrointestinal nervous system has been called the second brain with a large semi-autonomous nervous system. But, it could not perform its job without the constant communication and actions of the single layer of intelligent intestinal epithelial cells that line the gut. In the intestine the internal lining of the gut is just one cell thick with a thin layer of connective tissue below it. One layer of cells divides 1000 trillion microbes from the body's tissues. This single cell layer performs critical functions including very elaborate communication with friendly microbes, as well as immune T-cells, B -cells and macrophages.

The epithelial barrier cells maintain the mucous and antimicrobial proteins, communicating with and regulate both friendly and enemy microbes. When not functioning properly, the barrier activates immune responses that increase metabolic disease and viral infections including HIV and hepatitis. Responses between the barrier cells and the microbes are important in diabetes, multiple sclerosis and arthritis. When the system breaks down, inflammatory bowel disease and other illnesses can occur. One signal is the reactive oxygen (ROS) that can kill microbes, but can also signal for the repair of the epithelial barrier.

Dr. Paul Kautchakoff MD., of the Institute of Clinical Chemistry Switzerland, showed that the cooking of food was the cause of leucocytosis. Leucocytosis is the name that medical pathology gives to the excessive augmentation of white blood corpuscles in the blood in response to some "threat." According to Paul Kautchakoff MD., only food which has been unaltered from its natural state can be eaten without engaging the immune response. Even water heated above 191°F (88°C) causes a change in the composition and number of the white blood corpuscles. The boiling point of water is 212 °F (100°C).

There is no situation with greater complexity for the immune system than the border zone of the epithelial cells, the trillions of microbes, and the immune system just below. The 100 trillion bacteria and 1000 trillion viruses in the gut are critical for digestion, producing vitamins, boosting or decreasing immune function, modulating weight, affecting stress, and releasing neurological factors that influence the brain such as — GABA, serotonin, dopamine, acetylcholine and norepinephrine, as well as stimulating **Brain-Derived Neurotrophic Factor** (BDNF).

BDNF is active in the hippocampus, cortex, and forebrain—areas vital to learning, memory, and higher thinking. BDNF helps to support the survival of existing neurons and encourages the growth, regeneration and creation of new neurons and synapses. BDNF has been shown to play a role in neuroplasticity, which allows nerve cells in the brain to compensate for the injury, new situations or changes in the environment.

Unlike other nutrients alcohol is absorbed directly into the bloodstream through the stomach lining and the small intestine. Heavy alcohol consumption can damage the mucosal lining of esophagus, and increase mucosal defects such as inflammation and tearing and cancer. Alcohol promotes increased intestinal permeability as well as small intestinal bacterial overgrowth. One remedy for alcoholism is Oat grass juice which contains an antioxidant called **tricin**, that exerts smooth muscle relaxing properties, making it beneficial in gastro-intestinal cramping.

COLON HEALTH AGAINST CHEMTRAILS

If there is chemtrail spraying in your area, your liver is bound to be overwhelmed by the task of detoxifying the heavy metals, plus the toxins secreted by the various microbes. Heavy metals contained in the stool can be reabsorbed into the body if the colon is sluggish. Exercise, sunning and grounding will help waste material move along faster to be eliminated and not reticulated back into storage in the body. The cleaner the body the stronger its defenses!

The GI Tract is much more than a food processing tube it houses about 85 % of your immune system, due in large part to the 100 trillion bacteria that live there. Healthy intestinal bacteria can stimulate immunoglobulin A (IgA) production to enhance your immune response. When gut bacteria are happy they send messages to your mitochondria that increases the energy production of your cells, and increased energy production, means increased cellular detoxification. The greater diverse range of microbes, living in your gut the skinnier the person.

Having a healthy and varied diet, rich in different sources of fiber and raw fruit and vegetables, has been shown to create a more diverse range of gut microbes. When your gut bacteria are happy you are! If we want to FEEL healthy, we need to do whatever it takes to get there. The ultimate diet for health would be picking food directly from your own permaculture food forest and veggie garden. The closer to harvest the more lifegiving the food. Food grown outside of natural ecosystems (with rain, soil and sunlight) can never have the life-giving force nor disease-resistance that food in nature or permaculture systems. The complexity achieved through the diverse interspecies planting of permaculture design systems is healthiest for the plants and animals and healthiest for humans. By using Nature's design, we can realize the perfection of our own design.

The gut is much more than a food processing tube — it houses about 85 % of your immune system, due in large part to the 100 trillion bacteria that live there. Healthy intestinal bacteria can stimulate immunoglobulin A (IgA) production to enhance your immune response. When gut bacteria are happy they send messages to your mitochondria that increases the energy production of your cells, and increased energy production, means increased cellular detoxification. Having a healthy and varied diet, rich in different sources of fiber and raw fruit and vegetables, has been shown to create a more diverse range of gut microbes. The greater diverse range of microbes, living in your gut the skinnier the person. When your gut bacteria are happy you are!

Much of contemporary culture makes us SICK (*stupid, ill, crazy, killed*), then we take drugs and antibiotics that decimate the 100 trillion intestinal bacteria that comprise 85 % of our immune system, leaving us ever more weaker with each round of Flu, or each heavy chemtrail day. Countering the inevitable brain damaging effects of chemtrail heavy metals is going to require lifestyle optimization. Not just heavy metal cleanses and fasts, but an ongoing lifelong detoxifying diet, to encourage the body to "continually" eliminate the environmental toxic load.

THE ORDER OF GI CLEANSERS:

It is important to adopt the ideal sequence of taking substances to deep clean the GI tract during a chemtrail cleanse, heavy metal detox, fast or weight loss program. Find your own "system" and a schedule that works for you, it may go something like this:

1. Roto Rooter—Oxy cleanser: Potassium Bicarbonate and Vitamin C powder in a glass of water. Take ½ hour or more before brooms.

2. Magnesium citrate—A saline laxative thought to work by increasing fluid in the small intestine; can be combined with the Roto Rooter.

3. Enzymes and Vitamin C mixes—including Papaya Smoothie and Green Smoothies. Chlorophyll drinks. Take Enzymes before meals for digestions or between meals for cleansing.

4. Medicinals—Cleansing and tonic herbal formulas and teas. Take between meals. Tinctures and Bitters take before meals.

5. Brooms—Fibers, brans, pectins, and clays, PM Cleanser. Take brooms before bed or 1 or more hours after meals.

6. Activated Charcoal—You can take activated charcoal at any time, before or after meals, or anytime you feel an energy slump and suspect toxins might be the culprit. Charcoal only works to quench toxicity in the presence of the toxin. For example taking activated charcoal directly before or after alcohol acts to reduce its damaging effects.

7. Food-grade Zeolite or Diatomaceous Earth—Taken with water once a day. It's best used on an empty stomach at least one hour before or two hours after eating.

These are taken ½ hour or more apart…and for a full-on cleanse you would do 2 or 3 repetitions of this sequence per day. If you are chelating heavy metals as well you would take the EDTA and other chelators before the brooms. Eat lite as food will obviously interfere with the cleansing process by taking metabolic energy away from detoxification. Drink as much water as seems comfortable or reasonable to you – perhaps 8-10 glasses of distilled Shungite-charged water or spring water per day.

ELIMINATING TOXIC DEPOSITS

In metamorphic alchemy, following the Chaos (massa confusa) of the Nigredo stage, the alchemist undertakes a purification or Albedo, which is referred to as "Ablutio," or the washing away of impurities.

An unharmonious mind leaks vital energy in a continuous stream of negative thoughts, worries and skewed perceptions, which trigger disturbing emotions and degenerative chemical processes in the body. Buried feelings never die and are a source of disease. Autointoxication from poor diet and unhealthy gut bacteria leads to general malaise, and lack of focus and ambition, so that every effort in life is a burden. A fugue of mental depression results, often bordering upon melancholia. The melancholia of dysbiosis! Add the secret covert geoengineering aerosol spraying of various nano-particulate metals (aluminum, barium, strontium, lithium, etc.) being conducted worldwide — and the people get confused, gullible, and easily manipulated with very compromised immune systems. Whether you are suffering from depression, anxiety, insomnia, chronic pain, brain fog or other concerns, optimizing your gut function is key to restoring your health. Gut bacteria produce vitamins, hormones, neurotransmitters, enzymes and other molecules that can impact every cell and organ in our body.

The body sequesters heavy metals and other toxins within plaques, fecal mucoid plaque, nano-bacteria deposits, fatty tissue, biofilms, joints, tumors, cysts, and arthritic and arteriosclerotic calcium deposits. We must remove these metabolic sedimentary detritus if we are to free our body-mind and our energy metabolism from the harmful effects of ever increasing heavy metal accumulation.

A basic cleanser for recovery from Metabolic X and cancer: Sacred Bark, Sarsaparilla, Burdock, Yellow Dock, Dandelion, Elderberry, Guaco, Cuachalalate, Cocolmeca, Quassia, Verbena, Shavegrass, Piedra, Bitter Melon, Urtica, Sea Moss.

In order to effectively eliminate the heavy metals and other toxins that are being moved out of tissues by the chelating agents we must first remove the black Mucoid plaque, or Biofilm that lines the colon. Microorganisms growing in a biofilm are highly resistant to antimicrobial agents. The GI Biofilm is largely composed of the body's defensive mucus and candida, so the yeast/fungi must be addressed at the same time as the removal of the black tar. Bloating will reduce once the fasting and mucoid plaque removal is undertaken. The mucoid plaque must first be removed in order to get the "good stuff" in and the "bad stuff" out! Reticulation of heavy metals and other toxins is inevitable if the pathways for them to leave the body are blocked and devitalized.

Since cooked food contains no enzymes the body's enzyme stores are used up which in time leads to even further reduced digestive power, resulting in the degeneration of all Gastrointestinal functions. Cooked-food cannot be fully digested, assimilated or eliminated because it takes more enzymes and energy to digest, assimilate and eliminate it than the body gets out of it.

It is the end products of this ineffective digestion which leads to the unnatural build up on the colon walls and throughout all tissues. The membrane of the colon produces a protective layer of mucus in response to food which is denatured or harmful to the body. Normally pancreatic juices would strip off this mucus and residual feces within a few days. But since we eat denatured food with every meal the residue starts building layer upon layer. Peristalsis is impaired by the accumulated bulk and parasites take up residence in the decaying matter.

Mucoid plaque is created by the long-term consumption of excessive acid forming foods (red meat, dairy, eggs and bread, sodas and other sugar drinks, high-protein foods). Limiting animal products is beneficial for health by preventing the body becoming too acidic. Mucoid plaque is also produced when consuming processed foods, taking drugs, when you are under stress, or living in toxic environments. Causing the body to secrete mucus into its' alimentary canals and hollow organs to try and protect itself.

When the lymph system is overwhelmed with toxicity it becomes congested with mucus and impairs the immune system. If the lymph nodes become clogged it is a sign that the person is overwhelmed with toxins, pathogens, pollution or waste matter. Most probably the intestines are lined with a layer of impacted mucoid material which prevents effective assimilation and elimination. Lymphatic failure causes a buildup of toxins in the blood which become deposited in the tissues, organs and in the plaques lining the blood vessels and intestines.

This rubbery mucus coating that has been stuck to the inner walls of your bowels for many years, creates a breeding ground for parasites and unfriendly organisms, and inhibits efficient digestion. Clogged lymph nodes means the lymph flow is backed up or reduced so the cells which defend the body from invaders, cancer cells and toxins cannot do their job as effectively. Pathogens and cancer cells can then outgrow the body's ability to control them. If toxins cannot be removed fast enough from the body due to a backed-up lymph system, they may be encased in lymph fluid and stored in the tissues creating edema or bloat and contributing to obesity. When the lymph nodes are unable to produce enough lymph to deal with the accumulated toxins they slowly harden and lose their ability to function. This condition not only impairs the immune system but can eventually lead to cancer.

Toxins and waste accumulations in the body prevent the free flow of chi (energy) and can short circuit the nervous system. It is the power or vibration level of the electromagnetic (etheric) field of the body which determines cell division, healing, cellular vitality and the spirituality of the individual. If the chi is blocked by a congested lymphatic system which fails to cleanse the blood and tissues the cells literally starve of nutrition, energy and oxygen and die off in the poisons of their own waste.

Parasitic worms as well as unfriendly bacteria and yeasts thrive on the toxins, junk food and the mucoid layer and until it is removed it is unlikely that these pathogens can be gotten rid of. The book "Cleanse and Purify Thyself" by Rich Anderson explains how the removal of this mucoid matter can be done. Fasting on the Arise and Shine cleansing system becomes easy when you start to see all the old toxic residue come out of you. I don't know of any other fast or method of removing this destructive impacted mucoid layer from the entire digestive tract. You being to see noticeable improvement in your health after just a few days on this fast.

Make your own raw juices, do not use bottled juices and drink the required amount of water. It is important to drink the vegetable broth and take the minerals on this fast to aid in the elimination of the toxins and prevent acid build up making you feel sick. Fresh spring water, ionized water, alkaline water, Shungite water or Philosopher's water will help wash the toxins out of your system and prevent acidosis while detoxing. Drink at least 8-10 glasses of water per day or constipation may result. An important component of a colon cleansing program is the use of probiotics to help replenish the population of friendly bacteria which resides in your colon.

Regularly do colonics or enemas to clear the colon of impacted waste that causes heavy metal reuptake, plus prevent stagnant bowel wastes escaping into the blood. But colonics will not remove the black tar biofilm mucoid layer in which the parasites reside, so they will not get to the root of the problem, but merely provide temporary relief. Colonics save lives, however colonics can only remove impacted mucoid layers on the walls of the colon if used in association with cleansing program is undertaken which incorporates fasting, raw juices, psyllium/Bentonite, liquid minerals and cleansing herbs. The introduction of water alone will not remove much of the black tar. The body has to be in a state of deep cleansing before it will release the mucoid lining and then changing to a raw foods diet is the only way to avoid the re-accumulation of this toxic layer.

It is advised to eat plenty of vegetables and kelp for months before doing this fast to build your mineral reserves and reduce body acidity. When taking a large amount of cleansing herbs it is best to commit to raw juices, smoothies and water for the duration of a full-on cleanse. Anything that is not raw fruit and vegetables will slow down the cleansing cycle. If you see undigested food coming out in your feces you will need to grind or grate your food to make it more digestible. When coming off a fast, stop the cleansing herbs and finely grate, puree or juice the first fruit and vegetables you eat so they can be adequately digested. After a fast, chew well and don't eat too much at one time.

MUCOID PLAQUE FORMULA: An Intestinal Cleansing Formula in tablet or capsule form that softens and loosens the hardened mucoid plaque lining the intestines can be purchased (such as from Arise and Shine) or you can make your own. 6 X capsules or more as needed taken between meals, or at least 90 minutes after a Psyllium shake during the mucoid plaque cleansing process.

Cascara Sagrada Bark, Rhubarb Root, Plantain Leaf, Yellow Dock Root, Dandelion Root, Barberry Bark, Sheep Sorrel Leaf, Red Clover Blossoms, Cayenne, Peppermint, Fennel Seed, Ginger Root, Myrrh Gum Resin, Red Raspberry Leaf, Cayenne, Goldenseal Root, Lobelia Leaf, Alfalfa Leaf, Moringa, Horsetail, Chickweed Leaf, Marshmallow Root, Rose Hips, Slippery elm, Hawthorn Berry, Licorice Root, Kelp Leaf, Irish Moss.

IMPACTED COLON REMEDIES

• **Avoid** eating mucus producing foods red meat, dairy, eggs and bread.

• Eat **raw enzyme** rich foods with every meal, or fermented foods like miso and sauerkraut.

• Take **warming herbs** to strengthen digestion: Cinnamon, Cardamom, Cayenne, Ginger, Anise, Cloves, Fennel. Ginger helps digest any fat or oil in the meal.

• Use **detoxing herbs** to clear the body of accumulated mucus: Comfrey, Chickweed, Horehound, Sow Fennel Root, Verba Santa, Thyme, Mustard Seed, Mullein, Yucca Root, Black Cohosh, Juniper berries, Licorice, Cat's claw, and kelp. Guggulu with Triphala is the main Ayurvedic cure for Ama.

• Eat plenty of **fiber rich and raw foods** to speed transit time, sop up cholesterol and cleanse the colon. Thus we need a lifestyle fix back to the **Natural Hygiene** of living on the land.

• In general, **colon cleansing** options include oxygen-based cleansers, laxatives, herbs and supplements, enemas, bentonite or other cleansing clays, and colonic hydrotherapy.

• Anything that introduces **more oxygen** into the bowels will facilitate the removal of hardened deposits and rejuvenate the cells: Chaparral, Wheat Grass,

Raw vegetables, Pau d' Arco, Hydergine, Exercise, Deep breathing, Massage, Coenzyme Q10, Liquid oxygen products, Vitamins E, B2, B15. Earth's Bounty - Oxy Cleanse Oxygen Colon Conditioner.

• **Magnesium citrate** is a hyperosmotic saline laxative that pulls water from surrounding tissues into the intestine to stimulate intestinal movement and empties the colon.

• **Probiotics and prebiotics** help restore good gut bacteria and soothe symptoms! Latero Flora containing BreviBacillus laterosporus for easing gastrointestinal symptoms and eliminating Candida from the digestive tract.

• **Spirulina** promotes digestion and bowel function. It suppresses bad bacteria (including E. coli and Candida albicans yeast) and stimulates beneficial flora.

• The **inulin** in Chicory Root is a prebiotic that feeds the healthy microflora that boosts your immunity and encourages implantation, survival, and growth of freshly consumed probiotics. Roasted Chicory root and Chaga tea makes a great coffee substitute.

• **Licorice root** soothes the GI tract, reduces inflammation, soothe and heal ulcers and stomach inflammation, controls blood sugar, balances hormones, and is a potent antiviral agent.

• **Larch bark powder** and white oak bark for intestinal reconstruction.

• **Prickly Ash Bark Powder** stimulates the circulation, lymphatic system.

• **Elephant Foot Yam** (Amorphophallus paeoniifolius) ameliorates inflammation and oxidative damage in colon. It helps with diarrhea and abdominal pain and gas, and boosts your immune system and prevent colon cancer.

• **Apple pectin** tends to increase acidity in the large intestines and is advocated for those suffering from ulcer or colitis and for regulating blood pressure.

• **Marshmallow root powder** — The mucilaginous (gel-like) marshmallow offers a unique composition of about 37% starch, 11% mucilage, and 11% pectin. In the colon marshmallow gel softens hardened fecal plaques helping to remove them from colon walls.

• **Slippery elm** is a mucilaginous herb effective coating and soothing mucous membranes while also absorbing toxins. As part of a normal diet, the inner bark of slippery elm can be ground and eaten as porridge.

• **Clay/Psyllium Sludge Drink** — Bentonite clay with psyllium draws out poisons and sweeps the intestines clean. When bentonite clay absorbs water and swells, it stretches open like a highly porous sponge. Toxins (including pathogenic viruses, herbicides, and pesticides) are drawn into these spaces and bound through electrical attraction. 2 tsp in 10 oz of water before bed.

• **Epsom salt foot bath**, followed by rubbing Castor oil on feet and covering with socks.

• By increasing blood flow and circulation through exercise your gastrointestinal system, including the colon, gets more oxygen. The recommended amount of exercise to protect against colon cancer is estimated to be between 30 to 60 minutes of moderate to vigorous physical activity per day. Ten minutes of yoga stands out as one of the best types of daily exercise to keep your digestive tract moving and prevent constipation. Adopt 5 or more yoga poses especially for the digestive system.

DISSOLVING MUCUS AND FAT DEPOSITS

• Drink **Nachi Green Tea** to help dissolve and discharge animal fats and reduce high cholesterol levels.

• **Barley or Wheat Greens** is good for removing fat, cysts, and tumors from the consumption of too much animal foods.

• **Daikon and radishes** are helpful to eliminate excess mucus, fat, protein and water from the body.

• **Daikon and Carrot juice** or grated and simmered 5 minutes to make a tea will help eliminate excessive fats and dissolve hardened accumulations in the intestines.

Place 1 Tablespoon of fresh grated daikon in a cup with 1 teaspoon of miso, pour over some hot Bancha tea. Drink before bedtime for 5 days.

• Put the j**uice of half a lemon** plus a pinch of cayenne pepper and a teaspoon of maple syrup or raw honey in a glass of hot or cold water. This is called the master cleanser and will reduce mucus and improve circulation.

• **Enemas and colonics** will help cleanse an impacted colon.

• **Papaya enzymes** help to cleanse the intestinal walls of waste matter. These enzymes aid in the digestion of proteins thus avoiding accumulations of mucoprotein becoming trapped in the interstitial spaces between the cells.

• The amino acid **N-Acetyl Cysteine** (NAC) breaks down mucus deposits, however when using it remember to use twice as much vitamin C as the Cysteine to prevent developing kidney stones.

MUCUS ELIMINATORS:

Echinacea, Boneset, Goldenseal, Sage, Kelp, Comfrey, Chickweed, Sow Fennel root, Horehound, Verba santa, Thyme, Horseradish, Mustard seed, Mullein, Yucca root, Black Cohosh, Fenugreek, Ginkgo nut, Garlic, Licorice, Marshmallow, Yarrow, Hyssop, Savory, Guggulu with Triphala. Copious quantities of fresh Ginger Tea.

COLON CLEANSERS:

Use the intestinal and mucus clearing herbs: When ground up and taken internally, flaxseed soluble fiber is an effective laxative. Black walnut, hibiscus flowers, Triphala, horsetail (shavegrass), licorice root, alfalfa, borage, burdock root, cascara sagrada, senna, rhubarb root, pumpkin seed, yucca root, Irish moss, passionflower, marshmallow root, violet leaves, mullein leaves, aloe, slippery elm, cayenne. The tannins in Witch hazel bark and Schisandra berry are cytotoxic against colon cancer cells. Japanese Knotweed also contains a chemical known as emodin, which has the ability to regulate bowel motility and is a natural laxative. Buckthorn Bark is both laxative and stimulates peristalsis and mucous secretions in the intestines. Chamomile tea helps calm gastrointestinal discomfort such as upset stomach and gas. Ginger root tea is effective for stomach ache, nausea, and diarrhea. Milk Thistle Seeds can be ground up and soaked in water overnight to make a delicious raw porridge the next morning, sprinkled with cinnamon.

FOOD STAGNATION AND WEAK DIGESTION: Spleen and stomach weakness can produce excessive appetite. Poria cocos fungus, Green citrus peel, Peppermint, Magnolia bark, Cardamom seed, Caraway seed, Ginger root, Dandelion root, Slippery elm, Atractylodes, Wild yam root, Lovage, Rue.

BLOOD AND INTESTINAL CLEANERS: Rhubarb root, Burdock root, Cascara sagrada, Senna leaves, Triphala, Goldenseal, Borage, Psyllium, Yucca root, Bentonite clay, Cayenne, Yarrow, Chickweed, Irish moss, Plantain, Dandelion, Elderflowers, Blue Cohosh, Fenugreek, Red clover. Irritant laxatives are addictive and dangerous. Rotate herbs as the intestines lose their ability to contract and propel stool normally when irritant laxatives are used long term.

INTESTINAL BROOMS: Psyllium is high in soluble fiber, which means it is unable to remove hardened material from the colon walls. Insoluble fiber has a scrubbing brush cleansing effect while Soluble fiber works more like a sponge absorbing toxins. A combination of flaxseed, oat bran, and acacia gum provide a blend of soluble and insoluble fiber. Raw vacuum packed rice bran from certified organic brown rice can be bought from http://rhapsodynaturalfoods.com. Keep refrigerated. The tough outer husk of brown rice does not break down in the digestive tract, making it a good source of insoluble fiber. Buy vacuum packed, refrigerated and organic rice bran.

ASSISTING PRACTICES FOR CLEANSING:

• Sweat lodge type rituals with dancing and drumming

• Ocean swimming, spas, clay baths or clay packs, saunas and steam baths

• The hand held infrared wands are great for increasing circulation and detoxing

• Body brushing and lymphatic drainage massage

• Massage the abdomen daily before sleep, especially effective on a slant board

• Exercise, stretching and deep breathing

• Meditation and visualizations will reduce symptoms and speed integration

• Colonics and enemas followed by wheatgrass implants

• Taking a toxin absorber like Bentonite clay and a bulking agent such as psyllium as in the Arise and Shine system

• Using papaya, wheat grass juice, aloe or clay on sores, eruptions and internally.

• Chamomile, marshmallow and slippery elm to soothe and protect the GI tract

• Remineralized fruit and vegetables will provide the alkaline minerals for the bile, pancreatic and intestinal juices, along with bitter herbs such as Gentian, Dandelion and Turmeric to stimulate an increase in their secretion

• If the cleansing is just too intense you can slow it down by eating some pureed vegetable soup or ground millet.

• Cleansing takes energy so keep warm, keep moving, rest and relax.

• Grounding and sunshine have an exponential effect on detoxification.

• Put shungite stones or discs over areas of the digestive system that are weak or in discomfort. Shungite reharmonizes the energy so the organs can heal and become more efficient, thus relieving pain.

BITTERS: Bitter herbs are the cornerstone of herbal medicine. A range of physiological responses occur following stimulation of the bitter receptors of the tongue. The bitter taste stimulates the specific bitter taste buds at the back of the tongue to stimulate the parasympathetic nervous system to trigger a number of reflexes. These reflexes are important to the digestive process and general health. Bitters are useful prior to large meals, and during parasite cleansing. You can use these bitters 15 minutes before a meal to prepare your body for the full utilization of the food and efficient waste elimination and reduce in cravings.

Bitters stimulate the endocrine glands, digestive juices, liver pancreas and peristalsis. By stabilizing blood sugar bitters can be a useful part of your anti-candida, anti-pathogen treatment. Friendly bacteria produce small amounts of lactic acid and acetic acid that help to maintain your stomach acidity. When they are killed by the antibiotics, your gut becomes less acidic, more alkaline, and a perfect environment for Candida to grow and take over your gut. Because bitters increase the production of digestive enzymes like hydrochloric acid, they improve your digestion and help to raise the acidity of your intestines to slow Candida growth and re-balance your gut flora. Bitters tincture can also be put into sparkling mineral water, with ice and a slice of lemon as an aperitif prior to meals.

COMMON BITTER HERBS: Elecampane, Gentian, Dandelion leaf, Yellow dock, Barberry root bark, Mugwort, Blessed Thistle, Chicory, Chamomile, Goldenseal, Oregon Grape root, Andrographis and Yarrow.

NEW ZEALAND BUSH BITTERS: Harakeke (Flax), Kareao (Supplejack), Kumarahou, Kawakawa and Horopito (Pepper-Trees), Pukatea, Koromiko, Kohekohe, Puriri, Kowhai, Karama, Manuka & Kanuka, Korokia.

BERBERINE: Herbs containing Berberine such as Barberry root, Barberries, Bloodroot, Oregon Grape Root, Chinese Goldthread, Goldenseal root, act as an herbal antidepressant and a neuroprotector. Berberine has glucose-lowering effects, improves diabetes-induced memory impairment, as well as increasing the number of serotonin transporters available in the brain, enhancing the reuptake of serotonin and reducing the breakdown of acetylcholine, crucial for memory and cognitive function. Berberine is also showing promise in fighting cancer, reduces oxidative stress and lipid peroxidation, and improves glutathione levels. Berberine has strong antimicrobial ability on a range of pathogens, parasitic gut infection or Small Intestinal Bacterial Overgrowth. Berberine has remarkable abilities to heal a leaky gut by strengthening the tight junctions between cells, thereby reducing intestinal permeability.

ASSISTING CLEANSING: When changing to a raw diet the body starts to deeply detox. During this time you can feel cold and hypersensitive for 2 years, and need to incorporate things that help your detox organs like saunas, running, hot & cold, massages, rebounding, grounding and meditation. Toxic diets with cereals, sugar, transfats etc... produce numbing endorphins and inflammatory heat in the body. This repression of consciousness and loss of sensation is one of the reasons why we get addicted to the bad stuff and that we only start to feel the repercussions of life-harming substances after we stop and start withdrawing from them. When cleansing it is a good idea to assist the body in preventing the released toxins from harming tissues as they exit the body.

TEETH

The Canadian dentist **Weston A. Price** used a combination of cod liver oil (Vit A and D) and grass fed butter (K2) as a healing protocol to stop tooth decay and heal cavities. After the pancreas, the salivary glands contain the highest source of K2, which reduces bad bacteria overgrowth in the mouth and activates proteins to ensure that calcium is deposited in the bones and teeth where it is needed. K2 is essential for osteocalcin function, and is a crucial nutrient to preventing osteoporosis, heart disease and treating type 2 diabetes. Found in Natto, fermented soy, goose liver pate, free range egg yolks, Dutch Gouda, grass fed butter and other grass fed products. www.westonaprice.org/

Vitamin K2 is essential to reduce overgrowth of oral bacteria. Besides Vitamin K2 and D3 other tooth strengtheners include calcium phosphate, eating eggshell, and silicon from bamboo sap and horsetail. Acemannan (aloe) promotes tooth dentin formation by stimulating primary human dental pulp cell proliferation, differentiation, extracellular matrix formation, and mineralization, while significantly eliminating oral inflammation. If you cut the gel out of an aloe leaf and put that in your mouth, even sleeping with it around the infected tooth, this will cut the inflammation. Propolis is the most powerful anti-infection substance for teeth; you can suck on a lump of propolis, or use propolis tincture.

Straight **Helichrysum essential oil** in a dropper bottle applied throughout the day reduces infection, itching and inflammation. This is a powerful antiseptic oil for chembug sores, Morgellons, cuts, or acne. Helichrysum seems to work better than clove oil and is more pleasant. Chlorophyll or propolis on gums when you sleep relieves pain and inflammation. You can also sleep with a cut garlic clove around the infected tooth, if the garlic is not too burny. Holding piece of shungite on the gums near a tooth that is infected or weak will normalize the electromagnetics of the mouth, and reduce brain infection/inflammation.

Hemp seed oil contains the perfect ratio of Omega 3: Omega 6, this can be rubbed on the teeth and gums prior to bed to protect the teeth overnight. Mix the Hemp seed oil with wild Oregon oil as it is recommended for repairing tooth enamel. Also if there is any sage or lemon balm in your garden, chew on the leaves of any such herbs throughout the day. If you can take up to 2 tsp of cayenne per day, this revives oral health by improving circulation.

Puritan Pride multi-minerals do remineralize teeth, and so does silicon. Take some of the young spikes of Horsetail in spring, split them longways and dry out, then grind to a powder. Use this to make strong infusion in a slow cooker, or the hotplate of a coffee maker. Sieve then keep this in the fridge to swish your mouth with several times a day to help regrow tooth enamel and strengthen teeth. If run through a coffee filter, this infusion is also great spray for skin hair and nails. Grounding, ie: going barefoot in nature, is essential for strong bones and teeth.

I doubt there are many advanced dentists out there that are using things like ORMUS, Near Infrared and the above, therefore this is the kind of thing we need to take full responsibility for ourselves. Stimulating the facial nerves, jaw and neck with an acupuncture pen is also important, as well are rebooting the immune systems—so a series of 3 day fasts will help. The teeth are like the canary in the coal mine that reveal the strength of your immune system at any point in time.

Brushing teeth with Deuterium depleted water may help keep bacterial overgrowth at bay. Bacteria build up can be eliminated by putting 2 drops of Lugol's iodine in a shot glass of Colloidal Silver and using this to gargle or brush your teeth. The **Ionic Toothbrush** System Brush by Dr. Tungs Products can be used with a shot glass of Philosopher's water with a pinch of salt to eliminate plaque and bacterial overgrowth.

TOOTHPASTE: Activated Charcoal and Shungite can be mixed with clay to make a healing toothpaste ingredients include: Clay, Bamboo Charcoal, Shungite, Himalayan Salt, Lugol's, colloidal silver and peppermint oil. Activated charcoal has the ability to help whiten teeth naturally by adsorbing acids, plaque and toxins from the mouth, killing bad bacteria and removing stains.

GUM INFLAMMATION: For gums you can make an amber bottle of colloidal silver solution and add a small amount of essential oils such as: oregano, peppermint, hyssop, savory, grapefruit, helichrysum, along with some Himalayan salt and magnesium chloride. Put some in a small spray bottle or dropper bottle to keep on your nightstand to put on your gums before you go to sleep and when you wake up. Helichrysum oil and Near Infrared (NIR) or red led light will help reduce oral pain. Both chlorophyll, and propolis are formidable allies for reversing gum recession. Put either of these, or both on your gums overnight. **Hydrogen peroxide** 3% in an eye dropper can be run along the gum edge. A miracle cure for oral inflammation is fresh wheatgrass juice swished as a mouthwash. Strengthening collagen with Vitamin C etc… is essential for strong gums and healthy teeth. Fasting, colon cleansing and a raw remineralized diet will help keep gum inflammation at bay.

Oil Pulling with Black Seed Oil — For toothaches, tonsil, and larynx pain use as a gargle. Also, swallow a spoonful of black seed and chase with warm water on an empty stomach every day. Rub the jaw and neck with black seed oil.

Yunnan Baiyao powder can be rubbed into the gums before sleep to heal and protect the mouth from bacteria overnight, and it is perfect for oral surgery to recover from the removal of teeth. Yunnan Baiyao inhibitions cell death in bone in diabetic periodontitis supporting the ligaments and bones associated with the teeth. Teeth and gum infections can affect the heart and brain.

Acemannan (made from Aloe) promotes tooth dentin formation by stimulating primary human dental pulp cell proliferation, differentiation, extracellular matrix formation, and mineralization, while significantly eliminating oral and GI inflammation.

Medical Mushrooms are the best for immunity in the mouth in stopping infection and allowing regrowth of bone (and enamel). Alternating different mushrooms every few months would be best. Cordyceps, Maitake, Reishi, Shitake. Make your own or use a high quality product such as *Fungi Perfecti, Host Defense, Organic Stamets 7 Extract.*

Birch Bracket Mushroom — *Fomitopsis betulina* fungus has a long tradition of being applied in folk medicine as an antimicrobial, anticancer, and anti-inflammatory agent. The mushroom contains valuable enzymes and other substances such as cell wall (1-3)-α-d-glucan which can be used for the induction of microbial enzymes degrading dental biofilm that promotes the development of tooth decay.

FLUORIDOSIS: Sodium Fluoride is a highly dangerous toxin which target the following organs: Heart, kidneys, bones, central nervous system, gastrointestinal system, teeth. The highly reactive, caustic Sodium Fluoride in our drinking water has an *exponential negative effect* in association with heavy metals and aluminum. Fluoridosis can be reversed by sunlight, grounding, circadian compliance, wheatgrass juice and other K2 sources. Vitamin K2 gets calcium into the bones where it belongs. Fluoride makes cells efflux calcium more from the mitochondria. Calcium influx/efflux determines how much free radicals the mitochondria produce. Sunlight, grounding, high negative ion and EMF smog free environments improves the redox to eliminate fluoridosis, osteoporosis and arthritis.

BONES: Strong bones are essential to strong teeth. We have already determined how important silicon is to collagen and bones. Other nutrients that support strong bones include, Hops, Strontium citrate, Vitamin D, L-Lysine, Vitamin K2, Boron, Manganese, Copper and Zinc. Phosphorus supports calcium in building strong bones and teeth. Vitamin D helps the body absorb calcium while boosting bone mineral density. One of the best ways of getting calcium is in raw greens, that way you get a dose of K2 also. Oat, wheat or rye grass juice are perfect bone and teeth strengtheners rich in antioxidants, minerals, K2 and beta-glucan, which helps stimulate immune functions. When you consume borax it works synergistically with magnesium, so keep your magnesium intake up whilst taking borax. Take Strontium at a different time than calcium as it competes.

ANTI-PARASITE PROTOCOL

To remove parasites you want to cut out sugar processed foods, alcohol, wheat, sushi and pork out of your diet. It is the acidity and high sugar levels in our bodies is what provides cancer and parasites with the terrain that they need to thrive and breed in. You cannot permanently rid the body of cancer and parasites until you fix the underlying terrain issue. Which is to heal and clean the lymphatic system and the blood, and detoxify poisons, acids and plaques, including the morbid black plaque in the colon. Regenerating the body beyond the cancer/pathogen terrain primarily involves the need to turn cellular energy back to aerobic ATP production.

ANTI-PATHOGEN/ANTI-CANCER TERRAIN SHIFT: Primarily there is the need to turn cellular energy back to aerobic ATP production. Oxygen, Hyperbaric oxygen chamber, Sunshine, Grounding, Wheatgrass Juice, Apricot seeds, Alkalinizing Raw-Remineralized Vegetable Juice, Turkey Tail Mushroom, Astaxanthin, Pycnogenol (pine bark), Resveratrol, Essiac Tea, Raw veggie and sprouted diet of ground up food and fermented foods, Ketogenic diet-coconut oil; Alpha Lipoic Acid, Propolis, IV Vitamin C and Glutathione: 50 gram/1 hr infusion Vitamin C, Krill omega-3 for mitochondrial membranes. $H2O2$, Budwig protocol, probiotics, Baking Soda/Epsom Salt baths, Kelp baths, Povidone Iodine in foot baths, Colonics, gold roast coffee enemas, Lymphatic massage, Rebounding, Relaxation Practices and Laughter. Candida Cleanse. Zeolite, food grade Diatomaceous earth, Montmorillite clay powder can also be used for heavy metal detox and parasite elimination.) Silicon/Colloidal Silver water and Lysine to build up collagen - http://jana-sovereignstate.blogspot.com/2018/01/philosophers-water.html

PARASITE HERBS: Thyme Leaf is a traditional powerful antiseptic and tonic which has been used by many cultures for its antifungal and antiparasitic actions. In Russian culture Thyme tea and garlic often consumed daily to ward off parasites. Aloe, Fo-Ti, wormwood, black walnut inner hulls, pomegranate root bark, and garlic, Neem, Oregano leaf, papaya enzymes, papaya seeds, pumpkin seeds, cucumber seeds, Bitter melon, Garlic, Myrrh, Graviola bark, Sage Leaf, Gentian, ginger, Knotweed, Fennel, Rue, Horehound, Oregano, Grapefruit seed, Uva ursi leaf, Chinese rhubarb root, Anise, Neem, Olive leaf, Propolis, Barberry, Oregon grape, Clove, Gentian root, Hyssop leaf, Cramp bark, Peppermint leaf, Frankincense, Bacopa, Triphala, Embelia ribes (Vidanga).

INTESTINAL PARASITE CLEANSING

Garlic—(*Allium sativa*) either raw or in capsule or tablet form has been shown to be active against roundworm.

Green Black Walnut—Black walnut hull has been used for centuries for its antiparasitic and antifungal properties. It promotes intestinal health and beneficial flora. It is thought to change the terrain oxygenating the blood and creating a state hostile to invasive organisms, promotes healthy sugar levels, melts away fatty materials and detoxifies the colon.

Wormwood—(*Artemisia annua*) has also been used for centuries as a herbal remedy for intestinal parasites particularly Ascaris lumbricoides and Schistosoma mansoni. Wormwood contains sesquiterpene lactones, which are thought to weaken parasite membranes.

Epazote Wormseed—(*Chenopodium ambrosioides*) or Jesuit's tea is a Mexican herbal remedy used in the tropics for expelling roundworms, hookworms and tapeworms.

Pumpkin Seeds—(*Cucurbita pepo*) have been used as a remedy for tapeworms and roundworms.

Papaya seeds and juice—This potent juice can have anti-parasitic effects.

Ayahuasca—The South American tea Ayahuasca (containing the potent psychedelic chemical DMT) is medically beneficial, as it clears the body of worms and other parasites. Its purgative properties induce intense vomiting and diarrhea thereby clearing the body of worms and other tropical parasites, and harmala alkaloids themselves have been shown to acts against infections caused by parasitic worms. Ayahuasca kills parasites and increases intestinal motility. Harmine is able to reverse diabetes through pancreas beta cell proliferation, increasing islet mass and improving glycemic control.

BLACK SEED OIL: (*Nigella sativa*) or Black Cumin Seed is a broad-spectrum cure, as it is a good topical antioxidant, anti-parasite, anti-inflammatory oil. Black seed oil quenches all forms of inflammation from arthritis, gastritis, heavy metals, pathogens, oxidation, and radiation. Nigella sativa not only rebuilds the immune system and destroys cancer cells; it reinforces the good cells to fight cancer. Nigella sativa has been shown to be effective against numerous cancers, such as pancreatic, colon, prostate, breast and brain cancers, and also reduced the tumors in the lungs and alimentary canal. Black Cumin oil was even proven to annihilate pancreatic tumor cells at the rate of 80 percent.

By reducing inflammation consciousness is more focused, depression lifts and sleep deepens. Try 1 tsp of organic cold pressed Black Seed Oil at night to squelch inflammation and hunger, this reduces brain "noise" allowing for a deeper more regenerative sleep. The thymohydroquinone found in Black seed oil is an acetylcholinesterase (AChE) inhibitor, which stops the breakdown of the neurotransmitter acetylcholine in the brain…thereby countering depression, apathy, autism, Alzheimer's and schizophrenia. Alzheimer's in addition to preserving antioxidant enzymes glutathione peroxidase and glutathione-S-transferase.

Black seed oil contains conjugated linoleic acid and phytosterols that decrease blood-glucose, triglyceride and cholesterol levels, boosts metabolism and speeds up your body's fat burning ability and Liver gluconeogenesis. N. sativa has a broad spectrum of healing properties including antidiabetic, anticancer, immunomodulator, analgesic, antimicrobial, anti-inflammatory, spasmolytic, bronchodilator, liver and kidney protective, gastro-protective, and antioxidant properties, etc. Black seed oil offers defense against superbugs, fungi, yeast-candida and cancer. On teaspoon daily would probably eliminate GI tract candida overgrowth.

Black Seed oil actually tastes nice after a while, and is a great base oil for topical essential oil remedies. It can be mixed with the essential oils like fennel, oregano oil, clove oil and wormwood. Grind seeds as a condiment. Take 1 teaspoon of blackseed oil three times a day. If you don't like the taste mix it with half a teaspoon of raw honey or freshly squeezed juice. The oil can also be used for oil pulling to overcome periodontal disease and cavities. Oil pulling with black seed oil removes bacterial overgrowth in the mouth, and keeps teeth clean for an extended period and reduces gum inflammation.

HERBAL SPRITZER: The aromatic anti-parasite herbs and spices lend themselves to the creation of bitters, tinctures and herbal liqueurs such as Polish vodka liqueurs (nalewka, literally translates to "tincture") which are alcoholic extracts from fruit, honey, molasses, spices, flowers or herbs. When counteracting MetaboliX, Chemtrail Flu, Fungi and parasites it is a challenge to consume enough herbs in teas, capsules and elixirs. Another way is to use your homemade herbal tinctures in cocktails with ice, a slice of lemon, and sparkling water. This way you can be medicating and treating yourself at the same time.

All degenerative diseases and even parasites and infectious diseases are encouraged by morbid acid-toxicity levels in our bodies. Parasites love morbid matter, they are the agents of decay that send everything back to dust. In order to elevate the body beyond the pro-pathogenic condition we have to address both parasites and microbes simultaneously.

Hilda Clark formulated a parasite cleansing tincture called "Clarkia" that contains Wormwood, Clove and Black Walnut Husk in brandy or vodka. Note Dr. Clark favored wormwood and cloves in whole-herb form over tincture form, such as Clarkia. She also incorporates an electrotherapy in her anti-parasite protocol with a simple battery operated electrical device called a ZAPPER. If we are generally depolarized and lacking lifeforce due to removal from nature and generations of cooked-depleted food, then low voltage blood zapping makes sense, especially if we are suffering from parasites, infectious diseases or cancer. drclarkstore.com

"Electricity can now be used to kill bacteria viruses and parasites in minutes, not days or weeks as antibiotics require." ~ Dr. Hulda Clark

Since parasites can only exist in devitalized tissue they will continue to infect us until we reach a level of dynamic health and wholeness. If you have parasites it is a sure indication that your body needs regenerating. By parasites I refer to everything from viruses, bad bacteria and yeast infection to worms. If tissues are not in robust health they are an open invitation to infestation with parasites that thrive in the mucoid plaque of the colon.

To remove this plaque we must work on getting rid of the parasites and vice versa. Simply attacking the parasite won't work, we must remove morbid matter and purify and revitalize the terrain. If you are having pain when you are cleansing it could be the parasites complaining that their home is being disturbed. Drink more water, get exercise, grounding, sunshine and assist your elimination organs.

CHECKLIST FOR PLAQUE AND PARASITES

Permanently removing parasites from our bodies is not just a matter of taking some drug or herb. We have to change our entire lifestyle towards greater vigor and aliveness. To eliminate both the plaque and the parasites we have to undergo a comprehensive program which will repair the balance to the bodies systems both chemical and structural.

- Increase enzymes (trypsin, bromelain and Papain) and alkaline mineral stores (K, Mg, Ca, Si).
- Improve breathing response, adrenal and thyroid function.
- Increase production of gastric, Pancreatic bile and intestinal juices.
- Obey the bulk/fiber, moisture, lubrication rule for meals.
- Avoid acid producing foods, cooked and denatured foods.
- Attend to mental and emotional stress and learn to relax.
- Use a herbal cleanser like Arise and Shine; Essiac Tea; Senna + Yerba Mate Tea
- Avoid excess of any kind especially sugars, cereals, fats and stimulants.
- Use raw-nutrition to rebuild strength and integrity of structures.
- Use vermicides (parasite herbs) pumpkin seeds, papaya seeds, diatomaceous earth; Fennel, Rue or Horehound tea..
- Encourage the growth of healthy bacteria by eating raw fruit and veges, especially fermented cabbage to add to salads.
- Take friendly bacteria supplements after colon hydrotherapy.
- And most importantly realign our life to a higher responsibility to Life and Mankind.

HERXHEIMER REACTION

Biological Warfare agents are microorganisms like virus, bacteria, fungi, protozoa or toxins produced by them. Neurotoxin overload is a common problem that affects those infected with pathogens. Infectious diseases secrete neurotoxins that are highly destructive to body functions and can result in stressed liver detoxification, lethargy and fatigue, muscle soreness, mental confusion, emotional instability, hypothalamus dysfunction, and much more. The source of neurotoxins may be heavy metals, viruses, bacteria, fungi, molds, parasites and protozoans. Some of the toxins actually target and even damage the nervous system and the detoxification organs. This can further impair and block the route for normal excretion, causing toxins to accumulate.

When the Lyme and other pathogens are being killed, they produce neurotoxins and free radicals in defense. This chemical warfare subsequently clogs the blood, lymph, liver and colon which slows down the detoxification pathways. And as long as the patient is in treatment for Lyme, detoxification needs to be ongoing. When the body is overburdened with a toxic load, the patient might experience a Herxheimer reaction, which is like a bad hangover, with fatigue, headaches, brain fog, nausea, flu-like symptoms, and a tingling sensation throughout the body. If you're consistently helping to provide your body with the nutrients it needs to detoxify endotoxins and pathogen toxins, a herxheimer reaction is less likely because the flow of toxins leaving the body is perpetual.

Brain fog can increase during fasting or when taking antifungal herbs and enzymes, because the candida presents a higher toxin load to the body because of the herxheimer die-off reaction. The symptoms of dizziness and brain fog due to candida can be reduced via methylation with N-acetyl cysteine (NAC). Methylation is used to metabolize the catecholamines dopamine, norepinephrine and epinephrine, to inactivate histamine, and to methylate phospholipids, promoting transmission of signals through membranes. Grate some ginger root and make 6 cups of ginger tea per day, it will cure the fuzzy head by settling the stomach and cutting inflammation in the brain.

DETOX ORGAN SUPPORT: Methods of assisting the detox organs during a healing crisis or cleansing reaction include Epsom salt bath, castor oil pack, dry skin brushing, saunas and a cold shower, exercise, sunshine on the skin, earthing, swimming in the ocean, lymph massage, rebounding, colon hydrotherapy, activated charcoal, bentonite clay, diatomaceous earth, zeolite, colon reflorastation therapy, parasite cleanse, Epsom Salt detox baths, Castor Oil, and coffee enemas. Drink more water and get some grounding and it should pass in about 20 minutes. Get regular exercise, fresh air and nature's energies. Only the biosphere can create the EMF frequencies essential to life. Exercise benefits the brain by reducing insulin resistance and stimulating the release of growth factors that promote the growth of new blood vessels and cells.

If colonics are not possible, there are a number of ways to increase bowel activity: magnesium citrate, vitamin C in crystal form, digestive enzymes, papaya-kiwi fruit smoothies or herbal supplements such as hyssop, turkey rhubarb, burdock root, Milk Thistle or Cruciferous Vegetables, Alpha Lipoic Acid, Alka-Seltzer Gold + Glutathione + Lemon, Apple cider vinegar, Dandelion, Red Root, Sarsaparilla, Asparagus, Red Root and Red Sage. Chlorella works best when taken on an empty stomach.

Manayupa (*Desmodium molliculum*) leaf, a perennial herb found in Peru and other parts of South America, where tea of Manayupa is used to treat almost everything. Manayupa extract effectively supports detoxification of your liver, kidneys and lymphatic system.

HANGOVER CURES: B vitamins, Vitamin C, Activated Charcoal, lots of water. A teaspoon of Zeolite in a glass of water on an empty stomach. DHM (dihydromyricetin) from the Japanese Raisin Tree. Rattan tea, made from the leaves of Ampelopsis grossedentata is antioxidant and liver protecting. Other hangover teas include ginger, peppermint, lavender, chamomile and green tea. Fresh squeezed cabbage juice. Grounding, Epsom Salt bath, Magnesium chloride spray on the back of the neck.

ANDROGRAPHIS: (*Andrographis paniculata***)** is known as "bile of the earth" or King of Bitters and indeed this herb has been shown to have a strong liver protecting and bile enhancing effect. In clinical studies it has been shown to be superior to Milk Thistle in healing toxic liver damage, poor liver function and hepatitis. Hempedu Bumi has immune enhancing and anti-viral properties, is preventative effect against the common cold and also protects the insulin producing cells of the pancreas, improving glucose metabolism and diabetic retinopathy. Andrographis reduces inflammatory cytokines and helps eliminate biofilms.

COFFEE ENEMAS: If you are experiencing cleansing reactions that create painful headaches and other symptoms of toxic overload as a result of killing spirochetes, candida, or cancer cells, you might consider doing coffee enemas for pain relief. Coffee enemas stimulate production of glutathione S-transferase (GST) in the liver. GST is a powerful enzyme that binds to, metabolizes, and removes toxic substances from the body. By detoxifying the liver and colon coffee enemas treat the emotional basis of disease, treating depression and mental illness.

The palmitic acid in caffeine increases the activity of glutathione S-transferase (GST) by 600% in the liver and a 700% increase in detoxification in the small intestine. Glutathione is the primary antioxidant is primarily synthesized in the liver where it is abundantly present. The liver thus uses glutathione to neutralize poisons, e.g., alcohol, caffeine, medications, nicotine, and remove them from the blood. Glutathione participates in leukotriene synthesis for White Blood Cell mobilization (leukotrienes are a family of eicosanoid inflammatory mediators produced in leukocytes). The enzyme glutathione S-transferase makes excess free radicals water soluble for easy elimination from the cells and the body and blocks and detoxifies carcinogens. The amino acid, Cysteine is the limiting factor as N-acetyl-Cysteine (NAC), in glutathione synthesis, ensuring an adequate supply of glutathione helps cleanse the blood of toxins and substances.

For A Life Overhaul Try Green Coffee Enemas one a day for a week, then 1 every two days for a week, then once a week. Use in association with a Kelp Bath—bring 1 cup of kelp powder slowly to the boil and put in a long hot bath. Cool the bath water for a day, and put on the garden and house plants. Use an organic gold-roasted coffee with high palmitic acid specifically for enemas such as from SA WILSON. Buy only organic light roast coffee beans, or green coffee beans and grind them fresh as much as possible. Four tablespoons of coffee per quart of water is a good rule of thumb for brewing most coffees for enema use. You can also put in chamomile to soothe the colon. It is usually recommend holding the coffee about twelve to 15 minutes before expelling.If colonics are not possible, there are a number of ways to increase bowel activity: magnesium citrate, vitamin C in crystal form, digestive enzymes, papaya-kiwi fruit smoothies, herb teas or herbal supplements.

AMMONIA AND ACETALDEHYDE DETOX

We must improve the detoxification of volatile phenolic compounds such as ammonia and acetyaldehyde in order to eliminate Lyme and other pathogens. Dr Jack Kruse warns us that vegan Omega 3 supplements are most often contaminated with aldehyde.

. The following help reduce and eliminate these metabolically disruptive toxins: Ozone converts ammonia to nitrates. Glutathione, Alpha lipoic acid, Glutamate, Arginine, Ornithine, Citrulline, Taurine, Tryptophan, Glycine, Creatine, Choline, B Complex, Lethicin, Fish oil, DMAE, DHA Omega-3, Calcium D-Glucarate, D-Ribose, Ca-2 AEP, Acetyl-L-carnitine, L-carnitine, SAMe, N-acetyl-cysteine (NAC), Cysteine. Selenium, Lugol's Solution, Magnesium phosphate, Magnesium, Potassium. Sulfur foods: garlic, garlic mustard and other cabbage family members, MSM, choline, inositol, betaine, methionine.

Bentonite clay and Psyllium, Fulvic Acid from Leonardite and Shilajit, Activated Charcoal, Zeolite, Diatomaceous earth and other clays. Acidophilus, Probiotics, Lactulose. Cranberries, Goji and Camu camu. Papaya enzymes and Bromelain powder. Spirulina, Wheatgrass juice, Kelp, Slippery elm, Chia seed, celery seed, fennel seed, caraway seed, fenugreek seed.

AMMONIA DETOX HERBS: Alfalfa, Aloe, Ashwagandha root, Cordyceps, Danshen (red sage root), Devil's claw, Dong quai, Grapeseed extract, Graviola, Green tea, Neem leaf, Parsley, Sarsaparilla, Yucca root, Larch arabinogalactan. One teaspoon of Black Seed Oil morning and evening on an empty stomach helps cut ammonia and acetaldehyde in the GI tract.

Plus supplements for blood sugar regulation, nerves, liver, kidney, candida, stress, antioxidants and estrogen detoxification. Use Milk Thistle seeds with beet, Oregon grape, dandelion, wild yam, yellow dock, licorice, ginkgo biloba, barberry bark, Gotu kola, ginger, schizandra berries for liver cleansing and support.

LIVER AND KIDNEYS

The Liver and Kidneys are the most important detoxifying organs:

KIDNEY SUPPORT: Weakness of the kidneys can cause the accumulation and retention of fluids. Foods that support the kidneys include watermelon, buckwheat, onions, beans, grapes, all berries, seaweed, watercress, green magma and barely. Beta carotene, B complex and Vitamin E. Warming herbs reduce mucus, revive kidney yang and stimulate immunity, they are good for people who suffer cold and retain water in their tissues. Hepatic Herbs: Anise seed, Bayberry, Buchu, Cayenne, Celery seeds, Cinnamon, Chilli, Cloves, Coriander, Cornsilk, Couch grass, Damiana, Dandelion leaf, False Unicorn root, Fennel, Garlic, Ginkgo nuts, Ginger, Goldenseal, Gorse flower kidney tea, Horseradish, Juniper berries, Parsley, Plantain, Prickly ash, Sassafras, Stinging nettle, Rehmannia, Rosehips, Sorrel, Marshmallow, Mugwort, Mustard, Uva ursi, Watercress, Wild carrot, Wild yam, Yarrow. Java tea - (also known as kidney tea and cat whisker plant), Solidago, Birch, Restharrow.

BOLDO: Boldo is a cholagogue (bitters), meaning it will increase bile flow, thereby diluting and reducing infection of the gallbladder and formation of gallstones. Cholagogues are often also called bitters and they are used around the world. Boldo has also been used to treat urinary tract (urethra, bladder, prostate, and kidney) infections. Other urinary antiseptic herbs are Uva ursi, Buchu, Juniper berries, Kava kava, Saw palmetto, Shepherd's purse, Goldenrod, and Pipsissewa.

CRATAEVA: *Crataeva nurvala* is a small tree, is perhaps best known in Ayurvedic medicine for alleviating edema, kidney and bladder problems, especially urinary stones. It has been called the "Ayurvedic drug of choice for treating urinary disorders." Crataeva combined with Eclipta Alba (False Daisy), Katuka (Picrorhiza kurroa) Black hellebore, and achillea (yarrow) are used in the Ayurvedic tradition as specific therapies for hepatic inflammation, a disorder which can have secondary effects on urinary secretion.

SUPPORT THE LIVER

For liver pain or to stimulate its processes, castor oil packs are very effective. Castor oil contains a unique fatty acid that stimulates the liver, reduces inflammation, and increases lymphatic circulation and NK killer cell production (NK cells are lymphocytes that play a major role in deactivating viruses and combating tumors). Use fresh Juices to Soothe the Liver: Burdock root, Beets and black radishes, carrots and green leafy plants such as spinach, kale, romaine, dandelion, chickweed and other wild herbs. Since the liver has to process fats, people on a healing program should eliminate all but Omega 3, coconut oil and olive oils and stick to a low-carbohydrate diet.

STIMULATING BILE: Cholagogue herbs stimulate production and flow of bile. Cholagogues include - Artichoke leaf, Barberry root, Bupleurum, Burdock root, Celandine, Dandelion root, Goldenseal, Milk Thistle, Oregon grape root or Pau d'arco, Rosemary, Sage, Turmeric, Wormwood, Yellow Dock root. Other herbal liver remedies are Clarkia tincture, Swedish bitters, Chinese bitters, Coptis and Gold coin grass. In most cases, Gold Coin Grass tincture softens gallstones and alleviates gallbladder pain within a few days.

LIVER SUPPORT: During heavy metal detox and treatment for infectious organisms, we must guard against lipid peroxidation in the liver with protectors like glutathione and sulfur amino acids (Cysteine) from cruciferous vegetables for sulfation and detoxification: especially broccoli sprouts. L-cysteine supports liver detoxification, it is a precursor to the body's main antioxidant, Glutathione which helps prevent the peroxidation of fats and counters toxins, drugs and carcinogens.

NAC cysteine that is reputedly effective at reducing mucus in the lungs and sinuses, and cysteine will assist mercury to cross the blood brain barrier on its way out. Cysteine is a sulfur containing amino acid and flooding the body with extra sulfur at the same time satisfies the body's other competing needs for sulfur and preserves the cysteine that is relatively expensive. Always take it with twice as much Vitamin C compared to Cysteine to prevent kidney stones.

You should also eat lots of garlic, onions and eggs that are naturally rich in sulfur and take heaps of MSM in your drinking water while detoxing. Cruciferous vegetables contain a compound called glucosinolate, which can help stimulate the production of enzymes in the liver that aid in detoxification. Cabbage: is a sulfur-rich, cruciferous veggie that increases the production of antioxidant and detoxification enzymes, and stimulates the production of glutathione for liver cleansing, meaning that it helps your liver break down toxins so they can be more easily expelled.

Amino Acids For The Liver Include: Glycine, L-carnitine, N-acetyl-cysteine (NAC), SAMe, Glutamine, Methionine, Taurine and aspartate (aspartic acid).

The major component of liver cells is lecithin, which is a complex mixture of fats, namely, phosphatidylcholine, phosphatidylethanolamine, and phosphatidylinositol as main components. Additional antioxidant nutrients such as Choline, Alpha lipoic acid, Beta carotene, Vitamins C & E, B Complex, Selenium, Zinc, Beta Carotene, hydergine. The liver stores 90-95% of our Vitamin A and zinc is required for mobilization of Vitamin A stores from the liver; take brewer's yeast, seafood, pumpkin seeds and kelp for zinc.

LIVER HERBS: Artemisia, Angelica root, Barberry, Birch leaves, Black cohosh root, Burdock root, Borututu bark, Bupleurum, Carrot, Chanca Piedra, Chamomile, Chlorophyll, Corydalis, Dandelion root, Dong quai, Fennel, Garlic, Ginger, Gentian root, Goldenrod, Grapeseed, Graviola, Horsetail herb, Parsley, Plantain, Licorice, Mandrake root, Milk thistle, Mugwort, Pine Bark, Red beet root, Rehmannia, Reishi mushroom, Schisandra berries, Turmeric, Uva ursi, Wolf berries, Yarrow, Yellow dock root..

To help the liver process accumulated toxins it is good to add lemon to your drinking water throughout the day, or to mineral water for a treat. Mouth ulcers, liver disease, gallstones, fluid retention and obesity are just a few of the traditional medicinal uses watercress. Considered a liver tonic, watercress was used by Greek and Persian soldiers to increase stamina and improve health. Dihydromyricetin (DHM), a flavonoid found in Hovenia dulcis (AKA the Japanese raisin tree), helps the body metabolize alcohol more efficiently and protect liver function.

185

SPLEEN: The spleen is where red blood cells are recycled and where white blood cells, called lymphocytes, are stored. The chinese formula Gui Pi Tang (Restore the Spleen Decoction); Ginseng, Ashitaba, Dong quai, Codonopsis root, Astragalus root, Longan Fruit, Jujube seed, Poria cocos fungus, Atractylodes root, Ginger root, Black pepper, Nutmeg, Cinnamon, Cardamom, Cloves, Garlic.

ANEMIA AND LEUKEMIA: If your nails are thin, curved, or have ridges, it's usually a telltale sign of anemia or an iron deficiency. Besides increasing oxygen in the body anemia and leukemia are assisted by friction rubbing on the Tibia (Shinbone) and the forearm bones and then massage with Siberian Sea Buckthorn oil. Taking Sea Buckthorn oil internally along with Lion's Mane mushroom is capable of killing cancer cells, shrinking tumors and supporting the immune system in a variety of different cancers, including lung, stomach, esophagus, large intestine and cervical cancer. Lion's Mane mushroom and Sea Buckthorn oil is a good combination to support mucus membranes, including for esophageal cancer. Lion's mane extract may protect against the development of stomach ulcers by inhibiting the growth of H. pylori and protecting the stomach lining from damage.

Vitamin B12 is needed to produce an adequate amount of healthy red blood cells in the bone marrow. Vitamin B12 is available only in animal foods (meat and dairy products) or yeast extracts (such as brewer's yeast). Vitamin B12 deficiency is defined by low levels of stored B12 in the body that can result in anemia, a lower-than-normal number of red blood cells. Ten micrograms of B12 spread over a day appears to supply as much as the body can use. B12, Folic Acid, Vitamin K2 and Vitamin D3 plus daily sunlight on the body while lying on the grass/ground/sand for electrons.

Food sources of iron needed for hemoglobin include rich dark leafy greens and microgreens and sprouts, blackstrap molasses, chlorophyll rich leafy greens like spinach and kale, beetroot, spirulina, local edible weeds, mulberry leaves, shellfish and organic liver. Magnetite or Shungite pendant, far-infrared, amethyst crystals and negative ions. Spinal healing with sound (didgeridoo or bowls).

Tapping of the Thymus gland while deep breathing. Bone Marrow Breathing. IV Vitamin C has been known to eliminate leukemia and other cancers. A study found DRIED GINGER is 6x stronger than chemotherapy for killing cancer stem cells. They used dried ginger for the trial, however the fresh root must also be just as viable or even more so. Drinking lots of ginger tea rapidly drops your bad bug load. Semi-rawish Thai food is a good way to get all the anti-inflammatory spices and coconut in our diet. Cut, Burn and Poison Cancer treatment is not a cure, but a cause of cancer. Chemo harms the immune system rather than making it more intelligent.

VISUAL ACUITY: When first waking in the morning good blood supply and oxygen to the eyes, combined with REM sleep chemistry increases visual acuity on awakening, which subsequently disappears on the gravity of standing and the habitual nature of the daily morning. Drinking Gorse flower tea, Borage tea, Goji, Blueberries, Ziziphus jujuba and taking brain oxygen enhancers like germanium, Vinpocetine, Ginkgo, Butterbur root, Astaxanthin: red algae carotenoid and spirulina will help strengthen visual acuity during the day. Gotu kola protects the blood vessels that supply oxygen to the brain. B vitamins also improve the amount of red blood cells in the blood stream therefore carrying more healthy oxygen to the brain cells. For a medicinal fix take 1-3 tsp of cayenne pepper per day...mixed with raw vege juice, put in capsules with other herbs, make spicy Indian and Thai food etc... Your visual acuity will improve immediately. NAC and garlic mustard in your smoothies greatly magnifies the vividness of eyesight and improves perception.

EYES: The corrosion of the eyes cannot be good for the health of the corneas. I think that fresh coconut water mixed with distilled water might be a good eye wash to use after you have been outdoors under chem-assault. I suggest everyone get an eye washing glass. Nostrils and eyes will need to be cleaned after being in out in a thick chemtrail stew.

Eyesight is destroyed by eating cooked, frozen, processed industrial foods. Destroys the bonding angles, electrical potentials, shapes of tissues in the body as it relates to water. Also impaired mineral assimilation, utilization, mineral deficiency—especially silicon, zinc, selenide. Oxidation of tissues, insufficient hydration of eye parts, inadequate nerve and blood supply, and now artificial light and EMF sources all contribute to weakening the eyes. Eating goji berries and fresh pumpkin seeds and raw vege juices is a start, but ultimately food must be grown through green alchemy-high biogenic principles to be of maximally regenerative.

The eye lens's major antioxidant substances are: Vitamins C, E, and A or beta-carotene, Astaxanthin, Vitamin K2, N-acetylcarnosine, carnosine, glutathione, cysteine ascorbate, Ornithine, Calcium pyruvate, and taurine, coenzyme Q10, Alpha lipoic, Gingko, Cat's claw, Goji berries for beta carotene, blueberries, all berries including blueberries and bilberries; Spirulina, B vitamins, riboflavin, DHEA, Hemp and other Omega 3, green tea. The retinas of the eyes contain the most amount of DHA Omega 3 in the body.

Blue light from computer screens and TVs blocks DHA production in the retina which prevents DHA being conveyed to all cells of the body. Horsetail, Oatstraw and Nettle teas for silicon, necessary for hydration, collagen and the lens's gel shape. Beer is also an important source of silicon made soluble from the grains through the fermentation process. Pine needle sun tea also contains phytonutrients protective of eye structures.

It's believed that lutein and zeaxanthin, the primary **carotenoids** concentrated in the macula of the eye act to counter the free-radical forming action of light and oxygen. Egg yolks and maize having the highest lutein content and orange peppers having the highest zeaxanthin content. Lutein in spinach, kale, dandelion leaves and other dark green vegetables. Eyes also need Kelp and the minerals selenium, zinc, potassium and most importantly magnesium.

FLOATERS IN THE EYES: Most eye floaters are caused by age-related changes inside the eyes where microscopic clumps of protein within the vitreous gel tend to clump and can cast tiny shadows on your retina. Internal remedies for Floaters in the Eyes: Stephania tincture, Chlorella, Zeolite, Carbon 60, Fenugreek sprouts, Hyaluronic acid, Glucosamine sulfate, Vitamin C, L-methionine, L-carnitine, Inositol, Silicon, Zinc, Copper, Chromium. Internal remedies for Floaters: Colloidal silver eye drops. Stephania Root decoction or eye wash is used to help heal Lyme eyes and stringy, twisty floaters in the eyes.

Magnetite Eye Pillow: A eye pillow filled with magnetite sand, in a velvet cover, can be placed over on the eyes or the forehead while meditating and also to normalize painful inflamed areas of the body. This little tool is great to take to bed to ease aches, pains and congestion anywhere on the body.

INSECT BITES WITH NANO VENOM

Since insects bio-accumulate nano aluminum and other toxins from the chemtrailed air, it is certain that those dangerous metals are going to end up in insect venom. This could make an insect bite elicit an exaggerated immune-inflammatory response similar to adjuvants in vaccines. Adjuvants keep the vaccine antigens in the body longer thereby increasing the adaptive immune response to the vaccine. These adjuvants probably affect antigen residence time, the spatio–temporal behavior of the antigen and the amount of the antigen that eventually reaches the adaptive immune cell receptors on T and B lymphocytes. An alternative theory the danger theory proposed by Matzinger suggests that adjuvants trigger innate and adaptive immunity via responding to **cell death or damage** rather than nonself molecules.

Insect Bites Natural Treatments Include: Oatmeal packs, Baking soda, Vinegar, ice, raw honey, Aloe vera, Helichrysum essential oil, Calendula, Cinnamon, Lemon balm, Turmeric juice, Garlic, Onion, Witch hazel, Chamomile tea, fresh Sage or Basil leaves, 3% hydrogen peroxide.

Treat insect bites immediately with essential oils of Savory, Clove, Oregano, Thyme or Sage. A paste of colloidal silver and cayenne pepper placed on the bite may help. A nano detox bath as soon after the bite will catch the poison before it sets in: 1/4 cup Epsom salt, 1/4 cup sea salt & 1/4 cup borax with essential oils and soak in hot water 30 min or so.

Bentonite clay mixed with activated charcoal, colloidal silver, Lugol's and essential oils will provide **immediate relief from bites**. (This is also a toothpaste recipe).

A tick and mosquito repellent can be made from the following essential oils diluted with a carrier oil such as Jojoba oil: Marjoram, Citrus Eucalyptus, Juniper, Wormwood, Helichrysum, Tea Tree and Citronella.

Consider making a foot oil with Neem oil, Caster oil, Blackseed oil and camphor essential oil. Rub this mix on your feet daily and wear socks. This is worth trying to help eliminate parasitic worms and insects. There appears to be a body invading insect component to the chemtrail holocaust. We are entering new territory with the dark side's high tech chimeras.

Grow a Herb Garden as we have to be ready to use natural remedies for whatever ailments arise because the allopathetic medical world will not even acknowledge the reality of the changing terrain of anthropogenic disease symptoms, nor admit to their causal origins.

BUILDING COLLAGEN

Collagens are extracellular matrix fiber molecules in skin connective tissue and comprise about 80% of the extracellular material, contributing to its strength and facilitating elasticity, tightening, and the cell integrity of the skin. Collagen is the most abundant protein in mammals, making up from 25% to 35% of the whole-body protein content. Collagen is a key protein and connective tissue component that supports and connects bone, muscle, internal organs, cartilage and skin. The dermis is a deeper layer of human skin that supports the blood vessels and nerves while maintaining other functions.

Major extracellular components of the dermis are the ground substance, collagen fibers, and elastins, all of which are important to maintain the physiological functions of the skin. More than 20 different subtypes of collagen have been identified, with Type 1 collagen being the predominant form in the human skin, accounting for 70–90% of the total. It is synthesized by fibroblasts. Reduction in the number and function of fibroblasts subsequently cause a decrease of the collagen content in skin and thus lead to signs of skin aging, such as skin thinning, wrinkles, and a decline in elasticity.

Collagen is rich in glycine, proline and alanine, and in the unusual amino acid hydroxyproline. Vitamin C catalyzes the post-translational hydroxylation of proline and lysine residues incorporated into various proteins found in supporting tissues such as collagen, bone and intercellular cement. Hydroxylation of these residues imparts tensile strength by allowing fibers to cross-link within the proteins. It is important to note that collagen which is synthesized in the absence of Vitamin C is insufficiently hydroxylated meaning the abnormal collagen cannot properly form fibers and, thus causes the skin lesions and blood vessel fragility that are so prominent in scurvy.

As you age, collagen levels decrease and collagen strength declines, resulting in the appearance of wrinkles and lines on your face and body. Your skin becomes thinner, drier and loses its elasticity. Weak collagen allows pathogens to dissolve tissue and to squeeze between epithelial cells and invade throughout the body. Vitamin C, Lysine and Proline are needed to build strong collagen to protect against the spread of fungal, bacterial, mycoplasma and viral infections. Lysine is essential for tissue growth and repair and it inhibits the hyaluronidase enzyme that candida and cancer uses to break down collagen in order for the fungi or cancer to spread throughout the body.

HYALURONIC ACID: The stronger our collagen the more resistant the body is against microbe attack and inflammation, creating a protective barrier against microorganisms. Hyaluronic acid is a type of carbohydrate that lubricates and hydrates the eyes and the joints. The polymer Hyaluronic Acid found in human skin assists in retaining moisture, providing cushioning, helping to repair damaged tissue, maintaining the collagen and elastin matrix. Foods such as leafy greens, root vegetables and soy products contain it, while homemade broths made from animal bones, skin and connective tissues are even better sources.

COLLAGEN SUPPORTING FOODS: Supplementation with glucosamine, glycine, proline, Lysine, vitamin C, copper, manganese, magnesium and zinc can help to restore elasticity and strength to connective tissue. Quinoa is a complete protein, which means it has all nine essential amino acids. Quinoa can delay visible signs of aging, like fine lines and wrinkles, by stimulating the skin to produce new collagen. The content of tryptophan and lysine in quinoa protein is three times higher than that in whole wheat; quinoa can be sprouted and eaten raw to preserve the proteins. The main component of connective tissue is collagen. It is structured as three protein strands arranged as a triple helix, and is the most abundant protein in the body. Sulfur plays a role in the formation of muscle, skin, hair and nails and is a major building block of collagen, the connective tissue that makes up cartilage.

Dark green vegetables, lycopenes, avocado, green and black olives, eggs, wheat germ (proline), legumes (lysine), garlic and garlic mustard (sulfur), Alpha lipoic acid, kiwifruit and other foods high in Vitamin C like citrus fruits, bell peppers, and Brussels sprouts. Legumes and lean meats are good sources of lysine; and egg whites, meats, cheese, and soy all contain proline. Shellfish, nuts, and red and lean meats are all sources of copper, as are leafy greens such as turnip greens, spinach, Swiss chard, kale, mustard greens and asparagus

Alpha Lipoic acid is a naturally occurring organo-sulfur compound that boosts collagen production and maximizes the effectiveness and performance of our cells. Alpha Lipoic acid actually and revitalizes the antioxidant power of vitamin C and other antioxidants. The anthocyanins found in deep-colored, red-blue berries, beets and red seaweed help the collagen fibers link together in a way that strengthens the connective tissue matrix and green and white tea help prevent the breakdown of collagen. A lack of zinc in your diet could be the reason your nails are weak, with white spots or not growing. Oysters are rich in zinc, as are pumpkin seeds, sesame seeds, lamb, beef, and oats.

For healthy skin, hair and nails take the B vitamin Biotin (B7) 2.5mg daily. Biotin is important to fatty acid metabolism and cell growth. It is found in egg yolks, almonds, and sweet potato, swiss chard, wheat germ, whole grains, and salmon. Vitamin A supports collagen formation. Carrots, spinach, tomatoes, sweet potatoes, mangoes and apricots are all good sources of beta-carotene which your body converts to vitamin A. Vitamin E provides protection against free radicals and premature aging caused by sun damage and environmental pollutants. Eat foods such as nuts, avocado, spinach, whole grains and seafood for your vitamin E intake. Hawthorn, Japanese Knotweed, Kudzu, Red Sage, Echinacea, Scutellaria and Selenium support collagen strength.

LYSINE: Lysine is an essential amino acid, meaning that it cannot be manufactured by the body and must be obtained through the diet. Because it has to be obtained in the diet L-lysine is the rate limiting amino acid in the production of collagen. Vegans often do not get enough in their diet and can end up being deficient. It helps in calcium absorption, to form collagen in the bones and connective tissue and to produce carnitine, a nutrient responsible for converting fatty acids into energy and lowering cholesterol. L-lysine deficiency interferes with the normal circadian release of serotonin, thereby increasing stress-induced anxiety.

L-lysine benefits include treating herpes, increasing calcium absorption, reducing diabetes-related illnesses and improving gut health. Deficiencies in L-lysine have even been linked to behavioral problems. Threonine and Lysine is found in cottage cheese and wheat germ, chicken, brewers yeast, eggs and other protein foods.

MARINE COLLAGEN: Collagen that is derived from fish scales has a high concentration of glycine, hydroxyproline and proline. The hydroxyproline peptides stimulate cells in the skin, joints and bones, and lead to collagen synthesis through cell activation and growth. Fish collagen peptides have the best absorption and bioavailability due to their smaller particle sizes compared to other animal collagens. This allows the collagen to be absorbed at a higher level through the intestinal barrier into the bloodstream and carried throughout the body. The collagen rich parts of the fish, mainly the heads, skin, bones, fins and scales, can be made into homemade fish stock.

SILICON: Silicon is the architectural element to the collagen molecule and essential to tissue hydration and youthfulness. Collagen provides the cushion for your bones and joints and it is strengthened, hydrated and youthified by silicon. Babies have 30 times the silicon in their bodies compared to adults, and silicon assimilation does down as we age and digestive fire is impaired. The body burns through collagen during kundalini awakening, so you need to increase your silicon for bones, skin, hair and ligaments. A silicon rich diet is thus important to counteract aging. Silicon is found in Horsetail, Oatstraw, Nettles, Hemp leaves, Eyebright, Cornsilk, Comfrey, Lemongrass, Ginger root, Alfalfa, Blue cohosh, Chickweed, Dandelion, Red raspberry.

OPC's: (Oligomeric Proanthocyanidins) are a set of bioflavonoid complexes that perform as free radical scavengers in the human body. These polyphenols are found in a variety of plants such as Citrus skin, Grapeseed, Pinebark, Cocoa beans, Apples, Cinnamon, Aronia berries, and Sea buckthorn berries. They have many healing properties such as improved Vitamin C utilization, skin hydration, UV protection, strengthens blood vessels, improves eyesight and supports the collagen and elastin of the skin.

HUMAN GROWTH HORMONE: Growth Hormone Release inhibits the formation of fat and mobilizes existing stores; it also increases the tensile strength of structural protein, collagen, preventing sagging skin. To increase HGH take Arginine, Ornithine, Tyrosine, B12, B6, Vitamin C. Also Creatine, Tryptophan. Choline from DMAE, lecithin and Alpha-GPA. 500mg Acetyl L-Carnitine with 30-100mg Ornithine HCl at bedtime at least 3 hours after last meal. Don't eat sweets, refined foods or alcohol within four hours of bedtime as these inhibit HGH release.

PANAX GINSENG: Panax ginseng, (also known as Asian ginseng, Chinese ginseng, or Korean ginseng), is the original source of ginseng. Sun Ginseng Increases Type I Collagen production for a firmer, more elastic skin. Ginseng contains a large number of phytonutrients that stimulate skin regeneration. Ginseng is a highly anti-aging, skin revitalizing root, packed full of phytonutrients and antioxidants neutralize free radicals. It also contains active compounds that can increase the production of collagen and elastin in the middle dermis layer of the skin, making your skin more firm, elastic, and more resilient to damage. Panax ginseng stimulate collagen synthesis, and protect human keratinocytes and fibroblasts from photo damage by modulating the cellular signaling involved in the UV-induced cell death and/or carcinogenesis. The anti-inflammatory and anti-oxidative effects of Panax ginseng on human keratinocytes is effective in protecting human skin against aging processes. (Alma (Emblica officinalis) and Lupinus albus also show similar effects).

191

UV PROTECTION

Exposure to Ultraviolet (UV) light erodes the collagen and elastin matrix responsible for elasticity. This damage can show up as wrinkles, hyperpigmentation, sagging skin or even cancerous melanomas. Eating antioxidant rich fruits and vegetables and is an excellent way to improve sun resistance. Eating red seaweeds also offers UV protection as it contains a variety of pigments, including chlorophyll, red phycoerythrin, blue phycocyanin, and carotenoids like lutein, and zeaxanthin.

Astaxanthin the pigment from Red algae has the unique property of protecting the entire cell because of the polar hydrophilic ends that span across the entire cell membrane. UV protecting oils include Sesame oil which resists 30% of UV rays, while coconut, peanut, olive, and cottonseed oils block out about 20%. Spray skin with chamomile and green tea after being out in the sun for prolonged periods.

An aloe-astaxanthin lotion would amplify effects of a colloidal silver topical 5G protection. There's plenty of natural SPF out there — in your food: tomato paste (rich in lycopene) served with olive oil increased the protection against sunburn by 33%, Carrots are rich in carotenoids, long-term intake of vitamin C, together with vitamin E, can reduce the sunburn reaction to UVB irradiation. Selenium actually works together with vitamin E, vitamin C, glutathione and vitamin B3 as an antioxidant to prevent free radical damage in the body. Omega-3s from flaxseed has anti-inflammatory properties and research suggests that they could protect the skin from UV damage.

POMEGRANATES: Due to the red pigment, when pomegranate extract was used in conjunction with sunscreen, it increased the SPF by 20 percent. Pomegranate seeds – the polyphenols in the pomegranate seeds, protect the skin from both UVA and UVB free radicals. They can enhance the sun protection factor of sunscreen by up to 25% and also inhibit hyper-pigmentation. Snack on the seeds or toss them into a salad. UVB radiation causes DNA damage, protein oxidation, glycation and induces matrix metalloproteinases (MMPs). MMPs are also thought to play a major role in cell behaviors such as cell proliferation, migration (adhesion/dispersion), differentiation, angiogenesis, apoptosis, and host defense.

EUPHORBIA PEPLUS: The sap of Petty Spurge (Cancer Weed, Radium Weed) has been used for treating Sun Spots, Moles, Warts, Corns and non-melanoma skin cancer (squamous cell carcinoma). This is done by carefully putting some of the milky latex sap extracted from the freshly cut stem onto the Sun Spot or Wart. The plant's sap is toxic and "burns off" any skin that it came into contact with, especially to rapidly-replicating human tissue. Apply the sap twice per day, after 7-10 days the scab heals and falls off. Put live/raw Aloe vera juice on after the blemish has been removed. Grow a container of Euphorbia peplus along with Aloe Vera so you always have it on hand to remove melanoma and blemishes.

SKIN SUGGESTIONS

• Spray skin and hair with silicon rich Philosopher's water or Horsetail infusion to strengthen and hydrate.

• Presently I am using clay masques, hyaluronic acid before moisturizer during the day, papaya skins rubbed on, or papaya enzyme powder at night.

• **Carrot seed oil**, Squalane oil or Rosehip Oil under eyes and on wrinkles.

• **Black Seed Oil** can be used as the base oil for essential oil skin preparations, or as a makeup cleansing oil.

• **Clove essential oil** is the most antiseptic, more so than Tea Tree oil.

• **Helichrysum** essential oil, has a strong ability to lower inflammation due to inflammatory enzyme inhibition and free radical scavenging. It is excellent for oral infections, even better than clove!

• **Wheatgrass juice** and bentonite clay powder face/body packs. * The wheatgrass-bentonite green mixture is very gentle on the skin and will oxygenate, is antioxidant and healing. Bentonite you could get from your health store. You can also add Fulvic acid or Leonardite to clay face packs.

• **Hyaluronic Acid** found in human skin assists in retaining moisture, providing cushioning, helping to repair damaged tissue, maintaining the collagen and elastin matrix and creating a protective barrier against microorganisms. Hyaluronic acid gel can be used as a skin humidifier both day and night.

• **Papaya skins** rubbed on the skin or skulp and left on overnight

• **Royal Jelly** mixed with Vit E/Vit A cream and left on overnight

• **Goop** from growing buckwheat sprouts is also great strengthener and soother if left on the skin overnight.

• **Hydrolyzed Collagen** combined with Calcium and Vitamin D improves bone health better than combining Calcium and D only.

• **Vitamin K2** found in wheatgrass juice also put capsules of K2 oil on skin (swansonvitamins.com)

• **Coconut Water** - Guaranteed instant youthifying is to put the sieved water of a young or white coconut in spray bottle and spray skin. This is good for hair conditioning and styling also.

• **Onion Skin/Chamomile Spray.** Gently made (low temperature ie: don't boil) infusion of ground chamomile flowers, sieved, put through coffee filter and put in spray bottle, keep in fridge and spray skin several times a day…good for hair also.

• **Urine** - The first urine of the day is an exceptional youthifier for hair and skin. Urine of a rawfoodest who eats fenugreek sprouts and B-vitamins is a great hair spray great for styling hair. You can leave a light spray on your skin while sleeping. Very good for chapped, cracked feet.

• **Apple Cider Vinegar** makes a great antiseptic, healing sores, cracked feet, toenail fungi and acne. Reduce excess bacterial/fungi with apple cider vinegar spray, but keep away from the eyes.

• **Clove essential oil** is one of the most antiseptic, more so than Tea tree oil.

• Drinking **schisandra berry** tea has a profound anti-inflammatory effect on joints, skin and eyes. Infusion can be sprayed on the skin.

• **Sulfur** - Various sources of sulfur as in cabbage, fermented cabbage, MSM, DMSO are also great for skin.

• **Christopher Hobbs** gives the following herbs for skin problems: plantain, aloe, calendula, Gotu kola, Oregon grape root, St. John's wort, chamomile and lavender.

• Probiotics, papaya smoothies, all the beta carotenes, goji berries, kelp and lemon water, red algae and spirulina and all silicon rich plants are great for the skin.

• You could also take lysine, proline, vitamin C and or collagen, lecithin, sunflower seeds, fenugreek sprouts and other connective tissue builders.

• L-carnitine, vitamin C, E and iron are necessary for the formation of healthy skin cells. However avoid animal food sources of carnitine to prevent the buildup of cholesterol in the inflammatory cells in the atherosclerotic plaques in our arteries.

• I buy my clay (and herbs etc) from herbalcom.com, you can also add papaya (papain) or pineapple (bromelain) enzymes to the clay paste. Enzymes dissolve tissue and speed regrowth. Papain is also a powerful mucus solvent that helps to cleanse the intestinal walls and tissues of waste matter. Papain has the ability to breakdown proteins and converts some of it into Arginine which increases Growth Hormone Release.

DEAD SEA MASQUE: The dead sea mud is so filled with minerals that it rapidly restructures the skin, so you can use it to get rid of blemishes, sores, wounds, scars, dark pigment spots etc... The dead sea mud is black with minerals, and is more caustic and faster acting than regular clay, it seems to eat through dead, damaged tissue and will eliminate scabs in a rapid but caring fashion. The dead sea mud is very medicinal you will have to buy online from ebay perhaps. Bentonite is good, but the black dead sea clay is many times stronger, so I have to mix it with bentonite to slow its healing effect as it kills necrotic skin leaving dark patches until they can be rubbed off as the new skin forms.

The dead sea clay will be stronger at repolarizing, don't forget to do under the jaw and down the neck. Mixing clay powder with fresh wheatgrass juice makes it twice as powerful as a skin masque. The Dead sea mud is so filled with minerals that it rapidly restructures the skin, so you can use it to get rid of blemishes, sores, wounds, scars, dark pigment spots etc... The dead sea mud is black with minerals, and is more caustic and faster acting than regular clay, it seems to eat through dead, damaged tissue and will eliminate scabs in a rapid but caring fashion.

LIGHTEN PIGMENTATION: Anything that holds water in the structures of the body, that moves things around will help. Kelp, silicon (horsetail/ nettle), enzymes (papain, bromelain), garlic mustard (methylation), bentonite clay internally and externally, MSM (sulfur), Dong quai (hormones), licorice root, inside papaya skins rubbed on face and left overnight, Aloe vera leaves, Fenugreek sprouts or tea. Kojic acid from Aspergillus oryzae used to ferment soybeans for miso.

NATURAL HAIR TINTING: For ladies (or men) who are blond and going gray or white, you can even out your color and condition your hair with the following recipe: 1/3 cup of ground chamomile flowers and the skin of 1 yellow onion. Put these in 2 cups of water in a crockpot and heat on low for about 8 hrs. Sieve, then run liquid through a coffee filter or fine mesh, and put into a spray bottle. With this you can spray all your hair and spray more-so into your roots and scalp to assist healing, as well as the areas turning white or gray. The mixture is also youthifying for your face, neck and decolletage. The same recipe can be used for brown hair by using red onion skin, chamomile and spent coffee grounds instead; while redheads can use red onion skin and marigold flowers. This recipe removes gray color and fizz, while promoting hair body, strength, shine and health. It works like magic. Keep the bulk of your spray in a bottle in the fridge, from which you fill up a small spray bottle this way it stays fresh for up to 5 days.

BUILDING STRONG BONES: To build healthy bones you need grounding, sunshine (D3), K2 from (wild) greens and exercise. Silicon is more important to bones than calcium and you can drink Philosopher's Water for that…even the spine elongates and is youthified. Silicon is the architectural keystone to the collagen molecule. Bones are made mostly of collagen protein, which provides a soft framework, and calcium phosphate largely makes up the mineral content that adds strength and hardens the framework. The ideal source of calcium in the diet is dark leafy greens. Eggshells provide calcium phosphate along with trace minerals magnesium, Boron, Manganese needed to build strong bones. Eggshells can be ground up and put on your vege garden or the soil of your sprouting operation. There's a story that Einstein often ate lunch comprised of hard-boiled eggs & chicken noodle soup, where he cooked them together in the pot to save time. If it is good enough for Einstein, it is good enough for us.

PAIN RELIEF

Pain is a cry for attention! Pain can be a sign of weakness, congestion, obstruction, lack of movement, lack of energy, fatigue, poor construction, separation from nature, neglect, dis-ease or disease, dysregulation, extremes and/or damage.

Sugar and cereals makes the nerves more sensitive to pain and weakens the protein structures in the body, it also encourages yeast which produces toxins that increase pain. Any increase in calcium/magnesium in the blood will reduce pain via alkalinizing. Silicon is transmuted into calcium in the body, silicon rich herbs are: Nettle, Oatstraw, Horsetail, Eyebright, Cornsilk, Comfrey, Lemongrass, Ginger.

DMSO-Magnesium spray, infrared wand, hot and cold, acupressure, and scenar devices help to relieve painful muscles and joints. For arthritic and inflammation pain alternate various painkillers such as frankincense, celery seed, CBD, Teasel root, Devil's claw, Turmeric, Cayenne, White willow bark, Valerian, Passion Fruit flowers, Kratom, Kudzu root, Lemon Balm, Celandine.

A histamine flush using 50mcg Niacin taken with ½ tsp D-Ribose in water will warm the body against pain. 1-3 tsp of cayenne pepper per day greatly reduces pain. Olive Leaf is essential for easing the sense of raw nerve pain by protecting nerve sheaths; plus lecithin and Omega 3 to build up nerve sheaths. Lion's Mane mushrooms contain a group of compounds that are able to regenerate the myelin sheath on the axons of neurons. Whole food sources of Omega 3 are Hemp seed, Flax seed, Chia Seed, Perilla seed, Moringa Leaf, wild salmon and Blue Green Algae.

Rhodiola rosea gives such a boost to the immune system and adrenals that it reduces pain…as does sunbathing (vitamin D). By aiding the adrenal glands licorice will also reduce pain, as will Gingko by improving circulation and oxygen supply. White willow (*Salix alba*) is the original source of aspirin. The bark of white willow has a longer half-life in the body than aspirin does.

The Beta-carotene in pumpkin, goji berries, papaya and other orange fruit and vegetables reduces pain. Papaya leaf/seeds and papain or bromelain enzymes will also reduce pain. You can also get significant pain relief with B complex, Alpha lipoic acid and vitamin C. Kelp will provide the minerals for enzymes and high integrity cells. The more mineral dense and antioxidant rich our tissues, the less pain we are in.

A happy liver is essential to a pain free body. By boosting both zinc and selenium this will increase free radical (antioxidant) protection thereby reduce pain. Milk thistle will help the liver to detoxify, once the liver is healed this helps all tissues to reinstate their integrity. Anything GREEN reduces pain and depression by increasing oxygen and by alkalinizing, remineralizing and detoxifying. Raw cabbage reduces pain very effectively by helping the liver, it can be added to daily vegetable juice intake

Anything that buffers and alkalinizes acids/toxins/free radicals will reduce pain. The ionic effect of clay does this, either taken internally or as a clay mask, body-pack, or bath. Baths made from a tea of ginger root, peppermint (is cooling and boosts energy), and catnip, chamomile, borage, comfrey, basil, burdock will reduce pain. Also 1 Tbsp of Caster oil added to the bath helps the body to gently detoxify and leads to a feeling of expansion. Mineral salts from thermal areas added to the bath will also reduce pain and provide energy. Get some pure rosemary essential oil and rub into your temples, neck, shoulders, spine, feet and calves. Grow rosemary and encapsulate it also, and use it as a tea or in food, it's a major antioxidant and nerve protector.

OTHER HERBS FOR PAIN: Aloe extract, Kava Kava, Sheep's Sorrel, Olive Leaf, Valerian root, Wild Yam, Garlic, Ginkgo, Lemon balm, Catnip, Chaparral, Chamomile, Yucca root, Borage, California poppy, Kratom, Marijuana, Mullen, Marshmallow, Slippery Elm, White Oak Bark, Elderflower, Licorice, Jamaican Dogwood, Indian Pipe, Peppermint. Cardamon, Dong quai and Angelica have warming, blood and chi moving properties. Sassafras/Ginger/Cinnamon stick chi would also be good for arthritis type pains, giving a warming grounding feeling. Feverfew might be useful to counter the effect of excessive opiate production, dizziness, brain and nerve pressure from an overactive nervous system.

INCARVILLEA SINENSIS: Trumpet Flower is an Asian herbaceous plant that shows tremendous promise for its relaxing and pain relieving properties. Extraction (tincture or tea) of the whole plant of *Incarvillea sinensis* is used for as an analgesic and anti-inflammatory for arthritis and cancer pain, headache, stomach ache, neuralgia, insomnia, restlessness and anxiety etc... Incarvillea may be used as a potentiator of similar herbs like corydalis, California poppy, prickly poppy and kava.

AKUAMMA SEED: In traditional African medicine, *Picralima nitida* seeds are used for the treatment of malaria, pathogens/parasites/protozoan and diarrhoea. It is used as a painkiller and for its anti-fever, anti-diabetic and anti-inflammatory effects. It is structurally related to both yohimbine and kratom. The fruit pulp, possesses hypoglycemic properties, and Akuammicine, a compound from the seeds has demonstrated to 'stimulate glucose uptake' thus overcoming insulin resistance, a causal factor in all degenerative disease.

OVERCOMING DEPRESSION

Depression is a cultural dis-ease or social disorder associated with captivity and the stress of futility.

The Left brain/Left body pain associated with "blocked" kundalini flow... is probably cultural. The leftbrain adaptive brain has reached the end of the rope with regard to narcissistic will over our personal and collective existence. The behaviors of displacement, diversion, dissociation, and self-gratifying addictions that are telltale signs of deep underlying depression are becoming so pervasive that our lives largely constitute a drive to escape our own existence. As Jordon Peterson and others say, we must "face into our suffering of the world forthright," to achieve meaning, merit, competency, responsibility and self-realization. If we heal our brain and develop binaural hemispheric equilibrium we can then overcome our suffering by opening up to suffering, and stop running from our own existence.

Psychological adjustment to the chemtrail holocaust requires accepting the reality of human evil, and then moving on to create the Best Life Ever, regardless of the cultural circumstances. The extra survival pressures, in contrast to the worldwide movement in social awakening provides a powerful opportunity to stop being our own worst enemy, and to get out of our own way and Thrive!

Depression involves burnout of the noradrenaline adrenergic receptors, along with serotonergic deficits. To rectify the serotonin deficiency L-tryptophan has been used for depression and as an adjunct therapy for brain disorders including OSD, ADD, panic and sleeping disorder, Alzheimer's, migraines, and food/drug/alcohol addictions, suicidal behavior and sexual dysfunction. Niacin, 5-HTP and melatonin are important metabolites derived from tryptophan.

Supplements that help restore emotional equilibrium include L-Theanine, 5 HTP (L-tryptophan), DL-Phenylalanine, B Complex, B-12, Choline/DMAE, omega-3, vinpocetine, DHEA, S-Adenosylmethionine (SAMe), Alpha GPC (choline), N-Acetyl Cysteine (NAC) and Phenylethylamine (PEA). Beta Carotene, Lithium orotate, Selenium and Zinc, Vitamin C, Alpha lipoic, Melatonin, Nerve Growth Factor agent Huperzine A, CALM formula. Through its multiple roles in producing ATP energy, NADH energizes the brain thereby reducing depression (take flush Niacin and D-Ribose). Chromium Picolinate cuts carbohydrate cravings in people with depression. Stress is synonymous with inflammation and both lead to depression. Depressed patients retain salt and fluid probably due to extra secretion of the stress hormone aldosterone (sodium retaining hormone) — progesterone reduces bloating and depression.

HERBS FOR DEPRESSION AND ANXIETY: Ashwagandha, Borage, Black cohosh, Burdock leaves, Bala, Caapi, CBD oil, Corallorhiza Maculata, Chamomile, Catnip, California poppy, Codonopsis, Comfrey, Cowslip, Evening primrose, Feverfew, Gelsemium, Ginger root, Ginseng, Gorse flowers, Gotu kola, Green tea, Hop flowers, Kava kava, Red Thai Kratom, Lemon balm, Licorice, Linden flowers, Motherwort, Maca, Mucuna pruriens with Banisteriopsis caapi. Muira puama, Oat leaf, Papaya, Passion flower, Peppermint, Red clover flowers, Rhodiola, Rosemary, Skullcap, Spirulina, Valerian, Yarrow, St John's Wort, Yellow dock, Yerba mate. Devil's claw is anti-inflammatory and analgesic. Garlic Mustard, Cabbage family and probiotics. Bacopa Monnieri activates GABA.

KRATOM: *Mitragyna speciosa* is a tropical evergreen tree, native to Southeast Asia in the coffee and gardenia family. In natural medicine as a stimulant (at low doses), sedative (at high doses), kratom offers relief from physical and emotional pain, depression, and anxiety. It is a medicine for diarrhea and treatment for opiate addiction. Kratom is perfect to relieve the underlying discomfort and disquiet of inflammation as we undertake our deep heavy metal cleansing, colon cleansing, fasting and pathogen/parasite routines. You need less than 1/2 tsp/day and it eliminates nerve pain, joint inflammation, depression and fatigue. However memory recall can be impaired if used long term, so it is best used episodically. I think it is best to use Kratom daily during the first month or two of systematic healing or life change and then switch to another painkiller like CBD oil or tincture, combined with herbal anti-inflammatories such as galangal, ginger and turmeric for chronic pain conditions.

Rather than suppressing pain we must first address the underlying reasons for pain, which are usually lack of grounding, cooked diet and toxic substance intake, alcohol, insufficient herbs and wild plants, PTSD, lack of exercise and insufficient grounding and sunshine. Kratom is good for forgetting pain and trauma for it makes one equanimous, carefree and more social. Not being on path with our highest calling or true vocation, or living in an unconscious community will also create underlying spiritual pain and emotional anguish. When we are more connected to our soul, our higher senses are more active, allowing us to feel more connected to the Universe and Creation. Cognitive communion involves good perception and goodwill towards others, where there is syntropy, rather than entropy; and people are not scheming to "get something out of" or to "get on top of" others.

BOBINSANA: *Calliandra angustifolia* (Leguminoseae, Mimosaceae) is a gentle healing plant that has been used for thousands of years by the people of the Peruvian Amazon to heal wounds of the heart, enhance love, empathy, compassion, clarity, and concentration. Bobinsana is also used for its potent lucid and colorful dream inducing effects. As an herbal remedy, bobinsana is most commonly used as a tonic for colds, rheumatism, arthritis and uterine issues. Bobinsana is thought to help support the immune system as well. Bobinsana can also be prepared as an herbal bath.

BALA ROOT: Sida cordifolia contains small amount of ephedrine alkaloids so is useful for weight loss, and boosting physical endurance and strength. Bala's name means "strength" alluding to its bitter stimulant, painkiller, and tonic that strengthens and energizes the body and increases stamina. Bala induces perspiration, and a diuretic, stimulates the central nervous system, is anti-asthmatic, and lowers blood glucose levels. It is also used to speed recovery from chemotoxicity. Bala is both good for pain and inflammation, however it is a stimulant and wakes up the brain. Bala Root is interesting for as soon as that kicked into my system I lost the body sensation of existential dread and body pain dropped and body sensation becomes smooth, soft and calm.

CALMING HERBS: Herbs for calming nerves, insomnia, neuralgia, pain, shock, Die-off and depression of the down cycles, for tea, baths or capsulation: Borage, Burdock leaves, Chamomile, Catnip, Gorse flowers, California poppy flowers, Comfrey, Cowslip, Evening primrose, Ginger root, Goldenrod, Hop flowers, Juniper berries, Kava kava, Lemon balm, Linden flowers, Lobelia. Peppermint, Magnolia bark, Meadowsweet, Motherwort, Mullein, Nettle, Oat Straw, Passion flower, Red clover flowers, Rosemary leaf, Skullcap, St John's Wort, Valerian, Yarrow, Yellow dock. White willow can be used as an anti-inflammatory for nerve pain and headaches. Wood Betony is good for all head, neck and face pain including headaches. For migraine headaches: Fenugreek, Thyme and Feverfew. Fever: Dandelion, Elder flowers, Parsley seeds, Nettle, Sage, Yarrow.

CALM SMOOTHIE HERBS: If you feel your energy is too sympathetically activated (eg: palpitations, heat, sweating, tingles, high blood pressure, insomnia etc...) then put some Reishi, Catuaba, Rhodiola, Maca, Kava kava, Caapi, Valerian leaf, Chamomile, Raspberry leaf powders, lemon balm into your smoothie base mix. (herbalcom.com) You might want to add D-Mannose to your smoothie base or add a couple of teaspoons of D-Mannose powder to your smoothie if you are going through radical kundalini events, especially when there is a lot of pressure or electrical activity going on in the head. D-Mannose helps to provide the neurons with extra energy and thereby reduces neuron death from excitotoxic damage by inadequate reuptake of the neurotransmitter glutamate and calcium. Cryptolepis root tincture (*Cryptolepis sanguinolenta) is* used for insomnia, and also is traditionally used in West Africa to treat malaria.

QUICK PICK ME UPS: 3% hydrogen peroxide sprayed on feet, Apple cider vinegar sprayed on feet and inflamed joints; turmeric and cinnamon in diet; clove and oregano essential oils for topical immune assist are some easy fixes, but they probably need to increase their Vitamin D. If you have access to a sauna/ infrared sauna it is a good idea to use it daily. Drink half your bodyweight in ounces of water per day — with pure drinking water + Lemon Juice + Ocean-Derived Ionic Trace Minerals. Plentiful Vitamin C, Alpha Lipoic and Selenium while detoxing Heavy Metals. Sunbathing, Grounding, Ocean, put feet in a fast running stream, Vibe Machine, Rebounding, Bodywork, Yoga and Infrared saunas, Saunas/Steam room and negatively ionized air are essential for rapidly removing Heavy Metals and toxic chemicals out of the body. Green juices/ smoothies, papaya garlic-mustard-banana smoothies, rosemary oil on the shins, running, grounding, sungazing, toning, meditation, music.

LITHIUM OROTATE: Lithium promotes brain health and mood and can grow brain cells and prevent dementia. It prevents brain neuron tangles and decreases the number of senile plaques. However since lithium is now being sprayed on us from the sky, it may be best to avoid supplementation. Lithium is apparently used in chemtrails to improve citizen compliance by increasing apathy.

AMBIENT GROOVES: For **Ecoshock and anti-chemtrail emotional fortitude** I suggest constant ambient music, (not pure frequences/single tone) like The Frequency of Light by Brian T. Collins, or any with Binaural music from Dr. Jeffrey D. Thompson, www.neuroacoustic.com/entrainment.html

Online radios: Echo; and Hearts of Space; and Pandora. Sounds of water, birds, whales, ocean and the forest…and sounds representing "green, yellow and orange" maybe cleansing.

The epic music of Phillip Lober is also inspiring. Listen to positive psychologist Martin Seligman on "Optimism and Hope,"and other visionaries in order to keep positivity, sovereignty and executive function alive. How to Change Your Mind: What the New Science of Psychedelics Teaches Us About Consciousness, Dying, Addiction, Depression, and Transcendence, by Michael Pollan, 2018

PSYCHEDELICS FOR BRAIN REPAIR: Micro-dosing psychedelic drugs like LSD, Ketamine and Ecstasy (MDMA) has been shown to stimulate the growth of new branches and connections between brain cells which could help address conditions like depression and addiction. This means psychedelics could be the "next generation" treatment for mental health disorders, which could be more effective and safer than existing pharmaceutical options. Ketamine provides such a rapid antidepressant effect it is not clear why other NMDA-receptor channel blockers do not produce similar response. Psilocybin mushrooms provide relief from cluster headache attacks and establishes new connections among various regions of the brain and may actually heal damaged brain cells and generate the growth of new ones. Brain patterns undergo a dramatic reorganization after treatment with psilocybin. The brains of patients treated with psilocybin become "hyperconnected" and demonstrate greater communications across the entire brain potentially treating depression and other neurological problems. Peyote and San Pedro cactus are powerful entheogenic plants containing mescaline used in the treatment of alcoholism, cancer, depression and grief.

OCCIDENTAL DEPRESSION

I went to a talk at Naropa University given by Benki Piyãko, a Amazon Shaman and creator of the "Yorenka Atame" Healing Center (Knowledge of the Forest) and planter of millions of trees. He embodied an exquisite clear transmission of what is important, the preservation the purity of the forest, food, water and air. Good news that UN in Brussels is endorsing his use of Ayahuasca in his healing clinic. Benki's talk was very intense—feeling his predicament, that his life is under threat because he is trying to preserve the pristine state of nature that the earth deserves and needs. As such the *"indians"* still living in harmony with nature are our "elders" teachers and healers.

Benki referred to the planet killing white man as the occidental, or western. A creature so far removed from pristine nature that the rape, pillage and plunger of mother earth has become the norm. And once removed from the sanity and sanctity of nature's embrace it is a downhill race to greater and greater degeneration, delinquency and madness. The Spirit of the land is what informs our spirit—and that relationship is what imbues us with divinity and purpose.

The Ashaninka Benki Piyāko of the Brazilian Amazon is the quintessence of Spirit, whereas the occidental who has laid waste to the planet has only an abstract or ideological relationship to Spirit. Benki's goals are huge — reforestation, food forestry, trash for food programs combined with a state of the art recycle plant, a retreat center for healing "occidental sickness" with spirit medicines and to build a city in the jungle that is non-polluting and lives in harmony with the environment.

Occidental culture is not misguided, it is off the rails. It is a supersonic train heading for a massive wreck. We cannot compete with, poison and impede Nature and expect to get off lightly. Under the God Mammon technology will be increasingly be used to prey on, spy on and corral people into subhuman lives. Already a human life is not worth living in this predatory, entropic culture. We must fight to our last breath to get out of this "hell domain" and into a genuinely HUman society.

Benki writes: *"My happiness gives me strength to face the world to help the planet by creating a strategic plan to develop a sustainable and balanced way for humanity. Our government's policies now make us even more apprehensive, with their enterprises for the construction of dams, for the destruction of the forest, the extraction of minerals, with its reduction of indigenous lands, its investment in cattle breeding and in planting monocultures with the use of poisons which will then destroy our rivers. What are we going to do if our government does not know how to reflect upon its socioeconomic plans, leading the country to a human disaster? We want all the nations of the world to alert and warn our government to wake up and to go back a little. So that it admits it has committed mistakes which are now killing us all. This message comes from the Earth, as a request for Humanity to understand that we are transient beings here and one cannot just look at one's own well-being. We have to look toward future generations and what we will leave for them. We have to think of our children and of the Earth. We cannot leave the country impoverished and poisoned, as it is happening now."*

INCREASING SEROTONIN

We can combat the stress of the chemtrail holocaust by increasing serotonin and alpha frequency and recovering circadian hygiene. The feel-good neurotransmitter serotonin, is crucial to feelings of well-being. Alpha animals have strong Serotonin levels supporting empowerment and Presence. Serotonin calms, elevates pain threshold, promotes sleep and feeling of well-being, reduces anxiety, depression, aggression and compulsive behavior.

Tryptophan (5-HTP) — The neurotransmitter serotonin is made from the amino acid Tryptophan. Serotonin neural circuits help counterbalance the tendency of brain dopamine and noradrenaline circuits to encourage over-arousal. It calms, elevates pain threshold, promotes relaxation, sleep and feeling of well-being, reduces aggression and compulsive behavior and increases confidence and concentration. It is better to take tryptophan as 5-HTP, because it is a natural extract from the seeds of the Griffonia simplicifolia tree from the West African countries of Ghana.

The stress hormone cortisol activates the enzyme tryptophan pyrrolase in the liver which breaks down tryptophan, so taking tryptophan while under high cortisol, stressed conditions might supply little extra serotonin to the brain. Vitamin B3 (niacin) activates the enzyme that converts tryptophan to 5HTP. Thus taking 100mg B3 several times daily with meals will also serve to enhance the effectiveness of tryptophan.

The pineal produces melatonin and serotonin. The amino acid precursor of serotonin (5-hydroxytryptamine, 5-HT) is tryptophan. Adequate levels of vitamin B6 are necessary for the synthesis of serotonin. Within the pineal gland, serotonin is acetylated and then methylated to yield melatonin. Taking 50mg vitamin B6 once or twice daily with meals will also augment tryptophan-serotonin conversion, since B6 activates the decarboxylase enzyme that converts 5HTP to serotonin, and is needed for the synthesis of GABA and dopamine as well. The phosphate ester derivative pyridoxal 5'-phosphate (pyridoxal-B6) is the bioactive coenzyme form involved in over 4% of all enzymatic reactions

Melatonin actually promotes increased brain serotonin through its ability to reduce cortisol levels, and reduced cortisol levels will lessen the activity of the enzyme tryptophan pyrrolase which degrades tryptophan in the liver. St John's Wort is a mild MAO inhibitor that reduces the reuptake of serotonin in the brain increasing synaptic levels and it is also a cortisol inhibitor. James South MA has a fabulous article on L-Tryptophan at http://smart-drugs.net/ias-tryptophan-article.htm

Malabar tamarind (*Garcinia cambogia*), contains a substance called hydroxycitric acid (HCA) which increases levels of serotonin. Apparently raw cacao beans provide MAO inhibiters, which increase the serotonin and other neurotransmitters circulating in the brain. Mood elevating Ginkgo biloba increases the brain uptake of serotonin and improves circulation. Serotonin (5-HT) is a vasodilator, therefore a deficiency of serotonin decreases blood flow due to relative vasoconstriction.

Herbs containing Berberine such as Barberry root, Barberries, Bloodroot, Oregon Grape Root, Chinese Goldthread, Goldenseal root, act as an herbal antidepressant and a neuroprotector. Berberine demonstrates glucose-lowering effects, as well as increasing the number of serotonin transporters available in the brain, enhancing the reuptake of serotonin and reducing the breakdown of reducing acetylcholine. Deficiency of the amino acid L-lysine interferes with the normal circadian release of serotonin, thereby increasing stress-induced anxiety.

Low levels of Omega-3 DHA cause reduction of brain serotonin levels and have been associated with ADHD, Alzheimer's disease and depression. CoQ10 Idebenone raises mood by increasing serotonin levels even when the diet is low in L-Tryptophan. Long-term supplementation with SAMe repairs cell membrane fluidity and enhances the sensitivity of prolactin receptors, as well as GABA and beta-receptors and probably serotonin and dopamine receptors as well.

Social status also plays a part in our digestive health and sense of well-being, for there is some evidence of high serotonin levels in leaders and Type A personalities. About 95 percent of the body's serotonin is to be found in the stomach or enteric brain. Both the pineal gland and the intestinal tract produce serotonin. The gut wall has at least seven types of serotonin receptors that facilitate the digestive process. Escherichia and Enterococcus probiotic species all produce 5HT-Serotonin, and **L.reuteri** produces the calming neurotransmitter GABA.

Serotonin, that feel-good hormone, is a precursor to melatonin. Disturbances in your ability to sleep can cause you to gain weight. Carbohydrate consumption, acting via insulin secretion and the "plasma tryptophan ratio," increases serotonin release. Serotonin release is also involved in such functions as sleep onset, pain sensitivity, blood pressure regulation, and mood control. Because dietary carbohydrates increase brain serotonin secretion we can become addicted to eating starches and sugars in an effort to feel better. Magnesium also helps lower the stress hormone cortisol. Stress from EMF & radiation pollution drains magnesium levels and increases adrenaline so baths with Epsom salt and Baking Soda help to normalize the body and increase serotonin. Magnesium oil (Mg Chloride) sprayed on the skin is also great for frequency normalization.

With the zeolite-cancer research they are finding that zeolite works to repair the serotonin chemistry, and serotonin of course is the "calming" neurotransmitter that helps to key you into Alpha and Theta waves, the Schumann resonance and circadian rhythms…thereby strengthening the normalizing organizational principles of the cells and helping to restore a disordered bio-field, "Bio-field Repolarization. The **Schumann Resonance** (extremely low frequencies around 7.83 Hz) signal operates by being resonantly absorbed by brain systems and altering the serotonin/melatonin balance. Alpha waves are neural oscillations in the frequency range of 7.5–12.5 Hz. Alpha frequency around 10Hz – enhances the release of the mood elevator serotonin.

Neuroscientists have discovered that increasing alpha brain waves through endocannabinoids, oxytocin, dopamine, serotonin and oxytocin.

DEPRESSION AND MITOCHONDRIA

Depression is a common mood disorder that negatively affects how you feel, the way you think and how you act. Depressive symptoms include sadness that doesn't go away, loss of interest or pleasure, feelings of guilt or low self-worth, feelings of helplessness and hopelessness, disturbed sleep or appetite, lack of enthusiasm, low energy, and poor concentration. If you suffer from depression, you may be feeling so tired and drained that you find it hard to get out of bed in the morning and have a hard time going about your daily activities. Other than existential mortification over the state of the world, dysfunction of mitochondrial metabolism may be a cause or effect of depression.

One of the primary functions of mitochondria is to produce metabolic water. This can be tested by walking and grounding for an hour in nature on a sunny day—after which you will urinate a lot more than usual. Mitochondria are the central source of cellular energy. Stability of cellular function requires the integrity of numerous complex enzymatic reactions. There is evidence showing that mitochondrial dysregulation and dysfunction in various brain regions is associated with depression. In patients with a mood disorder, regions demonstrating brain pathology included the medial prefrontal cortex, medial and caudolateral orbital cortex, amygdala, hippocampus, ventromedial parts of basal ganglia, cerebellum and anterior cingulate cortex. There was increased regional blood flow and glucose metabolism in the amygdala during wakefulness and sleep, which correlated with the severity of depression.

NMDA receptors are understood to regulate memory function in the brain. The activation of postsynaptic NMDA receptors in most hippocampal pathways controls the induction of an activity-dependent synaptic modification called long-term potentiation—the process of memory formation in the brain. Memory is promoted by stress or excitement, and impaired memory from mood disorder suggests that cellular metabolic damage may persist even though stability of mood has been achieved. Overstimulation of N-methyl-D-aspartate (NMDA) receptors by glutamate caused excessive calcium ion influx, which compromised mitochondrial membrane polarity. Glutamate overstimulation also caused an increase in reactive oxygen species and a cascade of apoptotic factors. Oxidative DNA damage caused by hypoxia and inhibition of mitochondrial respiratory complexes may contribute to neuronal dysfunction and progressive brain injury.

The amino acid glutamate plays a central role in both the normal and abnormal functioning of the central nervous system (CNS). Glutamate is recognized to be the main excitatory neurotransmitter in the CNS. In addition, Glutamate is also an excitotoxin that can destroy CNS neurons by excessive activation of excitatory receptors on dendritic and somal surfaces. Excessive activation of NMDA receptors (NMDA receptor hyperfunction plays an important role in the pathophysiology of acute CNS injury syndromes such as hypoxia-ischemia, trauma, and status epilepticus.

The NMDA glutamate receptor system becomes hypofunctional in either the normal brain or the Alzheimer's brain after having first gone through an early stage of hyper-NMDA receptor activity. NMDA receptor hypofunction that occurs as the brain ages may be partially responsible for memory deficits associated with aging. **Ketamine** is an NMDA antagonist, and its blocking of NMDA receptors has been effective in preventing opioid-induced neurotoxicity. Kratom also contains alkaloids (rhynchophylline and mitraphylline) which function as NMDA receptor antagonists. The best and safest supplement to use when trying to slow the development of tolerance is magnesium, a natural NMDA receptor antagonist.

Stress models of the brain have shown that elevated cortisol levels cause tissue changes, especially in the Dentate gyrusin the hippocampus. Toxicity from excess excitation may be mediated in part by entry of calcium into the cell; the high intracellular calcium level may open the membrane permeability transition pore, depolarize the mitochondrial membrane, release cytochrome c, causing apoptosis or cell death. Chronic unpredictable stress caused a significant decrease in the number of immunoreactive neurons located in the striatum, medial forebrain bundle, ventral tegmental area, and substantia nigra, and reduced the activity of superoxide dismutase and catalase in the cortex, striatum, and **hippocampus**. Sungazing and grounding improves pineal hormonal health.

Enhancing the body's antioxidant systems and mitochondrial health is a substantial method of treating chronic depression. The body's main antioxidant Glutathione peroxidase protects intracellular metabolism from oxidative stress, reduces lipid hydroperoxides and scavenges peroxides. Besides its immune boosting functions Vitamin C is also required for the synthesis of carnitine. Carnitine is a molecule which is essential for the transport of fatty acids into the mitochondria. It is the mitochondria which convert food sources (such as fats) into energy in the body. Therefore, Vitamin C is also indirectly responsible for energy generation. Both increased exercise, oxygen, detoxification and increasing ATP production help with depression.

Deuterium Depleted water, grounding and sunlight/sungazing are vital to efficient mitochondrial function.

THE INNER ARTS: THE THREE KINGS

The Three Kings are essential to all Inner Arts to turn on the vagal nerve and activate the Parasympathetic Nervous System or "off switch" in order to do "inner work." Dropping the muscles at the back of the Tongue, doing a Throaty Breath and an Inner Smile. Dropping the tongue into the belly and breathing is the fastest and surest way of breaking through the contraction and anxiety that constitute surface living. It also automatically reduces hyper-activation of the nervous system in people in our proximity. The parasympathetic mode promotes rest, recovery, healing, growing and visioneering. Dropping the muscles at the root of the tongue electrically connects us into the ground of consciousness within the (8Hz)-serotonin, enteric or stomach brain. This then marries the left and right brain hemispheres, plus the Heart with the prefrontal lobes and ultimately the body with the earth and planetary Schumann resonance (8Hz). The Inner Smile creates the endorphins needed to the relaxation of the HPA-axis overdrive and put us in a "growth" state. When we are actively engaged in growth, we don't have time for stagnation, regression, defense, self-destruction and death.

HAPPY HIPPOCAMPUS MEDITATION

When there is not much to be "happy" about in our lives we literally have to manufacture happiness from within. We can do this through The Happy Hippocampus Inner Art. The Hippocampus is located on the floor of each lateral ventricle of the brain, thought to be the center of emotion, memory, and the autonomic nervous system. The shape of the elongated ridges looks like a seahorse and is depicted as such in art, most often as a horse with a mermaid tail. The Happy Hippocampus meditation can be done lying in bed, on one's stomach with your head on its side, so that the arms and pillow arrangements allow support for you to press your dominant thumb onto your Third Eye.

Then you do The Three Kings (inner smile, tongue drop, throaty breath) and feel into your Hippocampus. Essentially imparting happiness into your Hippocampus with your meditation focus. Lying on your back and putting a piece of shungite on your Third Eye while meditating greatly amplifies the meditative function and results. You will have to repeat the word "Happiness" while you do this, because your inner Hippocampus seahorse is probably pretty unhappy and so you have to apply consciousness into it order to change its vibratory state and emotion, while pressing firmly into the Third Eye You may notice resistance to the happiness vibration change in your Hippocampus because this meditation uncovers the depth of death, sadness, loss, deprivation and unhappiness we harbor within our brain, however if we don't apply ourselves to brain change, we may go through life in deep dissatisfaction and grief with no means of changing our life circumstances to bring us joy.

Once you are able to easily activate the Happy Hippocampus, the meditation can be done while sungazing for added rewiring/frequency change; or using a piece of Shungite on the third eye to help wipe the slate clean and energize. Often with need various "assists" to palpate, touch and transform numb, comatose or insensate, inactive regions of the brain. Regular exercise releases endogenous opioids, enhances serotonin function, stimulates nerve growth factors, promotes cell proliferation in the **hippocampus**, and leads to a livelier, better-oxygenated brain. BTW the more alcohol that one drinks the more atrophy occurs in the brain's memory storing hippocampus.

THE HYPOTHALAMUS ASSURANCE BOOST

After you have generated happiness in the Hippocampus, you will need to generate "reassurance" in the Hypothalamus which the Hippocampus connects into. While meditating - look back through the optic nerve into the brain core and send reassuring light into the Hypothalamus. The Hypothalamus is region in the central core of the brain that coordinates both the autonomic nervous system and the activity of the pituitary, controlling body temperature, thirst, hunger, and other homeostatic systems, and involved in sleep and emotional activity. As social animals our sense of "security" or self-affirmation is socially generated, however in the competitive Borg society we are more likely to receive negative or subversive feedback which atrophies or starves our Hypothalamus... that is, our autonomic emotional regulator. As you focus your attention on the Hypothalamus send into it the light of reassurance while mentally repeating a supportive word such as comfort, encouragement, assistance, sustenance, help, relief, goodness, wholeness etc...

THE GOODIFYING EMEDITATION

This is the most important Inner Art from the Sovereignty 2 series. The Goodifying Emeditation (the "E" stands for emotional) overcomes the disenfranchisement of self-rejection and rejection from others. It is this toxic inheritance which is the main interference pattern to a sovereign command of one's life, and is the seed energy for all our methods of self-abuse, self-sabotage and self-negation. So first you need to get into the body to "operate it" and to do that do the Three Kings (tongue drop, throaty breath, inner smile).

Then in relaxed meditation, *look back into the brain* as though the forehead was a spotlight, you will focus feeling directly into the judicial center, ie: the ACC and corpus callosum. You may feel an unfathomable hunger in this area, as though it is bruised and needy. As you breathe into the neediness and focus the mind's light on this area, repeat the word "Goodness" and self-absolve yourself of any sin implicated onto you by the unlawful, selfish needs of others. As you shine the mind's eye through the forehead, into the core of the brain, you will notice that the Adam's Apple area of the throat starts to pulsate in unison with the diaphragm. This is a rhythmic orgasm of sorts that arises from the Goodifying focused energy of the brain meeting the opened grateful heart. You know you have made contact with the limbic brain and brainstem when you see a warm golden red glow inside your brain core.

The Goodifying Emeditation can be practiced in bed, or lying on the grass, and can also be incorporated into sungazing sessions, baths, bus rides, or walking etc... If you sit by the rapids of a river, with your bare feet on the ground or in the water. The negative ions from the rapids acts to enhance the field force of your meditation and facilitate rapid healing/wholing. There is significant immune enhancement via doing the Goodifying emeditation near river rapids. I was doing the Goodifying Emeditation down by the river and noticed increased warmth/chi under the jaw as the immune system gets a boost, reflecting the increased yogic-tantric action of being around high negative ion sources... Homes, yoga studios and temples need to be built around high negative ion generators in nature.

My spiritual exercise book one: "The Inner Arts Practicum" Lulu.com.

9

OPTIMIZATION

YOUTHIFYING AND PEAK PERFORMANCE

MITOCHONDRIAL ENHANCEMENT

Mitochondrial enhancement which will help both prevent depression and repair brain tissue in areas where mitochondrial dysfunction is causing depressive symptoms. **Mitochondria,** the energy-producing structures in cells, exist in networks that dynamically change shape according to energy demand. Their capacity to do so declines with age, and there is a causal link between dynamic changes in the shapes of mitochondrial networks and longevity.

Intermittent fasting and dietary restriction, exercise, cold temperature and DHA increased AMP-activated protein kinase (AMPK), maintained the mitochondrial networks in a fused or "youthful" state. In addition, they found that these youthful networks increased lifespan by communicating with organelles called peroxisomes to modulate fat metabolism. Toxins, such as aluminum, mercury and other heavy metals, can severely damage the mitochondria and as metabolic energy falls we accumulate more and more toxins because we don't have the energy to adequately detoxify. A high enzyme diet means maximizing ATP production with a minimum of exhausting the body's resources for digestion, maintenance and repair. Deuterium depleted water improves mitochondrial efficiency and reduces wear and tear on these organelles.

INCREASING ATP ENERGY PRODUCTION: Supplements that are known to help increase the energy your mitochondria produce include: Spirulina, Omega-3, Flaxseed Oil, Lecithin, Kelp, Iodine, Green Tea, Black pepper, Cayenne, Astragalus Root, Cat's Claw, Grape seed, Yerba mate, Motherwort, Mushrooms (Lion's Mane, Maitake and Cordyceps), Yohimbe, Goji, Ginger, Resveratrol, Gotu Kola, and Rhodiola. Acetyl-L-Carnitine, L-Arginine, L-Carnitine, Creatine, N-Acetyl Cysteine (NAC), L-Glutamine, Alpha lipoic acid, NADH, Niacin-B3 + D-Ribose, B complex, Co-enzyme Q10, Ca-2 AEP, DHEA, D-Ribose, Resveratrol, Citrulline malate, Apples-malic acid, Magnesium Malate, Sodium Phosphate and Potassium Phosphate, Magnesium ascorbyl phosphate, Chromium & Vanadium. Plus powerful water/fat soluble antioxidants and zinc and selenium to protect mitochondria.

DR. JACK KRUSE: See Dr. Jack Kruse's YouTube videos on improving mitochondrial function. He says the most important things for improving the electrical potential of the cell are conditions that support the body's redox potential: Compliance to circadian rhythms, DHA-Omega-3, reduce Blue Light exposure,   deuterium depleted water, deep sleep, cold exposure, stress reduction, grounding, stress reduction and exercise.

RAISING KUNDALINI: Kundalini is the amplification of Spirit which breaks through the repressive metabolism of our enculturated bodymind and awakens us to levels of perception, sensation and aliveness we never knew were possible. Spirit is a river flowing back to its oceanic self, pretty much everything Flatland humans do prevents this full cycle of return. The more we turn to Nature to heal and whole us, the closer we come to Goodness, Godliness and Holiness. Only intact nature's energy can revive our dis-eased energy and metabolism and deliver us to the fullness of our deeper Self.

The fire of life burns by itself if given the conditions to do so. Raising kundalini (Chi) amounts to increasing cellular energy (ATP), unblocking the flow of energy and increasing movement (physical – mental – spiritual). After kundalini is raised we must pay equal attention to protecting tissues, and integrating and substantiating the energy of consciousness. To maintain an awakening we need total dedication to what Spirit seeks to convey through us, for it is hard to fit the largess of Spirit into the naysaying Hindbrain world. If we are not focused on our universal mission we will crash back down into our small self in the humdrum world.

Rawfoodist communities would have the largest number of kundalini initiates as bodies weighed down with cooked food cannot generate the cellular energy necessary to spark up the metamorphosis process. Fasting and becoming a rawfoodist is an essential first step to eliminating narcissistic self-centrism and opening up to grace. Simply changing to a raw diet will likely initiate a kundalini awakening by removing the metabolic impediment to the light. The raw diet also keeps the blood alkaline with raw vegetables, the body's water ionized and bio-structured while providing the antioxidants to prevent nerve damage. Sprouted greens and a green smoothie liquid diet will allow the energy blockage and somatic repression to loosen its hold. DHEA, ginseng and other sex hormone enhancers, adaptogens and nootropics provide the neurohormonal foundations to elevated light flow. Only raw is REAL: Check out David Wolfe, Gabriel Cousens, Dan MacDonald (the Life Regenerator), Markus Rothkranz, Tony Wright, and Brian Clement on YouTube.

Other initiatory practices that fuel the flame are calorie restriction, fasting, and all methods of detoxification. One of the best secrets to raising kundalini is sungazing, in which you meditate on the rising or setting sun for 15 minutes/day. The sun provides unlimited energy for defragging and enlightenment. Plants also provide a direct link to God through the "Soma," or the 108 entheogenic plants that are associated with the consciousness raising. Another traditional method of reaching for Godhood via transcendent masculine means is the "Philosopher's Stone," ORMUS, monatomics or White Powder of Gold, Magnetic trap water, and living-water. While more the down to earth feminine pole is addressed via earthing through the use of clay baths, clay packs, taking clay internally, mud baths and making pottery.

Flexing the nervous system with alternating hot & cold, that is plunging temperature changes such as sauna, cold shower, or nude-sunbathing then jumping in cold water. To get energy moving you can use movement and vibration such as dearmoring bodywork, binaural music, toning, mantra, singing, hanging, running and some stretching like yoga, meditation, breath of fire, holotropic breathing, trance dancing, drumming, Guru devotion and shaktipat. Reconnect to the Cosmos by camping out under the stars, vision quests, exercising in nature, earthing/grounding, the Inner Arts, Qigong and martial arts in nature. Novelty, change, challenge, travel, play, beauty of nature, camping, extreme experience, intensive physical and mental training creates the neurogenesis and plasticity, which permits the nervous system to ripen, pop and expand—just like popcorn!

Romantic love, tantra, sex, the Hieros gamos, Courtly Love, Chivalric love, transpersonal non-relationship, celibacy and interaction with unique, authentic people, peer companionship, new places and novel experiences can spark off a Kundalini awakening. Snake dreams, sex dreams and atom bomb dreams are some of the spontaneous stimulatory agents involved in awakening Chi. These dreams are both the "cause and an effect" of the metamorphic chemistry. These and other kundalini symptoms may occur outside of a full-blown awakening and do not necessarily mean a full awakening is on its way. Abiding in the liberation of the expressive power of the Muse opens the faucet to continued illuminated expression and unfolds your the grand adventure of your unique spiritual quest.

INCREASING OXYGEN: Increasing oxygen levels may be primary means optimize ATP production: Ginseng, Ginkgo Biloba, Gotu kola, Hydergine, Vinpocetine, Spirulina. Magnesium helps stabilize ATP; in fact 80 percent of the magnesium inside the cell is complexed with ATP. The amino acid L-Citrulline helps the body rid itself of ammonia and recover after exercise, freeing ATP energy for other uses. The structured water, electrolytes and sugars of young/white coconut water ups your ATP production. You can also filter fresh coconut water and put it in a spray bottle for your skin and hair. *Coconut oil is readily converted to fuel for ATP and doesn't get stored as fat in the body.

MITOCHONDRIAL REPAIR: NAD+ precursors like Nicotinamide riboside and Nicotinamide mononucleotide (NMN) also help to ensure proper oxidative conditions in our mitochondria and as a result enhance our ability to hold charge or light. Niacin, Chlorophyll, CoQ10 is hydrophobic while MitoQ and PQQ are hydrophilic, Alpha lipoic, Gold, Platinum, Uridine, Benfotiamine, Idebenone, Pterostilbene, Resveratrol, Pantethine, Pantothenic acid, Megahydrate, Cell Salts, Krebs chelated minerals, Succinic acid, Oxaloacetate, Alcar, Quercetin, Rutin, Grape Seed Extract and L-Arginine Alpha-Ketoglutarate.

Older organisms have more molecular damage in them, which causes an animal that eats them to age faster than one that eats younger organisms with less molecular damage. A diet of older organisms shortens lifespan by 13-18% due in part to the increase in molecular damage, fewer enzymes, and reduced silicon etc.…Plus there are different nutrients in the tissues from old animals and plants compared to young animals and plants.

Longevity or Continuity = Maximum ATP (energy) with a Minimum of Free Radical production.

ANDROGENS FOR TESTOSTERONE: In order to overcome depression and raise our energy, focus and power to execute our survival protocol and thrive in the chemtrail holocaust, both men and women will need to ensure that their testosterone levels are strong. Testosterone levels decline about 1 % per year after age 30, but there is a lot we can do with herbs and supplements to maintain our zest, drive and executive functioning. Establishing high functioning hormonal agency will allow us to keep up the good fight well into our 90s. We will need all the courage and energy we can get to halt the decline of civic culture and to build civilization next! Androgen's are necessary for empowerment, sovereignty and executive, prefrontal lobe function. Dopamine has a close relationship with androgenic hormones, it works by upregulating the androgen receptors, suppressing prolactin, and increasing the rate of steroidogenesis by stimulating GnRH release in the hypothalamus.

As cortisol levels increase there is a decline in the anabolic adrenal hormone DHEA (a precursor of testosterone) which increases depression and leads to increased vulnerability to the catabolic tissue-breakdown effects of cortisol. DHEA, the most abundant hormone and precursor to many other hormones seems to balance the effects of cortisol by improving the body's ability to cope with stress. It can boost energy levels, strengthen immune function, improve memory, and reduce body fat. DHEA acts as a "mood elevator," preventing depression and protecting important neurons in the brain. Dopamine the libido driver is synthesized from L-Dopa (Mucuna pruriens) and its amino acid precursor Tyrosine.

FOODS AND HERBS TO BOOST TESTOSTERONE: Pomegranate, Extra virgin olive oil, Coconut, Oysters, Wild Salmon, Eggs, Bromelain enzyme in pineapples, Cruciferous Vegetables, Asparagus, Spinach, Whey Protein, Garlic, Pumpkin seeds, Nettle leaf, Fenugreek, Vitamin D, Citrus, Red grapes, Ginseng, Tribulus Terrestris, Horny Goat Weed Blend, Maca, Saw Palmetto, Ginseng, Mucuna Pruriens, Polypodium Vulgare, Muira Puama, Tongkat Ali, Fo-ti, Forskolin, Ashwagandha, and Arginine. The herb Mucuna pruriens is a potent androgen enhancer. It contains fairly high amounts of this thing called L-Dopa (levodopa), which is a precursor to the brain neurotransmitter/hormone; dopamine.

IMPROVING SEX HORMONES: Sunlight on the skin is essential for healthy hormonal balance, as sex hormones are made from cholesterol in the skin. Sungazing increases the happiness neurotransmitter Dopamine which improves our libido and assertiveness. Pollen is rich in aspartic acid, an amino acid involved in rejuvenation of the sex glands. Forskolin is a herb that increases Cyclic AMP, which is essential to synthesize and regulate thyroid hormones, growth hormone, cortisol, DHEA, testosterone, melatonin and other hormones. Omega 3 and DHA increases NO, L-Arginine, Ornithine, Histidine, Choline, B-5, B-6, Niacin, zinc, selenium, magnesium, boron, manganese and iodine.

HERBAL ANABOLIC STEROID PRECURSORS: Ashwagandha. Black Cohosh. Blessed Thistle, Blue Cohosh, Chasteberry, Damiana, Dodder Seed, Dong quai, FoTi, Ginkgo, Ginseng, Gotu kola, Horny Goat Weed, Huanarpo, Huang Qi, Long Jack, Licorice root, Maca, Mucuna pruriens, Muira puama, Raspberry leaf, Sarsaparilla, Saw palmetto, Tribulus, Wild Oat, Wild Yam, Yucca. Viraloid, extracted from Wild Yam, is a new super anabolic/anti-catabolic from Australia that causes massive protein synthesis and muscle build up by increasing testosterone levels and "opening up" more testosterone receptor sites.

INCREASING ANABOLISM: Increasing Human Growth Hormone (HGH) is essential to turn the body around to an anabolic building state. Arginine stimulates the pituitary into producing Growth Hormone which increases the size of the Thymus gland thus increasing T cells and B cells. Immunity improves along with tissue regeneration, muscle toning, wound healing and cancer inhibition. Growth Hormone Release (GHR) inhibits the formation of fat and mobilizes existing stores; it also increases the tensile strength of structural protein, collagen, preventing sagging skin. To increase HGH take Arginine, Ornithine, Tyrosine, B12, B6, Vitamin C. Also Creatine, Tryptophan. Choline from DMAE, lecithin and Alpha-GPA.

OTHER ANABOLIC AGENTS INCLUDE: Fulvic acid, Chromium picolinate, Borage, Gumar, Yerba mate, Sarsaparilla, Rhodiola Rosea, Fenugreek, Wild oats (Avena sativa), Stinging nettle root, Sea buckthorn (Rhamnus frangula), Spikenard (Aralia), Rhaponticum, Schizandra, Shilajit, Ashwagandha, Maral Root-Rhaponticum carthamoides (Leuzea), Licorice and Ginseng: Eleutherococcus and Siberian ginseng.

AVOID ANIMAL FOODS: The vegetarian diet increases metabolism and offers protection from heart disease. The researchers found that within 24 hours of carnitine consumption—eating a sirloin steak, or taking a carnitine supplement—certain gut bacteria metabolize the carnitine to a toxic substance called trimethylamine, which then gets oxidized in our liver to trimethylamine-n-oxide (TMAO), which increases the buildup of cholesterol in the inflammatory cells in the atherosclerotic plaques in our arteries, increasing our risk of heart attack, stroke, and death. Apparently the choline in eggs, poultry, dairy and fish produces the same toxic TMAO as carnitine in red meat. The body makes all the carnitine we need without supplementation or meat eating.

CELL PROLIFERANTS: Aloe, Basil, Comfrey, Calendula, Elderberries, Mullein, Papaya, Pollen, Royal Jelly, Raspberry, Sage, Slippery elm, Watercress, Yellow dock. Food that is high in enzymes, young and fast growing such as sprouts, plant shoots and asparagus increases your enzyme load and cell growth, regeneration and repair.

OVERCOMING INSULIN RESISTANCE

The Metabolic X, Cancer, Diabetes, Heart Disease etc… phenomena is the result of 12 thousand years of the progressive deterioration of the optimum human diet. The SAD diet (high glycemic/grains/sugar) induces cells to become insulin resistant, and to compensate for this the pancreas produces more insulin, which leads to an increase in circulating insulin levels, or hyper-insulinemia. This compensatory high level of insulin and insulin resistance may support cancer growth, for insulin is an important growth factor in the body.

Insulin may signal cells to proliferate through a variety of mechanisms: directly signal growth, as well as signally other more potent growth factors (insulin-like growth factors, or it can make cells more sensitive to other growth factors. When the body is given plentiful food insulin increases and it drops dramatically during a fasting state. Reducing cancer proliferation therefore requires the reversal of insulin resistance, plus the reduction of insulin levels, and the stabilization of blood sugar through lifestyle changes, prevention of obesity, increasing physical activity, raw Paleo diet, herbs and nutritional supplementation.

The antimutagenic lifestyle restores healthy terrain. Cancer is caused from immune system overwhelm and chronic inflammation to toxicity without adequate resources to deal with the toxins, emotional conflict or environmental mutagenic. Due to body terrain changes the cancer cell loses the ability to produce energy via aerobic respiration and so it defaults to the more primitive anaerobic fermentation energy mode. Cancer cells need 19X more glucose than a normal cell to survive because they produce energy (ATP) anaerobically via fermentation which is much less efficient than aerobic respiration. The only way for the cancer cell to satisfy its high appetite for glucose is to trigger the cell to have more insulin receptors to convey more glucose into the cancer cell than a normal cell. If we create a body terrain that inhibits anaerobic respiration and Glycogenolysis, ie: the breakdown of glycogen to glucose (blood sugar), then we reduce the cancer cell's ability to generate enough ATP energy to feed itself.

LOWERS INSULIN RESISTANCE: Chromium, Chaga and Agaricus Mushrooms, Blueberry leaf, Fenugreek, Ginkgo biloba, Bilberry, Green tea, Red raspberry leaf, Nettle, raw coconut oil, Vitamins K and D. Other ingredients that promote healthy blood sugar levels, include the minerals chromium picolinate and vanadyl sulfate; green tea (containing EGCG), which has been shown to have both insulin-enhancing and blood sugar-suppressing activities. Allied in their effects are the powerful antioxidant (and insulin mimetic) Alpha lipoic acid; the bioflavonoid quercetin; the amino acid derivative N-acetylcysteine; herbal extracts of Mulberry leaf and Goat's rue; and Vitamins B6, C, E, and K2.

INCREASE INSULIN SENSITIVITY: Sunlight exposure and avoiding blue light from computer and cell phone screens improves insulin sensitivity. Avocado, Maitake Mushroom, Caper, Cinnamon, Fenugreek, Ginger, Coleus forskohlii, Chromium, Ginseng, Alpha Lipoic Acid. Fatty acid availability, uptake and oxidation all play a role in metabolic flexibility and the inflammation/insulin resistance axis. To counter inflammation we need to eat wild, fatty fish like salmon, young tuna and halibut and oils high in EPA and DHA. Release of insulin is strongly inhibited by the stress hormone norepinephrine (noradrenaline), which leads to increased blood glucose levels during stress.

• Insulin functions best within the pH range of 7.79-8.02. All process in the body are pH specific. The pH even governs the oxygen supply to determine the rate of metabolism. At 7.46 pH the blood is able to transport the most amount of oxygen and carry off the most amount of metabolic wastes.

• Exercise improves insulin resistance, increases insulin sensitivity and raises glucose uptake, as well as increasing the levels of the glucose transporter protein GLUT4. Oxygen increases insulin sensitivity, Nitric Oxide increases oxygen to the tissues.

• Extra B vitamins, folic acid and Vitamin C are needed when drinking alcohol.

• Coconut Oil—Raw coconut oil protects against 'insulin resistance.'

• Vitamin D and Sunshine—Manage testosterone aromatase conversion to estrogens with Vitamin D from sunlight exposure.

• Omega 3—Eat wild, fatty fish like salmon, young tuna and halibut and oils high in EPA and DHA. Buy flax seeds and grind them as needed.

• Bioflavonoids—Use the white of oranges, pomegranate, acai and berries in smoothies.

• Probiotic Foods—Sauerkraut/Cabbage Cider is a great digestive aid and cancer inhibitor.

GYMNEMA SYLVESTRE: Gurmar has long been used in the Ayurvedic medicine of India as a treatment for diabetes. Gurmar has been shown to enhance the ability of the pancreas to produce insulin in laboratory animals and to rejuvenate dysfunctional pancreatic cells. *Gymnema sylvestre* has an anticancer, anti-candida effect by curing diabetes. This herb has even been shown to boost the number of pancreatic beta cells in the pancreas that release insulin. Inula racemosa has been found to increase the sensitivity of insulin. Drink a ton of Dandelion root and Gymnema sylvestre tea for its anticancer effect. www.herbalcom.com

ASIAN GINSENG: Asian Ginseng (*Panax ginseng*) daily reduces fasting blood glucose measurements, and makes you feel better and thus able to exercise more. Ginseng reduces blood glucose levels, cholesterol and triglyceride levels as well as reducing oxidative stress.

CEDAR BERRY: (*Juniperus monosperma*), six cedar berries three or more times a day. Juniper berry (*Juniperus communis*). Cedar berries contain high levels of insulin, this may be a helpful herbal remedy for pancreatic function in diabetics. Cedar berry with its toning properties, helps in the inflammation of gout, ureteritis, and hemorrhoids. Cedar Berries reduce inflammation on the skin and in the joints, making them useful as an alternative treatment for psoriasis and arthritis.

ADAPTOGENS AND RASAYANA THERAPY

Rasayana literally means "the path that plasma takes." Rasayana or adaptogenic herbs, like ashwagandha, Safed Musli and Panax ginseng, nourish the whole body by strengthening the primordial tissue, and are considered both a renewing kidney Yang tonic and Chi (Qi) activator. It is generally recommended to undergo "rasayana therapy" after a detox or cleansing regimen, when the systems of the body are more receptive to assimilation of higher doses of rasayana herbal supplementation. Rasayana administered without prior detox and purification is said to be like seed sown on barren land, from where no good results can be expected. Rotating adaptogens and herbs in general is a good idea as the body's response weakens over time and the herbs become less effective.

If we mapped chimps foraging schedule over a year we would probably observe that their herb usage is aligned with the sun, moon, potency of the plants, and needs of the various organs according to day, week and month. With advanced sensitivity training and a regenerator's permaculture garden we may be able to recover this superpower that wild chimps never lost—a biochemical merger with their environment. Working with nature we can regain the bliss and peace of the garden of Eden. Safed Musli (*Chlorophytum borivilianum*) is a Rasayana herb with little white flowers from Indian Medicine supposedly used as an aphrodisiac and adaptogen. Safed Musli is an all in one natural treatment for sexual weakness and impotence. Safed Musli is the most potent herbal pro-erectile agent, sometimes mixed with the inclusion of equal parts Mucuna Pruriens

ADAPTOGENIC HERBS: Adaptogens are herbs that help cope with stress by restoring hypothalamic cortisol receptor sensitivity. Rotate the use of various adaptogens after fasting, cleanses and chelation. Perhaps the most well-known adaptogen is Ginseng of which there are three types: Asian (Panax ginseng) for stimulation, American (Panax quinquefolium), which soothes and Siberian (Eleutherococcus senticosus) for stamina. Adaptogenic herbs include: Astragalus, Ashwagandha, Ashitaba, Bacopa in combination with Ginkgo biloba, Blue lotus, California poppy, Cordyceps, Cat's claw, Codonopsis, Chaga, Devil's claw, Dong Quai, FoTi (He Shou Wu), Goldenseal, Gotu kola, Green tea, Hawthorn extract, Hops Flowers, Jatamansi, Jiaogulan, Kava kava, Gynostemma, Licorice, Holy Basil, Maca, Maral, Magnolia bark, Manchurian Thorn Tree extract, Muira puama, Nopal cactus, Rehmannia, Rhodiola rosea, Reishi, Schizandra, Shatavari root, Damiana with Suma, Shilajit, Tayuya, Tibetan ginseng (Rhodiola crenulata), Valerian.

Jiaogulan, or Southern Ginseng, (*Gynostemma pentaphyllum*) is an adaptogenic herb known as "immortality tea" and said to be more powerful and less expensive than Ginseng. Jiaogulan is a herb that has been shown to restore homeostasis. It has been shown to increase glutathione production and reduce nitrate levels.

SUPERFOOD LIST: Superfoods are nutrient-dense foods that have health-promoting properties such as reducing one's risk of disease or improving any aspect of physical or emotional health. Superfoods increase energy and vitality, regulate cholesterol and blood pressure and may help to prevent or fight cancer and other diseases. Superfoods in combination with sunbathing provides the most amount of regeneration with the least amount of toxic byproducts.

Examples of Superfoods include: Dandelion leaves, garlic mustard leaves, nettle, Moringa leaf, alfalfa leaf, duckweed, water cress, spirulina, kelp and dulse, blue green algae, kale, spinach, parsley and cilantro, arugala, wheatgrass juice, broccoli sprouts, microgreens and sprouts of all kinds, blueberries and berries of all kinds, Incan berries, jackfruit, kiwifruit, passion fruit, papaya, acai, pomegranate, Amla Indian Gooseberry, Mulberries, Camu Camu, fresh olives, olive leaf, avocado, raw coconut, home grown vine-ripened tomatoes and peppers, bamboo sap, wild salmon, New Zealand bee pollen, propolis, raw cacao (chocolate), maca, goji berries, aloe vera, pine seed, hemp seed, pumpkin seeds, sprouted, Brazil nuts, walnuts, quinoa pilaf, poppy seeds, real Essene bread, dehydrated chia/flaxseed crackers, sprouted seed hummus spreads. Purple Corn is #1 in anthocyanin antioxidants - even more than blueberries. Shiitake and other medical mushrooms.

Sang Hwang mushroom, or the *Phellinus Linteus* mushroom in Latin, prefers to grow on mulberry trees to other trees. Asians have used the mushroom for hundreds of years to treat diarrhoea, gastrointestinal dysfunction, haemorrhage, cancers and other ailments. Asians use it in skin care to eliminate wrinkles by strengthening the collagen and elastin matrix and enhance the layer of fat beneath the skin for a visible anti-aging effect Sang Hwang mushroom decreases the formation of oxidative stress by almost 90% and inhibits tumour growth at a rate of up to 96.7%.

OVERCOMING METABOLIC X

THE BASIS OF DEGENERATIVE DISEASE

Our industrial efforts to ensure the longevity of our food leads directly to shorter and shorter lifespans for ourselves!

Industrial grown and processed food is 100% crap! Bodies built from industrial food are not build to generate energy from food because the fats in the mitochondria organelles are the wrong kind. Homo sapiens is radically deficient in Omega-3 DHA fat which is required for the brain, and for the cardiolipin fat in the cell membranes of the mitochondria and electron transport chain which creates ATP the energy storage molecule. If you cannot "burn" fuel due to having the wrong fats in your mitochondria you just end up as an obese diabetic blob — and have children that are also obese diabetic blobs.

Lack of Cardiolipin (DHA-Omega 3) in the tissues that support the electron transport chain in the mitochondria…is one of the main reasons why Homo sapiens is becoming increasingly insane. The **Essential Fatty Acid Ratio** between Omega-6 to Omega-3 became grossly unbalanced with the advent of cereal agriculture 12,000 years ago. Basically dysmetabolism and degeneration of the human species arose due to lifestyle and diet changes as we moved from the Paleolithic period to the Neolithic age, which ultimately led to inadequate DHA-Omega-3 fatty acid in the brain and in the membranes of the cell's mitochondria powerhouses.

Humans evolved on a diet with an equal ratio of Omega-6 to Omega-3 essential fatty acids, whereas in Western diets the ratio is 15/1. Our Omega-3 to Omega-6 ratio should be 50:50. Now Omega-6 is 20X too much and inhibits DHA-Omega 3 needed for mitochondrial energy production and brain fat. The ratio has been in decline since the end of the Paleolithic Age, and now with transfats, it is no wonder humanity is insane and terminally aggressive.

The loss of mitochondrial membrane structure and function, especially with regards to CARDIOLIPIN, which is largely composed of DHA Omega-3, caused the disruption of energy generation in the cell's power centers. The consequent loss of cellular voltage can be seen as the underlying cause of all human distress, disease and dysfunction…acting as a catalyst on all other causes in all domains (body, mind, soul, social, cultural, environmental). Rectify this one deficiency and any solutions we implement are amplified geometrically and synergistically.

The decline of Borg civilization due to chemical agriculture and cooked food has to do with the increasing disease and mental illness as a consequence of the collapse of cellular energy generating system. The degeneration of Homo sapiens started with the Neolithic age, agriculture and cereal growing — for since the end of the Paleolithic age we have had an accelerating lack of DHA-Omega 3 for the brain and the cardiolipin walls of the mitochondria. Hence our cellular energy production has gone down. Our degenerative diseases reflect this loss of metabolic fire - creating sclerosis, toxic plaques, poor detoxification and mutagenesis.

A high intake of trans fats is one of the best predictors of aggressive behavior. It is worth noting that trans fats probably contribute to the problem because of their inhibitory effect on Omega-3 metabolism. Main sources of trans fats are: junk food, fried food, doughnuts, cookies, cakes, & almost all processed foods & those made with hydrogenated vegetable oils. Violence associated with criminal behavior can stem from specific nutritional deficiencies, including deficiencies of Omega-3 fatty acids, magnesium, and zinc. Such nutritional deficiencies impair brain development, contributing to brain inflammation, hyperactivity and cognitive dysfunction.

Quench Inflammation and Enhance Metabolic Efficiency — When you reduce inflammation (especially in the brain) and repair mitochondrial function you generate more ATP and burn more energy — then metabolism, detoxification and neurohormonal function improve and the body doesn't hold onto excess weight. Dr. Jack Kruse recommends an Epi-Paleo diet, that is steering away from carbohydrates to more of a fat based diet with emphasis on seafood for the DHA necessary to make cardiolipin…the special DHA based fat in the mitochondrial membrane that supports the electron transport chain that makes ATP. There is no way to save the species Homo sapiens without reversing the damage done to our body, mind and soul from 12 thousand years of degenerative culture. By reducing calories while adopting a superfood nutrient-dense diet loaded with raw enzymes and colorful phytochemicals…along with significant daily exercise the Metabolic X basis for infectious and degenerative disease is overcome…and the dehumanization of the species halted.

***It is best to take Omega 3 from whole food sources due to aldehyde toxin contamination of Omega 3 supplements.

OMEGA 3 WHOLE FOOD SOURCES: Omega 3 needed to build super intelligent mitochondrial and cell membranes. To avoid rancidity go for whole food sources rather than oils. Plant sources include: Moringa leaf, Purslane, and the seeds/oils of Hemp, Flax, Chia, Kiwi fruit, Pomegranate, Perilla, Walnuts, Sacha Inchi, Camu camu, Borage Spirulina and other Bluegreen algae. The highest herb sources of Omega 3 are basil, oregano, cloves, marjoram, tarragon, spearmint and capers. Super antioxidants, chlorophyll and colorful plant pigments (phytochemicals) and olive leaf will protect the Omega-3 and allow its healthy incorporation into cells. Ideally should be taking Parent Essential Oils (PEOs) from seeds and nuts and the body will make all the Omega-3 it needs.

Also containing Omega 3 are Organ meats, Grass fed lamb, Eggs from chickens feed on algae, fish and Omega 3 containing plants. Wild fish (Salmon, Mackerel, Tuna, Halibut), Krill oil, Ratfish oil. *Krill oil is better than fish oil, because the high levels of natural antioxidants in Krill prevent the oil from going rancid. Fish Oil/Omega 3 is no longer recommended as supplemental fish oil is proinflammatory, and much of the ocean is polluted with radiation, heavy metals and other toxins.

Overcoming Metabolic X requires a rebalancing of this ratio by eating fish and seafood and other high Omega 3 containing foods to rebuild the membranes of cell and mitochondria, thereby repairing production and regenerating the nervous system. The body cannot even detoxify itself without enough energy and so metabolism gets corrupted by the build up of wastes. To cure Metabolic X we must avoid the cooked and hydrogenated fats, transfats, polyunsaturated oils (soybean, corn, safflower, canola etc…), sugar, salt, cereals and processed foods.

Metabolic X Syndrome is characterized by having the following symptoms: insulin resistance, hypothyroidism abdominal fat, obesity, high blood sugar levels, high triglycerides, low good cholesterol, high blood pressure and adrenal exhaustion. Metabolic Syndrome causes heart disease, risk of a heart attack or stroke and diabetes, underlies all degenerative disease, and makes the body vulnerable to infectious disease.

Once the cells walls have become desensitized to insulin (Insulin Resistance) glucose floats freely in the blood elevating blood sugar and dropping Mitochondrial energy production. This sugar is then sent to the liver where it is converted into fat and circulated via the bloodstream throughout the body in a process that can lead to weight gain and obesity. Free-floating insulin in the blood can damage the lining of the arteries and contribute to the development of atherosclerosis plaque on the artery walls. Increased insulin and glucose levels reduce the kidneys' ability to remove salt, as well as increasing the risk of blood clot formation.

Furthermore we must regenerate the thyroid (iodine, raw coconut oil), adrenal glands (adaptogens licorice root and Vitamin C), detox the digestive system and repair its lining, detox/rebuild the liver, increase methylation with sulfur rich vegetables, support digestion with enzymes, remineralize, use herbs to overcome insulin resistance, ie: help glucose get into the cell and lower blood sugar. Plus incorporate mega anti-pathogen, antioxidant, anti-inflammatory foods and supplements into our diet, along with getting adequate exercise in nature.

One of the weight loss secrets of the raw food diet is lipase, a fat-splitting enzyme found in foods that are live and raw such as sprouts, fresh fruit and vegetables. Lipases are associated with fats in their natural state, thus bean sprouts, nuts and seeds contain lipase, amylase and protease. In the raw, sprouted form the oil in nuts and seeds contain a significant amount of lipase to help with their own digestion into smaller units. In living or fresh foods the fats are still fresh and "sweet." Living and germinated fatty foods (within reason) do not cause insulin resistance, diabetes or obesity. The key is to keep fat around 10% of calories and to make sure that all fat that enters us is still living and intact. If in doubt—SPROUT!

By reducing calories while adopting a superfood nutrient-dense diet loaded with raw enzymes and colorful phytochemicals and Omega-3…along with significant daily exercise the Metabolic X basis for infectious and degenerative disease is overcome…and the dehumanization of the species halted. By shifting from quantity to quality with superfoods we can adopt the calorie restriction or intermittent fasting lifestyle, which will promote vigor, vitality and increase our lifespan.

The most important food we can eat is "sunlight!" The more disconnected from the earth and deprived of sunlight that we are, the more food we have to eat to get enough electrons to create the cell's energy molecule ATP. When producing ATP we get 1/3 of our electrons from food and 2/3 from sunlight. Sunlight hitting the eye is also necessary for the creation of thyroid hormones and endorphins, so it is no wonder there is an obesity epidemic. See the YouTube videos of **Dr. Jack Kruse**.

As each of us unleashes our full cellular energy we can overcome the sadomasochistic patterns of dominance and submission that are holding the species back in a primitive, disempowered state and generating disease on all levels. With ideal ATP production to power our genius and enterprise we can begin to redeem our species karma, regenerate the earth and do the right-thing under universal law We can even begin to know the true meaning of fun! Once full energy generation is achieved we can live a life of unity with Source, whereby all that is false and destructive falls away allowing the epigenetic de-repression of our humanity to begin. Anything that increases consciousness, communication, communion and intimacy - or the power of the flow of Spirit's ordering information and informing order will reduce cancer and other Metabolic X symptoms. Synergizing solutions will stop the descent into the complexification of problems, making possible the redemption of the human species through accelerating conscious "humanization."

See: CARDIOLIPIN ~ The Heart of the Matter http://jana-sovereignstate. blogspot.com/2011/07/

EXITING MUTANT BORGLAND

You cannot get help to transcend the predatory zeitgeist, from within the therapeutic framework of the predatory zeitgeist.

I have been trying to find the words to describe the oppositional defiance and denial of reality that infects those with a resistance to what is actually going on. When those who are lucid describe the circumstances we find ourselves in (chemtrails, scorched earth fires, weather warfare, global cull) those who insist on remaining deluded call the obvious reality a "conspiracy theory. "This would be funny, if it weren't so serious, for without a worldwide awakening to reality there is little hope of turning things around for the better. We know the type of deeply HUman world we want to live in, and this is not it. All those who are awake need to band together to work-play on solutions (soul actions).

The Borg soap opera is the Hindbrain hijacking the neocortex. The drama of which keeps us glued to the mainstream circus. To stop wasting your time with the Thanatos culture you have to turn your back on the Borg circus, and to do this you need to commit to raising your energy and consciousness to the mystic, shamanic, creative and executive-prefrontal levels. Ultimately by focusing on becoming a sovereign HUman instead of a pre-personal assimilated Borg we free ourselves from the machinations of the mainstream satanic, luciferic realm.

The Borg is the energetic sleep of our psyche and soma through cultural systems of addiction, denial, avoidance and resistance to facing our shadow. The Borg is the separate-self-sense; of being alienated from body, soul and cosmos and forming a homogenized mass of lost individuals, preying on and feeding off of each other in a vain attempt to get to the top of the pile. If for any reason we are cut off from the sensation of the God within, that is our connection to our Kosmic nature and infinity, then we live in existential fear. This is the real-fear of the cells of the body expressing their genuine plea for the organism to adhere to a code of Life!

To prevent or cure cancer you need to exit the "mutant terrain" of cancer—cooked food, demineralization, lack of enzymes, carbos-cereals-sugars, hypoxia, loss of zeta-potential, acid blood, animal protein diet, trans and altered non-living fats, loss of aerobic ATP energy production, smoking,

218

chemtrails, radiation etc… Overcoming insulin receptor resistance—the main signifier of MetaboliX Syndrome—is essential to maintain the correct hydrogen bonding and osmotic properties needed for superconducting and superfluid quantum coherent water in the nanospaces of the body's tissues. Reducing insulin resistance is essential to eliminate the MetaboliX terrain that promotes cancer and is an ideal environment for pathogens. Thereby allowing the ideal liquid crystal structure of water in the body can provide the ideal matrix for the generation of DNA and other biological structures.

Diabetic tissues are accompanied by characteristic yellowing from Advanced glycation end-products (AGEs) of the collagen matrix that decreases in collagen hydration and heightens collagen breakdown. AGEs (Advanced Glycation End products) - accumulate in long-lived structural proteins, such as collagen and elastin increasing the stiffness of blood vessels, joints and the bladder, and impairing function in the kidney, heart, retina and other organs. People with diabetes have an increased risk of dehydration as high blood glucose levels lead to decreased hydration in the body. By restoring insulin receptivity and lowering excessive blood sugar, the osmological differential between inside and outside the cell is improved and the aquaporins can operate more effectively to keep the cells adequately hydrated.

The combination of hydration and collagen integrity has significant importance to the body's EMF-morphogenic communication system. This relates to the "holism" and "depth" of consciousness achievable, especially with regards to biological intelligence and psychic and spiritual consciousness—. as is evidenced through the study of quantum consciousness and the atomic structures of living things such as Mae-Wan Ho's fabulous research. In her paper *"The Acupuncture System and The Liquid Crystalline Collagen Fibres,"* **Dr. Mae-Wan Ho** says "water associated with collagen shows a surprising degree of order. Could they be the super-conducting channels that enable every single cell within the body to intercommunicate for perfect coordination?

Connective tissues contain a lot of water; these soft connective tissues (apart from bones and cartilage) are typically 60 to 70% water by weight. The proteins together with the water form a liquid crystalline matrix in which every single cell in the body is embedded, which makes connective tissues the ideal medium for intercommunication. A colleague and I proposed in 1998 that the acupuncture meridians may be the structured water aligned with collagen in the connective tissues and that the Qi may be positive electric currents carried by the jump-conduction of protons through the hydrogen bonds of the water molecules aligned along the collagen fibers." www.i-sis.org.uk/Collagenwaterstructurerevealed.php

The water associated with collagen acts like a *liquid crystal* capable of communication via quantum coherence. This liquid crystalline continuum mediates hyper-reactivity to allergens and the body's responsiveness to different forms of subtle energy medicine. **Bound water** layers on the collagen fibers provide proton conduction pathways for rapid intercommunication throughout the body, enabling the organism to function as a coherent whole. We propose that the acupuncture system and the DC body field both inhere in the continuum of liquid crystalline collagen fibers that make up the bulk of the connective tissues.

See YouTube: Mae-Wan Ho - *Conference on the Physics, Chemistry and Biology of Water 2014*

DNA REPAIR

Light flow in healthy DNA is coherent and superluminal—that is it is faster than light or nonlocal. The great German researcher in biophysics, Dr Fritz Popp, said that in health, the light in the DNA is coherent. This light appears to emerge from the DNA and pass on the DNA's information to the cell, and thereby to control the cell. As a consequence constant exposure to the destructive effects of UV radiation, ionising radiation, EMF smog and electrical radiation along with toxic chemical substances and processes, the cell has to work harder. With cumulative damage cells can no cope with the ever-increasing amounts of destructive energy thrown at it, our DNA can be distorted and trigger all manner of disease. The theory of cumulative damage assumes that a stress cycle with an alternating stress above the endurance limit inflicts a measurable permanent damage.

Aluminum readily passes the blood brain barrier (BBB) and accumulate in the brain, especially when it is nano. It is easy to get in, and much harder to get out. Aluminum can also disturb DNA transcription and replication to result in abnormal metabolism and protein synthesis. In addition, Aluminum interferes with cellular energy generation, create inflammation and free radicals and bring about changes in the cholinergic neurotransmitter acetylcholine. The degradation of the integrity and function of the Blood Brain Barrier leads to dementia and other degenerative diseases.

In the field of environmental pollution, heavy metals such as mercury, cadmium, lead, chromium, copper, cobalt, nickel, tin, arsenic, aluminum, etc. Such pollutants are not easily be degraded by microorganism and may even undergo bioamplification. Industrial pollution consisting of the 'heavy' metals, is not only causing dementia, but also altering our DNA. Based upon the increasing evidence that DNA methylation changes occur in AD brains and in response to particulate matter inhalation... Environmental factors are known to induce several epigenetic modifications such as DNA methylation and acetylation or methylation of histone proteins.

Of these, the most well characterized epigenetic modification is DNA methylation. DNA methylation regulates gene silencing and mounting evidence suggests strong correlation between environmental exposure to air pollutants and altered DNA methylation. The process of epigenesis or DNA methylation occurs when methyl groups are added to the DNA molecule. DNA methylation is essential for normal development and evolution, and is associated with a number of key processes including genomic imprinting, X-chromosome inactivation, repression of jumping genes, aging and carcinogenesis or mutation.

Nature is geared towards repairing DNA, while humans are geared towards destroying it. Aging can be largely attributed to the accumulation of DNA damage. Damage to DNA mechanisms that synthesize proteins results in faulty proteins, which accumulate to a level that causes "fatal" damage to cells, tissues and organs. Colostrum is one of the most powerful, broad-based DNA repair agents; Naringenin a flavonoid in Grapefruit repairs DNA; Folic acid and SAMe and Fulvic acid boost DNA repair; selenium is involved in DNA repair. DNA repair is promoted by all flavonoid rich plants including Moringa oleifera, Cat's claw, Gingko and all colorful fruits, vegetables, herbs, grains, legumes, nuts, and teas. Significantly lower levels of DNA breaks occur on a raw diet with a high ORAC antioxidant capacity.

The hydrogen bonds in the bound water around the DNA molecule play a major structural and functional role in the helical shape of DNA. The enzymes and proteins involved in DNA replication and repair make extensive use of hydrogen bonds. The neutron in the hydrogen atom of Deuterium (H+) destabilizes DNA and is associated with mutation damage and cancer through the mechanism of hydrogen bonding. The bonds created by heavy water (deuterium) are stronger than normal hydrogen bonds. Tighter deuterium bonding stiffens proteins and requires more energy to break during metabolic reactions. Deuterium affects the shape of molecules, including the shape of enzymes—many of which are involved in DNA synthesis and repair.

The presence of deuterium in these enzymes slows DNA replication, it causes errors in transcription, and it hinders DNA repair. Deuterium-depleted water can reverse DNA damage, stabilizing DNA and providing DNA protection from radiation damage. Improving mitochondrial function is an important mechanism of extending lifespan, as decreased mitochondrial function, impaired ATP generation and increased free radicals levels have been implicated in driving the aging process. Mitochondria dysfunction (due to being damaged from the presence of deuterium (Heavy hydrogen, H+) etc…) is what kicks start cancer and genetic dysfunctions. **Because fungi has a deuterium retaining pump it actually grows faster in the presence of heavy water. This is no doubt why candida is correlated with cancer, reduced, immunity, mitochondrial dysfunction, insulin resistance and metabolic disease.**

When mitochondria become dysfunction due to deuterium damage the cells turn cancerous; that is they change to metabolize glucose anaerobically via fermentation to attain energy. This shift to inefficient anaerobic ATP production is the main reason why those with cancer have low energy. The answer lies in mitochondria DNA (mtDNA), which accumulates mutations at a faster rate than DNA in the nucleus. In skin, for instance, mitochondrial mutations are thought to be responsible for the gradual loss in the quality of collagen, the skin's scaffolding, which is why skin loses its shape and forms wrinkles. If we ever find ways to protect or repair mtDNA, this new discovery means that we could significantly delay aging. www.vrp.com/articles —Mitochondrial Theories of Aging, by **Ward Dean, MD**

Damage in mitochondrial DNA leads to the generation of toxic reactive oxygen species (ROS), which produce further damage in mitochondrial DNA setting up a vicious cycle of mitochondrial dysfunction. The accumulation of mutations in mitochondrial DNA leads to progressive bioenergy deficiency, cellular damage, degeneration and eventually death. Since mitochondrial DNA is more susceptible to damage by ionizing radiation, UV, electro-smog, nanometals, deuterium and free radical oxidation…*the secret to anti-aging and chemtrail thrival is to protect, preserve and enhance our mitochondrial DNA.*

The vortical ORMUS trap water machines (www.cherokeegold.net) may be "spinning off" via centrifugal vortex the heavier deuterium water molecules, resulting in the collection of deuterium depleted water that has a lower surface tension and life-promoting properties. A sign that Magnetic Trap water IS Deuterium-Depleted Water is that when sprayed on the skin it very easily penetrates the skin and significantly enhances mitochondria activity and ATP production, as is evidenced by the "heating effect" of Trap water on the skin. The fact that ORMUS trap water immediately enhances the mitochondrial activity of the skin, points to the fact that it must provide the correct hydrogen bonding matrix for mtDNA enhancement and repair.

TELOMERES

Aging is caused by the accumulation of damage to the cells. Some of the causes are unavoidable such as ultraviolet radiation, free radicals, and genetic effects; others involve environmental, behavioral and cultural influences. Telomere length is reflective of our biological age and accurately indicates the speed at which we age. What's important to the speed of aging that makes cells stop growing is the shortness of telomeres, not the average telomere length. The genotoxicity of Nano Metal Oxides in DNA damage resulting from oxidative stress on telomeres will significantly foreshorten the lives of all those who do not adopt an antioxidant rich diet and ongoing heavy metal detoxification. Moving to locations with less genotoxic exposure from chemtrails may be something to consider for young couples wishing to start a family.

Longevity scientists may run into trouble stimulating cell division in elderly with regards to cancer and so you have to remove the acidic/hypoxic cancer terrain, and stimulate stem cells. Research shows that psychological stress—both perceived stress and chronic stress—is significantly associated with higher oxidative stress, lower telomerase activity and shorter telomere length. Stress hormones increase oxidative stress damage, in part by exhausting antioxidant enzymes. The fact that stress lowers telomerase activity indicates that chronic stress increases telomere shortening and thus cellular aging. Telomere length itself is related to elevated stress hormones (catecholamines and cortisol).

People living in false power, exploitive and violent/aggressive societies have shorter life spans. While those living in regenerous, non-entropic cultures live longer lives and the civilization itself is more sustainable (stable). In social structures that are affiliative, compassionate, giving, fun and humorous there is a greater sense of personal control, self-expression, health, and consequently higher levels of telomerase—the enzyme that elongates telomeres at the ends of DNA strands. Meditation, exercise, mutuality, music and other forms of stress reduction increase the lifespan of telomeres. Maintaining telomere strength is important in generating maintaining sovereignty for youthfulness is essential to self-empowerment. Longer telomeres give you super health, sovereignty, independence and the potential for a self-created life.

Deep soulful social connection is highly important to youthifying. Telomerase is higher in social relationships that are reciprocal, compassionate, giving, fun and humorous, where there is a greater sense of personal control, self-expression and health. Meditation, exercise and other forms of stress reduction increase the lifespan of telomeres. Love or opening builds coherency, while fear disrupts it. Promoting restful sleep has an important role in reducing tenseness, restlessness and improving tissue repair, mood and longevity.

The thyroid gland ties into the prevention of both infection, oxidation and inflammation, and how pH and oxygen levels are boosted by maintaining iodine and glutathione levels in the body. Thus increasing cell voltage and disease resistance. Healing and anti-aging requires a cell voltage of -50mVs in order to generate "new" cells. Since cell voltage reduces with age we can say that high cell voltage is concurrent with telomere conservation, while the oxidative entropic effects of low cell voltage lead to telomere decay and cell death. There is accelerated telomere shortening in response to life stressors, along with a drop in cell voltage, free radical oxidation, adrenal exhaustion and fatigue.

By the time the human reaches adulthood, the body consists of close to

100 trillion cells. Cells have only a "limited number" of cell divisions possible in a human lifetime. By the time you're 40, there are maybe only 30% of your possible cell divisions left. When the cells use up their natural allotted cell divisions, the end is death. The mechanism that controls this cell division lies with the telomere, which is a cap-like structure on the end of each of the 23 pairs of chromosomes.

Each time your cells divide, your telomeres at the ends of DNA strands get shorter, such that after a certain number of divisions the telomere disappears, and the end of the chromosome begins to fray and stop dividing. Over time, this cumulative cell death leads to aging. To grow biologically younger instead of older by repairing the telomeres we need a telomerase activator, to reawaken telomerase just enough to rewind the clock of cellular aging without causing an undue risk of runaway cells and cancer.

As the countdown clock of the telomeres run down cell division stops and your life ends. Accelerated telomere shortening occurs in response to life stressors due to increased oxidation by free radicals. The enzyme "telomerase" acts to repair damage to the telomere, and helps to maintain its length and stability. Theoretically by raising telomerase we may be able to prolong cell life and slow down or even reverse the aging process.

As a consequence of the foreshortening of the telomeres, the worn-out cells either commit suicide or merely stick around without further dividing. The problem with these inactive cells is they *secrete inflammatory chemicals* that damage other healthy cells leading to the trail of aging, senescence, and degenerative disease. The aging process can be reversed by reactivating the telomerase enzyme, thus stopping the shortening of the telomeres, thereby leading to the repair of damaged tissues and reversing the signs of aging, substantial restoration, including the growth of new neurons in their brains. As long as we maintain a raw diet and high oxygenated lifestyle the potential of getting cancer with telomerase reactivation is negligible.

TELOMERE REGENERATION

Telomeres ordinarily shrink by 1% annually, from birth to death. The telomeres of people with unhealthy habits have much faster shrinkage, while those of people with healthy lifestyle and good habits their telomeres shrink at a slower rate, thus enabling such people to live to approximately 100 years. Progressive DNA damage and mitochondrial decline are both considered to be prime instigators of natural aging. DNA damage is directly linked to compromised mitochondrial biogenesis and function.

Telomere shortening may be influenced by obesity-related inflammation and oxidative stress, and obesity-associated gene (FTO) gene-involved pathways. Telomeres, through tumor suppressor-p53, act to regulate overall metabolic function. The p53 protein (also known as TP53) is a DNA-binding protein that, together with proteins p16 and p21, acts as an emergency braking system for the cell cycle. Once activated, p53 can promote arrested growth and repair, cell death, and most importantly for aging, cellular senescence or apoptosis.

Telomere dysfunction and shortening of telomeres results in measurable decline in mitochondrial number and alterations in function. Lengthening the telomeres is the key to anti-aging—so for anti-aging you must cut inflammation, reduce oxidation, live in biological architecture, eat raw food, green plant protoplasm, adopt a reduced calorie remineralized diet with periodic fasting, engage in the yogic and Inner Arts; and incorporate various youthifiers such as aloe vera, depleted deuterium water, ORMUS trap water and monatomics, and then you have the fountain of youth. Only if your life has a higher purpose that is.

Other longevity agents include supplementation with a combination of melatonin, 5-HTP, vitamin B6, Passion flower, St. John's wort, Magnolia officinalis bark, lemon balm, hops and valerian root helps to support sleep. The adaptogenic herbs Astragalus, Ashwagandha, Siberian ginseng, Schisandra and Manchurian Thorn Tree and Rhodiola rosea help to reduce stress induced fatigue by supporting the adrenal glands and normalizing stress hormones.

CALORIE RESTRICTION, KETOSIS AND NAD+: The ketogenic diet and Ketosis provides the benefit in life extension, lowering inflammation and boosting NAD+. Calorie Restriction has also been shown to increase NAD+ levels in the body, and can extend longevity by 30–50% in many mammals. Lowering blood glucose levels minimizes the inflammation that consumes NAD+. Burning Ketones for fuel instead of glucose requires 1/2 as much NAD+. Our bodies produce less NAD+ as we age, thus impairing the communication between the Mitochondria and cell nucleus. Over time, decreasing levels of NAD+ impairs the cell's ability to make energy, which leads to aging and disease and perhaps even the key factor in why we age. Supplementation with Nicotinamide MonoNucleotide (NMN), the immediate precursor to NAD+, boosts NAD+ levels..

NICOTINAMIDE RIBOSIDE: Vitamin B3 is also known as niacin (nicotinic acid) and has 2 other forms, niacinamide (nicotinamide) and inositol hexanicotinate, which have different effects from niacin. Nicotinamide Riboside and NAD+ are expensive, so for those who want a cheaper longevity fix you can take B3 and D-Ribose instead. Niacin requires adequate D-ribose to form NR and thus NAD+. NR and NAD+ has benefits such as potentially supporting muscle mass and function being a potential treatment for Alzheimer's Disease, improving the function of stem cells, increasing lifespan and lowering the risk of cancer. To improve niacin's conversion to Nicotinamide riboside in the body take about 1 tsp of D-ribose along with 100 mg of immediate-release niacin three times a day. If you don't like the flushing kind take nicotinamide instead. If you have a serious degenerative disease condition, schizophrenia, autism or dementia you could slowly build up your dose to 1000mg and 3 tsp of ribose several times a day for a large male.

RESVERATROL AND ALPHA LIPOIC are two approaches currently being studied for their life-extending propensities. Japanese Knotweed is a more reliable source of resveratrol than red grape skins and red wine. impact on your body's production of telomerase, the enzyme that "rebuilds" your telomeres. Resveratrol also induces apoptosis of various tumor cells and inhibits their proliferation, thereby exerting antitumor effects.

ADENOSINE MONOPHOSPHATE: AMP is a purine nucleotide that is a cell-communicating substance with anti-inflammatory and anti-irritant effects, it is great at fighting viruses, calming the central nervous system and even speeds hair growth. AMP is involved in protein synthesis, and is a precursor to the energy carrier molecule ATP. The ATPase levels in overweight subjects is 22% lower, however by supplementing with AMP this stimulates ATPase production thereby correcting low energy levels due to mitochondrial dysfunction. It is also a key component in certain enzyme reactions necessary for proper fat and carbohydrate metabolism. As well as improved metabolic function, AMP reduces oxidative stress and improves exercise performance, body composition, cognitive function and slows aging. Adenosine monophosphate and L-Carnitine that boosts cellular energy and improves metabolic function!

ZINC SULFATE: Zinc sulfate contributes to promote telomere length extension via increasing telomerase gene expression and activity. Oysters contain more zinc per serving than any other food.

OMEGA-3 from krill oil, southern hemisphere squid oil (calamarine oil), flaxseed or chia seed reduces telomere aging. Chia reduces the glycemic load and reduces inflammation. The special magic combo is Omega-3, Vitamin A - retinol, Vitamin D, Vitamin E - mixed tocotrienols, vitamin K1 and vitamin K2. The sleep hormone Melatonin, is an antioxidant/free radical scavenger that appears to prevent the shortening of telomeres associated with aging; and may act similarly to fight degradation of the cells in the retina. We should consider Ratfish oil as having MAJOR telomere restorative properties. The ultimate antioxidant supplement of all time is ratfishoil.com/ from Norway. It will improve your fat metabolism by detoxing the liver. It is radiation protective—and perhaps the most antioxidant substance on the planet.

MAGNOLIA BARK: The telomere caps at the ends of chromosomes determine how long we will live. Current thinking is that every time a cell divides its telomere caps get shorter. Once the telomeres get short enough cells have a hard time dividing and perhaps become senescent. It has been found that chronic stress appears to speed up this process. Magnolia bark is a traditional Chinese medicine used to treat menstrual cramps, headaches & migraines, anti-stress, aphrodisiac, antioxidant, antibiotic, digestive, diuretic. It controls the body's primary stress hormone, cortisol, increases levels of the calming neurotransmitter -acetylcholine, and eases digestive disturbances caused by emotional distress and emotional turmoil. Magnolia bark contains two compounds that decrease cortisol levels induced by anxiety which hinder a male's sexual power and reaction. Magnolia bark also contains alkaloids that relax tense skeletal muscles, without any change in motor activity or muscle tone. When cortisol is present for long periods of time and in excess quantities, it becomes extremely toxic and can do extensive damage to the immune system. It can also diminish muscle mass, and lead to shrinkage of our vital organs and thinning of the skin.

Our brain cells, or neurons, are extremely sensitive to the effects of cortisol, which in excess can cause brain cells to die. Magnolia Bark Extract lowers the stress response, anxiety and depression—almost immediately, without side effects. Magnolia Extract promotes enhanced survival and growth of injured brain cells, counteracts adrenal fatigue, reduces inflammation and pain, protects against seizures, acts as an antidote for pesticide poisoning and plays a significant role in alleviating asthma.

Magnolia Flower Essential Oil: Treats depression, flu and nasal congestion, aids sleep, heals wounds and burns faster, relieves pain, itch and inflammation.

BUCKMINSTERFULLERENE C60: Our DNA have membranes that allow water to flow through and clear impurities. Because structured/clustered water is smaller than bound water, it flows more easily through cell membranes and is more efficient in removing those impurities. The larger, bound water does not flow easily through cell membranes, and therefore the impurities remain and can eventually result in illness. Shungite charged water which is six-sided, crystal-shaped, hexagonal clustered water molecules form a supportive matrix of healthy DNA. Shungite contains Carbon 60 which regrows telomeres.

ASTRAGALUS: The Chinese herb Astragalus is rich in saponins which have shown activation of telomerase. A company called Geron developed a drug TA-65 from Astragalus that activates the Telomerase enzyme. But apparently, just taking the herb itself will not give you the same results, as there is very little TA-65 produced in the regular processing of this herb. Astragalus is considered an adaptogen useful to reduce stress and to enhance memory, learning and brain function in general as well as to increase energy metabolism.

ASHWAGANDHA: Ashwagandha has powerful antioxidant properties that seek and destroy the free radicals, plus raise levels of the antioxidant enzymes catalase and glutathione peroxidase. Ashwagandha has powerful antioxidant properties that enhance the telomerase enzyme that regenerates the telomeres and prevents their oxidation. Exercise, grounding and sunshine maintains telomere length. Calorie restriction conserves telomeres by reducing the free radical load.

COCONUT WATER: The biggest cause of DNA malfunction is dehydration! Coconut water is far more structured, electrical, pure and energizing that bottled or tap water. The core of a cell's DNA is a column of structured hexagonal water. Raw coconut oil boosts the thyroid and speeds metabolism. This coconut water kefir recipe combines the probiotics and enzymes of water kefir with the electrolytes and vitamins of coconut water. Other waters that assist DNA repair include silicon rich water, fresh coconut water, structured water, watermelon, distilled water, ionized alkaline water, octagonal water and H3o2.

REJUVAMATRIX: The frequencies at which human DNA vibrates are in the 54 to 78 GigaHertz range. The RejuvaMatrix consists of a mat composed of a copper screen covered with crushed quartz or sapphire crystal, placed between two one inch foam pads. The Tesla coil generates a field of 50 to 75 decibels at 54 to 78 GigaHz for total body immersion. The RejuvaMatrix appears to not only stop the shortening of telomeres but lengthens them. After 10 months of use of the device, average telomere length had increased 2.9%. http://www.rexresearch.com/shealy/shealy.htm

EXERCISE STRENGTHENS TELOMERES: Experts believe that telomere length may be linked to inflammation and oxidative stress, both of which exercise has been shown to ease over time. A study in 2008 found people who exercised vigorously 3 hours/week had longer telomeres and were biologically 9 years younger than people who did under 15 minutes. That is the people who got the most physical activity had telomeres that appeared nine years younger than those who were sedentary. EWOT Bio Hack is Exercising with an Oxygen Mask.

NEUROLOGICAL REPAIR
AND BRAIN ENHANCEMENT

People don't understand that what is happening to the trees — is happening to their BRAINS!

There is something definitely wrong with the cogno-moral faculties of contemporary humans. The ruination of the upper atmosphere and the destruction of the ionic/electromagnetic environment for life - through the water cycle and food, means the breakdown of DNA. Inflammatory foreshortening of their telomeres is the prime candidate amongst potential determinants of mortality, capability and cognition up to extreme old age.

The East, West and Middle East are at loggerheads not because of a clash of civilizations but due to the repression of humanization to that of Hindbrain dominance. On both sides of the fence we have brain damage from religious indoctrination, combined with a lack of education and the almost complete disregard for the development of creativity, executive-sovereign decision power and human potential. As a society goes through an idendity crisis there is often a frenzy of mythic symbolism, polarization and divisiveness before the catharsis of an evolutionary jump.

Divisiveness, fragmentation and reductionism are a surefire road to ongoing destruction. While we wait for humanity to wake up and become sane, there is much we can do to support our existence and preserve our humanity within the chemtrail, EMF and GMO holocaust. Massage, yoga, sungazing, meditation, Inner Arts, OUT breathing, raw plant based diet of permaculturally grown food, engaging in the regenerative Arts, taking up a spiritual-humanitarian vocation and most importantly - extensive time in Nature will help reverse the damage done by Hindbrain chemo-industrial civilization.

SUNLIGHT: Strength and sanctity can be maintained by recovering a sense of the sublime spirituality ((energy) of our consciousness in connection to the sun as the circadian biochemical oscillator that determines our "depth" and connectedness through synchronizing with solar time. Slave-time doesn't compute with Solar-time.

Sungazing at dawn and dust will provide similar painkilling and anti-depressant benefits to CBD oil. By resetting your circadian clock and your "spiritual" chemistry sungazing is an amazingly rapid fix to much of what ails us in this discombobulated, disconnected culture. By making like a Sphinx on the grass (or ground) at sunrise and sunset the sunlight hitting the eyes makes thyroid hormones, beta endorphins, DHA-omega-3, cellular ATP energy and cell voltage, dopamine and sex hormones.

DHA-Omega-3 is the main fat in cardiolipin, the structural fat that holds the electron transport chain in the mitochondria. Borg culture has become increasingly deprived of DHA-Omega-3 since the Paleolithic age. It has been 12 thousand years since taking up agriculture and the creation of cities. Now with toxic blue light from computer screens and 5G EMF toxicity, the need for sungazing and grounding becomes essential. 5G inflammation will speed the trajectory of all diseases, and exacerbate the decline of the metabolic X basis of the Fall of Man.

A drop of Lugol's iodine in a gallon of drinking water brings the protons in the water closer together, and this draws the respiratory proteins in the mitochondria closer, making ATP creation more efficient. High DC current in the body regenerates the tissues and generates powerful consciousness! Sunlight also builds a strong immune system, distributes DHA to all the cells of the body, rectifies hormonal and neurotransmitter imbalances, builds strong bones, decalcifies the pineal gland and removes fluoridosis of teeth

STRESS REDUCTION: "Moshe Szyf PhD, found that many of the stress-dampening genes in the hippocampi of the unhappy people were switched off. Although the unhappy people possessed all the right genes to dampen their stress response, the genes were methylated, which suppressed their activation. Szyf calls these suppressed genes "frozen assets," because while they are present in the brain, they are not accessible to its owner, the methylation of the mood area was a response to the unhappy childhoods that the schizophrenics had suffered." 250, *The Genie in Your Genes*, Dawson Church.

NERVE REGROWTH: Regular exercise releases endogenous opioids, enhances serotonin function, stimulates nerve growth factors, promotes cell proliferation in the hippocampus, and leads to a livelier, better-oxygenated brain. Dendrites, the tentacle-like branches of the nerve cells, create connections between neurons and transmit information from one to another--socialization and varied sensory experience grow more dendrites in the cerebral cortex. The brain makes the most neural connections when it is actively involved in learning, therefore, learning should be multisensory and interactive. Substances that raise acetylcholine have shown benefit for Alzheimer's disease. Recent animal studies show that NGF protects acetylcholine activated neurons, showing positive implications for treatment of Alzheimer's.

NGF is essential in the development and survival of neurons in both the central and peripheral nervous systems. Ways to increase NGF include strenuous exercise, stress reduction, uplifting social interaction, falling in love, travel, Sauna/Heat Shock. Nerve growth factor (NGF) promotes growth, maintenance, and survival of neurons and axons and helps repair myelin sheath, the coating around the axons.

Potential nerve growth enhancing effects have been found with Butyrate, PQQ, Lithium, DHA-Omega 3, Vitamin A, Phosphatidylserine, Alpha-GPC (choline alfoscerate), Acetyl-L-carnitine arginate, Uridine + Choline + DHA + omega-3.

HERBS FOR ENHANCING NERVE GROWTH FACTOR: The following are herbs that have multiple reports of potential benefits in neuron protection and repair: Ashwagandha, Ginger, Gotu kola, Ginseng, Grapeseed, Vinpocetine, Curry, Forskolin, Genistein, Chinese spikenard, Magnolia officinalis, Green Tea, Licorice, Forsythia, Lonicera, Sage, Milk Thistle, Gotu kola.

Ashitaba stimulates the production of Nerve Growth Factor (NGF). Ashitaba dry powder increases Nerve Growth Factor (NGF) by 20% after only four days!

Skullcap root (Huang qin) is a powerful anti-inflammatory that protects nerves by diminished inflammation in glial cells and lowering nitric oxide (NO) production.

Scute Root (Scutellaria baicalensis)also prevents excitotoxic injury by N-methyl-D-aspartate (NMDA). Scute root contains a yellow bioflavonoid called baicalein, which is similar to quercetin, used to treat allergy, asthma and digestive system inflammation.

Lion's Mane mushroom crosses the BBB to increase the Nerve Growth Factor and repairing nerve myelin, and has significant anti-anxiety and mood elevating benefits, and may facilitate weight loss by improving fat metabolism.

Milk Thistle Extract was found to grow more neurites (branches of nerve cells necessary for their normal function and that aid in the regeneration of new cells), but it also helped nerve cells alive longer.

Turmeric with black pepper decreased lipid peroxidation, inflammation, mitochondrial dysfunction, and apoptosis.

REMYELINATION: The myelin is a protective fatty layer that insulate nerve fibers in the central nervous system and enables them to quickly transmit impulses from the brain to other parts of the body. Myelin is 75 percent fats and cholesterol, and it is 25 percent protein. Ashwagandha, Red sage, Cat's claw, Bone set, Olive leaf, Flaxseed, Evening Primrose oil, Coconut oil and Grapeseed oil helps nerve cells via supporting the cell membranes and myelin sheaths. B Vitamins, B12, choline, inositol and lecithin protect the myelin sheath from damage. Lecithin- Dietary sources of lecithin include egg yolks, soy beans, sunflower seeds, wheat germ and liver. 5-HTP, GABA, Acetyl-L-Carnitine, Magnesium, Potassium, Cacao, Probiotics, fermented foods, Kimchi, Natto, Chinese Pu-Erh tea, Pollen, PADMA BASIC Tibetan Formula. Hops, Ashitaba, Lion's Mane Mushroom. Omega-3, flax, chia and hemp seeds, nuts, avocado, Olive leaf, Olive oil, grass-fed butter and coconut oil, Vitamin D, sunlight, grounding.

Vitamin K2 protects mitochondria and the cells that synthesize myelin against damage caused by free radicals. Heavy Metal Detoxification helps to remove accumulated toxins that may play a role in myelin sheath deterioration. Copper assists in maintaining healthy myelin, since the myelin sheath is primarily composed phospholipids and copper activates cytochrome-c-oxidase, an enzyme important to phospholipid production. Copper is also needed for neurotransmitters. Consume beef liver, shellfish, nuts and lentils to boost your copper intake and support myelin production. Thyroid hormones help your cells activate genes, triggering the production of specific proteins such as myelin basic protein (MBP), an essential component of the myelin sheath. You can prevent an iodine deficiency by consuming kelp, shellfish, fish, beans and Lugol's. Sleep doubles the production rate of immature oligodendrocytes which are an insulating material known as myelin that protects the brain's circuitry.

REBUILDING NEUROTRANSMITTERS: Neurotransmitters (all 37 of them except one), are made from amino acids. Neurotransmitters are produced on-site in the neurons of the brain from their amino acid building blocks some of which can readily cross the blood-brain barrier. Sufficient amino acids plus vitamin and mineral cofactors must be present to produce adequate neurotransmitter levels. Symptoms for deficiency of the B vitamin Choline include kidney failure, high cholesterol and high blood pressure. Choline is a building block for Acetylcholine which is the parasympathetic nervous systems primary neurotransmitter. Acetylcholine is necessary for muscle control and tone as well as memory, long-term planning, mental focus, mood elevation, sexual activity and other functions. Pantothenic acid, B5 is needed for acetylcholine production. The protective coating for nerves, the myelin sheath is mostly lecithin (which is composed of Choline and another B vitamin Inositol).

Exercise, sunshine and grounding leads to more efficient use of insulin, thus reducing insulin resistance and decreasing the amount of food which is stored as fat. When the cells process nutrients better, they make neurotransmitters better.

MARMITE AND VEGEMITE: Researchers found that the vitamin B12 in Marmite increases levels of the neurotransmitter – GABA. GABA inhibits the excitability of neurons in the brain, with the chemical acting to 'turn down the volume' of neural responses in order to regulate the delicate balance of activity needed to maintain a healthy brain. Essentially Marmite may help reduce burnout and fatigue and consequently depression. Besides B12 Marmite and brewer's yeast also contains beta-glucans, ribonucleic acid (RNA), para aminobenzoic acid, and myo-inositol. Inositol, also called vitamin B8, is for the storage and metabolism of amino acids. It is also an important part of the citric acid cycle, or the main series of chemical reactions that leads to food being turned into energy within the body. inositol also benefits the immune system and the production of hair and nails. For addressing mental health concerns inositol is recommended in nutritional supplements along with tryptophan and omega-3 fats for bipolar disorder patients, panic disorder, depression, schizophrenia and obsessive-compulsive disorder and binge eating.

NOOTROPICS FOR BRAIN POWER: L-Pyroglutamic Acid, Coenzyme Q10, N-acetyl cysteine (NAC), Agmatine Sulfate, Glutathione, Carnosine, Phenylalanine, Taurine, Arginine, Trimethylglycine, Tyrosine, DHA-Omega-3, DHEA, DMAE and Centrophenoxine, NADH, Piracetam, Noopept, Theanine, Huperzine, Vinpocetine, Pyroglutamate, Acetyl L-carnitine and L, Lysine, Ribose, Phosphatidylserine, Sunflower Lecithin, Spirulina, Vitamin C, Magnesium Ascorbate, Lion's mane mushroom, Chaga, Artichoke. Plus 2 B-Complex a day. Mucuna is great, can be mixed with MAO inhibiting Banisteriopsis caapi and Bacopa for stressful days. Oxygen, movement, exercise, grounding, sunshine, mindful sleep, friendships and meaningful work are very important to brain function. Lecithin has specifically been found to be ineffective at treating dementia, while CDP choline (Citicoline) is regarded as effective for dementia and Parkinson's (presumably through increasing dopamine receptor density); and it's a uridine supplement as well. Alpha GPC is 40% choline by weight and is able to cross the blood brain barrier intact.

LION'S MANE MUSHROOM: (Hericium erinaceus) supports nerve regrowth and neurogenesis (via NGF), is a neuroprotective agent (by supporting myelination), reduces beta amyloid induced cognitive deficit and dementia and reduces anxiety and depression, while accelerating wound healing. Lion's mane is traditionally used as a supportive agent in cases of total physical exhaustion, neurasthenia, inflammations, ulcers or gastric mucosa inflammation.

http://stores.ebay.com/thebulksource/ —Hard Rhino Bulk source for NAC

https://liftmode.com/

The Mood Cure: The 4-Step Program to Take Charge of Your Emotions, by Julia Ross

HUMAN GROWTH HORMONE

Human Growth Hormone (HGH) is a polypeptide hormone secreted by the anterior pituitary gland that regulates tissue growth, cellular repair, energy levels, fat loss, and muscle growth. HGH levels are high during childhood for growth and for helping maintain tissues and organs throughout our lifespan, however, after 30 years of age the amount of HGH produced by the pituitary begins to decline. Prolonged stress and aging are associated with reduced secretion of HGH, thereby lowering quality of life and diminishing libido. HGH causes anabolic shifts in the body, causing it to go into a positive nitrogen balance, building muscle, promoting healing and increasing tendon, ligament and bone strength.

HGH helps to keep neurogenesis, or new brain cell development, moving smoothly right through until old age. HGH has the power to clear the neural pathways, rejuvenate and repair damaged tissue in the brain, and can restart new nerve cell development. HGH stimulates the necessary proteins to maintain both long term, and short-term memory retention, however when levels drop off this leads to a decline in general memory.

Human Growth Hormone is released during the first few hours of sleep, during fasting, in higher temperatures such as a sauna, during physical trauma and intense or prolonged exercise. Some studies show that every hour of sleep before midnight is equal to two hours of sleep after midnight, because the largest pulses of GH secretion occur naturally right before midnight. The sleep hormone - melatonin rises after the sun has set, and melatonin stimulates growth hormone secretion. So matching our circadian rhythm with nature's cycles increases HGH. The solar wind at dawn, stimulates the pineal gland, thus the sunrise period between 4-6 am is the best time to sungaze. At these times, the pineal stimulates the pituitary to secrete Human Growth Hormone. That's why sungazers experience rapid nail and hair growth, restoration of hair color, and general rejuvenation.

HGH is inversely related to serum insulin levels. Meaning the higher our insulin levels, from intake of high-sugar food and beverages, the lower our HGH levels. High blood sugar inhibits HGH production, so you should avoid sugary foods in general, but especially so before bed. HGH stimulates protein production and causes fat cells to release fatty acids and to increase the rate of fat burning in the liver. Because HGH levels slowly decreases after the teen years this often results in increased body fat, decreased muscle mass and lowered immune response as we age. It is the natural high production of HGH that keeps teenagers thin while indulging a big appetite. By increasing fat burning and reducing the size of fat cells, HGH can reduce body fat without decreasing caloric intake. Since HGH increases fat burning for energy this increases physical and mental endurance.

With special importance regarding thriving in the chemtrail holocaust, HGH stimulates the Thymus gland thereby improving the immune system! One of the leading factors in immune system decline is the reduced rate of GH as we age. The Thymus gland is the master programmer of the T-cells educating them to kill specific enemies. The Thymus gland is affected by HGH reduction and thus T cells decline in number. High HGH levels is insurance against degenerative disease as an alert T cell system is necessary for the prevention of plaque formation in the arteries and cancer prevention.

INCREASING HUMAN GROWTH HORMONE

• Don't consume sweets, refined foods or alcohol within four hours of bedtime as these inhibit HGH release. Spiking insulin levels retards the release of HGH. Obese people usually have a deficiency of HGH probably due to their insensitivity to insulin (insulin resistance) and the consequent higher levels of insulin in their blood. Avoid caffeine as it boosts insulin levels.

• The Thyroid hormone Thyroxine acts as an immune stimulant by causing the pituitary to release HGH which in turn increases the size of the Thymus and mobilizes immune activity. Kelp provides the iodine needed for Thyroxine production. Manganese is also needed for Thyroxine.

• *There are several nutrients that enhance HGH release these include:*
~The amino acids Arginine and Ornithine and cofactors B5, B6, C.

~L-Dopa, Mucuna and Vasopressin.

~Niacin, GABA and the Amino acids: Glycine, Phenylalanine, Leucine, Valine may stimulate HGH secretion.

~Papaya enzyme Papain, has the ability to breakdown proteins and converts some of it into Arginine which increases Growth Hormone Release.

~Adaptogenic herbs like goji berries, rhodiola, ginseng, reishi, ashwagandha and schisandra help increase HGH by lowering cortisol, and reducing stress and inflammation.

ARGININE AND NITRIC OXIDE: Certain amino acids are known to stimulate the secretion of HGH, including arginine, glutamine, lysine, and ornithine. Most of the substances that increase arginine and Nitric Oxide production also increase HGH! Thus many aphrodisiacs, sexual performance enhancers and HGH supplements will help sustain metamorphosis, regeneration and longevity by preventing the depletion of NO metabolism. Supporting both HGH and NO production keeps the nervous system in a hyperactivated metamorphic condition. A word of caution however, because of its ability to increase human growth hormone (HGH) people with any kind of cancer or chronic infection, should not take L-arginine supplements and avoid food sources of arginine including: chocolate, beer, grain cereals, meats, seeds, nuts, and beans.

OMEGA 3 or **EPA:** Alpha linolenic acid is found in fish and krill oils. The fish with the highest content of EPA are anchovy, salmon, herring and then mackerel. EFA's stimulate the release of Growth Hormone and alters the response of the thyroid gland to thyroid hormones. Omega-3s, have a potent impact on your body's ability to adequately produce Testosterone and other essential hormones. They also raise energy production in the mitochondria and act in the body's thermoregulation and calorie loss.

LECITHIN: Choline boosts HGH levels, especially in the form known as CDP-choline. CDP-choline (citicoline) is a nootropic compound that converts to both choline and cytidine upon ingestion. CDP Choline also can have a very powerful brain boosting effect. As a precursor to the neurotransmitter

Acetylcholine, choline plays a vital role in a number of cognitive processes like those integral to memory, learning capacity, and reasoning. Choline makes phosphatidylcholine, a component of cell membranes.

ALPHA-GPC: Another lecithin extract L-Alpha Glycerylphosphorylcholine is a naturally occurring phospholipid precursor and metabolite, found in plentiful supply in mother's milk. It increases in endogenous HGH secretion, contributing to improved mental focus and cognitive function, language, motor capacity, improved balance, coordination and muscle strength, raises fact burning functions in the liver. Alpha-GPC offers major cellular protection via osmotic pressure regulation and is a metabolic antitoxin and improves the overall quality of life. GPC is a major reservoir for cell membrane omega-3 phospholipids and helps keep choline and acetylcholine available to the tissues.

GABA: The neurotransmitter GABA is made from the amino acid Glutamic acid (Glutamine). GABA promotes fat loss and stimulates the production of Human Growth Hormone. GABA can be taken as a supplement, which produces a calming effect on people who struggle with temporal lobe symptoms like temper, irritability, and reduces anxiety, elevates the pain threshold, reduces the blood pressure and heart rate and reduces compulsive behavior. Because of the blood brain barrier it is best to take substances that stimulate the body to increase its GABA production, such as Ashwagandha, Blackseed oil, Chamomile, Jasmine tea, Green Tea, Kava Kava, Lavender, Lemon balm, Magnolia Bark, Skullcap, Valerian root, and Taurine. Sunlight, Exercise, Deep Breathing, Meditation and Yoga also increase GABA.

FORSKOLIN: (*Coleus Forskohlii*) activates the enzyme adenylate cyclase, which in turn, increases cyclic adenosine monophosphate (cAMP) in cells. Cyclic AMP is essential to synthesize and regulate thyroid hormones, growth hormone, cortisol, DHEA, testosterone, melatonin and other hormones. By increasing cAMP levels there is relaxation of the arteries and smooth muscles, lowering blood pressure, along with enhanced insulin secretion, which can help drive carbohydrates and protein into muscle cells for energy and recovery. Forskolin also increases thyroid hormone function, thereby raising metabolic rate, and significantly increases fat burning (lipolysis), which may translate into fat loss. It also stimulates digestive enzymes, allowing better digestion and assimilation of food.

SEXERCISE AND EXERCISE

Exercise 1 hour daily releases anti-inflammatory cytokines from the skeletal muscles, produces stress relieving endorphins, and moves lymph.

• With regular aerobic physical activity individuals tend to develop less cardiovascular disease than their sedentary counterparts thereby reducing senility. and signs of aging.

• Fitness benefits include improvement in the heart's pumping ability and the diameter and strength of the coronary vessels that supply oxygen to the heart muscle.

• Heightened sexercise increases insulin sensitivity, lowers excess cortisol, promotes weight reduction and can help reduce blood pressure and "bad" cholesterol levels in the blood.

• The protective effects of physical activity also help prevent non–insulin-dependent diabetes, hypertension, osteoporosis, cancer and reduces aging and dementia.

• The increased energy, blood and lymph flow removes calcium deposits from the joints and arteries, that would otherwise result in restricting the range of motion and eventually leading to arthritis.

• The Emancipator sex amplifier counteracts sedentary lifestyle and associated pelvic deadening, ossification and rigidity, and alleviates energy and lymphatic stagnation, thereby overcoming atrophy second-nature and neurosis of the pelvis.

• The Emancipator's ability to amplify sexual output for the same amount of effort means that it is an ideal healing aid for those who are incapacitated by a chronic illness or disability and for the elderly and those with chronic fatigue.

• Decontracts and opens the pelvis leads to improved spine and central nervous system health and more energy flow up the spine for deepening conscious awareness and substantiating spiritual growth.

***If you are an experienced international e-commerce entrepreneur looking for the next big product to sell contact me about licensing The Emancipator at jananz@hotmail.com

GROUNDING

Earthing is essential for mineral utilization in the body, and for the smooth operation of all metabolic processes. Negative Ions is what Earth herself offered us freely till we messed up her electromagnetism. Earthing is the single most important countermeasure to the damaging effects of heavy metal nano-particles, because the earth offers up antioxidant electrons that protect against free radicals and inflammatory damage, improves circulation, reduces pain, improves sleep, increases energy, recover faster from injuries, eliminates stress, numbness and back pain. Thus if you go barefoot and try and earth in nature which has been contaminated then you will just expose yourself to the oxidizing nanometals and radiation. We need to use the earthing mats etc, but we also need to create the technology for fully earthed floors in our houses.

Grounding/earthing is vitally important, but when the ground becomes saturated with nanometals and radiation, even regular grounding in nature is dangerous from contamination through the skin. If we can't adequately ground because of the nanometals on the surface of the earth, this means we are more vulnerable to the heavy metals and the infections. In places like the USA that have been chemtrailed and contaminated with atomic radiation you cannot take your shoes off, so we cannot readily use the natural antioxidant capacities of the earth.

I was thinking that you could set up a grounding station UNDERNEATH your house, for if there is soil there, it would be relatively "clean" compared to exposed places. But the nanometals get right into your house. I know, because they oxidize the surface of the soil in houseplants. We need more earthing technology for the home like universal mats, and earthing sheets, but most

234

of all we need to stop the vulgar bastards from destroying the air, land, water and ocean; and destroying humanity and all life on earth. Negative ions draw out radiation, charge and hydrate cells and flush toxins, hence the need for grounding and nature.

Do you have a piece of personal grass. You can sprinkle magnetite sand into it, over an area the size of your body. This will increase the piezoelectricity. Slightly damp earth also helps with earthing. Lie naked on the grass and wait for the sensation of your body being sucked into the earth, as your energy field feeds on the ions from the ground. It takes 40 minutes for the red blood cell's electric shields to repolarize so that the blood becomes uncoagulated (unsticky). This helps with circulation and oxygenation of the body-mind. Correctly polarized blood is also important for the immune system to fight off pathogens.

The surface of the earth offers up 100mV of free grounding energy whenever we put our bare skin or bare feet on the ground. You can amplify the charge from the earth to 200mV by hammering copper rods into the earth, which you can hook up copper electrodes (bracelets, foot bracelets) with copper wires. Perhaps lying on a copper plate hooked up to the rods would also work, similar to **Galen Hieronymus** and his "Eloptic Energy." Dr. James Oschman is great on grounding.

ANTENNAE TO DISSONANCE

"Our entire biological system, the brain, the earth itself, work on the same frequencies." ~ Nikola Tesla

Earth's electrical and magnetic frequencies are being overshadowed by the toxic cacophony of man-made EMFs, which we have to protect ourselves against. But our "spiritual" etheric body IS the earth and solar system itself, and so cutting ourselves off from cosmic resonance is not the answer. The answer is to educate, evolve and legislate against life-harming technologies in ALL their forms. The greater the life-harming technology that the Thanatos crowd throw at us, the more committed and creative we will be at coming up with work-arounds and life-promoting solutions.

Nothing could be more primitive than contemporary culture as it can only lead to the breakdown and death of all life on earth. We can barely even conceive of life beyond the Death Culture, and yet all of us are called to "do something" should we care enough to listen. Only the biosphere can create the frequencies essential to life. The atmosphere has changed and with that life on earth has changed. We are breathing air that is unnaturally ionized, while our body's EMF field requires air that is ionized as Nature intended. To compound the harmful effect of mal-ionized air, we also now live in an electromagnetic soup from EMF pollution. Study methods for reducing the impact of EMF smog on you and your family. www.emfanalysis.com/basic-steps/

Because our bodies are 70% water we naturally absorb EMF but because our blood has a steady flow it cools like a radiator in a car. Smaller waves pass through and as the blood circulates it cools fairly fast. Larger waves have less effect because we only catch part of the waveform. The range of 30 MHz to 300 MHz waveform matches the size of our bodies. The Eyes, Thyroid, and Testes have very low blood flow so they are more sensitive to EMF damage.

Besides the increased UVC and cosmic rays, the nuclear radiation from Fukushima, and chemtrails are the most widespread toxic, mutagenic agents against tree and plant growth. The wifi, cell phones and other EMF smog is amplifying the vegetation die off worldwide. In heavy chemtrailed areas everything is dying. Technically if you cannot grow food in your area, you will have to move to the countryside or to a different location on the planet where food growing is still possible. The reason being, that if conditions are so toxic that healthy plants cannot be grown, then it is obviously unhealthy for all life forms including humans.

Weather Wars, Disaster Capitalism. Chemtrails, HAARP, and the Full Spectrum Dominance of Planet Earth, by Elana Freeland

BIOELECTROMAGNETISM

MATra CAN BE WEAPONIZED TO CHANGE DNA: Magnet Assisted Transfection (MATra) is a gentle method to transfect cells cultures in labs. In this new technique, nucleic acids are first associated with specific magnetic nano-particles (MagTag®). Then using magnetism the DNA or RNA is then delivered into the target cells leading to efficient transfection without disturbing the membrane architecture, without leaving a hole in the cell membrane like other transfection technologies. Aluminum encapsulated nanoparticulates containing weaponized siRNAs and miRNAs can be uptaken by cells, where they can recombine or silence DNA. Cyclotronic resonance or high power WIFI microwave energy is the catalyst that opens ionic (plasma) cell wall membranes permitting weaponized RNA to enter the cell and recombine with healthy DNA. Cyclotron resonance itself also fractures healthy DNA creating spontaneous recombinations, ie: mutations. It really does look like they are either intentionally, surreptitiously or inadvertently attempting to recode our DNA, the operating code for our bodies.

MAGNETOCEPTION NAVIGATION: The brain has also been found to emit very low intensity magnetic fields, which could be related to what's it called "magnetoreception," how birds and other animals know which direction to travel, how to stay in harmony even in large flocks, and how to sense upcoming natural disasters before they happen. Can humans relearn to harness these same abilities? Magnetic fields have also been shown to be able to induce altered states of consciousness. There are five million magnetite crystals per gram in the human brain. Interestingly, the meninges, (the membrane that envelops the brain), has twenty times that number. The shape of these 'bio-magnetite' crystals shapes do not occur in nature, suggesting that they were formed in the tissue and groups of these crystals have the capacity to act as a system. Women have an 80% higher concentration of Magnetite in their inner ear fluid than men.

HAARP & WHALE NAVIGATION: When the Navy or the oil companies use their sonic, microwave or radar devices we can be sure that these frequencies interfere with the magnetite crystal navigation system in our brains, but also those of all navigational animals including birds and whales. The HAARP frequencies apparently travel through water, as we know that HAARP was invented to be able to communicate with submarines over the earth's horizon, so they must travel through water.

One researcher pointed out a huge array in the water off of Rothschild Island, which puts the Alaska HAARP array to shame. The beaching of whales in New Zealand, Australia and Chili could be due to the HAARP wave that comes out of underneath South America at the underwater facility at Rothschild Island, Antarctica. Watch the Total Precipitable Water - MIMIC-tpw Map online every three days and see if the chirper blast wave from the HAARP occurs and take a screen shot, to see how it changes the weather in the next few days. Within weeks you are likely to get a beaching of whales because no doubt the frequency destroys their navigational neurology, misaligning the magnetite crystals and damaging neurons.

The frequency pulses seen on the MIMIC-tpw map that often arise latitudinally (vertically) out of Antarctica are now also traveling longitudinally around the earth from various Hot Spot points on the earth's crust near the equator. These could be "core" emanations from the expansion of the earth's crust, which is associated with earth's relationship with the sun, moon and other planets (and the Nemesis solar system). Dutchsince says these are Very Long Frequency energy waves changing to Very High Frequency energy waves in the upper atmosphere. This frequency conversion creates electron cascades that build up and reflect other waves such as microwaves—which then show up on the Total Precipitable Water Map...MIMIC-TPW2. These "chirper frequency cascades are reliably predictive of upcoming earthquake and volcanic activity.

MICROWAVE FREQUENCY: 5G microwave (radar range) technology comprises of 86 bandwidths ranging from 600 to 4,700 MHz, whereas the frequency of a microwave oven is 2450 MHz. Microwave ovens work by electromagnetic radiation or microwaves which hit the water molecules inside your food and make them start wiggling around. When the strong microwaves produced by a microwave oven interact with metal object their electric fields cause the mobile electrons in the metal to accumulate at the tips creating a strong electric field in the surrounding air eventually resulting in sparks. We can expect the nanometals and heavy metals in our bodies to heat up our tissues when exposed to microwave radiation, and at the very least create ongoing free radical oxidation and inflammation. 5G is likely to cause changes in consciousness, such as level-shifting, breaking the train of thought, lack of focus and loss of conscious, and to make people electro-hypersensitive. 5Gdangers.com

ANTENNA TO EMF SMOG: Heavy metals and aluminum in the brain acts like an antenna to EMFs, and could produce constant buzzing in the head, brain fog, eye twitches and the inability to sleep and other symptoms. There is a diabolical synergy between computers and cell phones, heavy metal poisoning, EMF damage and infections. Heavy metals in the brain and body act like an antenna to EMF pollution to increase the damaging effects of both, and make us more electro sensitive. This then changes the microbes in the body and the intestinal bacteria so that they produce more damaging toxins. Grate some ginger root and make 6 cups of ginger tea per day. It will cure the fuzzy head by settling the stomach and cutting inflammation in the brain.

LEAKY GUT AND BLOOD BRAIN BARRIER: To make matter worse, the EMFs create a leaky blood brain barrier, which allows increased heavy metals, pathogens and toxins into the brain. Heavy metals and EMF also lead to leaky gut and dysbiosis so you cannot get adequate nutrition as well as becoming autotoxemic. Then if you have not upgraded your glutathione antioxidant levels and you detox from heavy metals and pathogens too quick the toxins will be recirculated back into the body instead of leaving the GI tract. Without adequate NAC and other glutathione boosters (like Alpha Lipoic Acid, Milk Thistle and Pycnogenol), the increase in "mucosal biofilm" blocks the body's ability to kill the pathogens and eliminate the toxins and heavy metals.

CELL PHONE BRAIN DAMAGE PREVENTS DETOXIFICATION: Fibrin is an insoluble protein formed during the clotting of blood. It forms a fibrous mesh of polymerized fibrin together with blood platelets to form a clot over a wound site thereby stopping blood flow. Heparin is a naturally occurring anticoagulant produced by basophils white blood cells and mast cells that prevents clots. Heparin inhibits the formation of fibrin. Fibrin must be prevented from building up in the brain from cell phone damage in order for the immune system to get in and remove damaged cells, plaques and infections.

INFRASTRUCTURE CORROSION: Wooden and metal power poles are deteriorating in the high oxidation/corrosion/rusting conditions of chemtrails + EMF smog + UVC. When 5G microwave (radar range) technology is implemented this will amplify the wood and metal deterioration still further—increasing the electrochemical corrosion of buildings, roads, bridges, houses, sculptures, skyscrapers, cars, planes, trains, train-tracks etc... The infrastructure of civilization is imperiled far more from 21st technology than it was during the 19th and 20th centuries—revealing to us that we are on the wrong track. Even rocks and stones are being rapidly oxidized creating a white patina and freeing up minerals to increase the growth rate of lichen and black mold.

SOLAR UV, EMF SMOG & 5G PROTECTION

The reason why I wrote a book on how to counteract the evil of chemtrails is that I am a horticulturalist/permaculturalist/reforester and I noticed all the vegetation here in Boulder was dying a gruesome death...from chemtrails + microwave frequencies. There is no chance for enlightened society, nor even enlightened individuals in a culture that is destroying the atomic and energetic basis for life's existence. We connect to the cosmos (God) via the ionosphere and magnetosphere when outside and grounded on the earth. I would modify that by saying...We connect to the cosmos when in wild nature, away from human settlement, the electric grid and microwave communications. (See Dr Jack Dr. Jack Kruse and Dr Graham Downing YouTube videos).

THE 5G NETWORK KILL TOWERS: For the large part, the California energy company Pacific Gas and Electric (PG&E) is owned and operated by the Rothschild syndicate, the head of the UN-NWO. PG&E is implicated in the anomalous California fires in 2017-2018 for Agenda 21-30 and the bullet train track. Since homeowners who lost their houses in the fires are most often not allowed to rebuild, the banksters will end up with the majority of land. In this way the Khazarian Zionists and friends will literally"own" America—and we can easily see how a 5G and chemtrail sickened population will quickly become captive under a feudal slave system. 5G will be the REAL killer, a coup d'etat for the ĒLite depopulationists—sensitive individuals feel like committing suicide almost immediately on exposure to 5G, and the damage accumulated overtime by microwaving the environment is almost unthinkable.

Dysnature Syndrome is the result of destroying frequencies, patterns, cycles and vitality of pristine Nature. You have to be insane to be at war with Nature! With thousands of 5G satellites from Space X, OneNet and others it is going to be very difficult to hold onto our sanity. Wireless Frequencies are now around 1-3 GHz, whereas with 5G the frequencies will be between 24-90 GHz. The military are using microwave frequencies at 95 GHz for crowd control and subduing protestors. A 5G system goes right through any wall, and when using both the 4G and 5G systems, and *the vector of 2 microwave arrays* is a death sentence in itself. The 5G millimeter-wave radio frequency beam" penetrates the skin's surface and causes an intense stinging or burning as though the body is "on fire." As far back as the 1980s, scientists began testing the millimeter wave energy as a non-lethal weapon, they called "the Active Denial System (ADS). This "non-lethal weapon system" being rolled out in cities across the world is a population control system which will "cook"everything in its range of exposure.

Symptoms Of 5G Exposure: EMR poisoning symptoms include brain fog and inability to focus, disorientation, inability to concentrate, confusion, fear, hot flushes, an instant type of fever, literally feeling as if you are cooking from the inside; inflammation and areas centimeters wide on the body that swell up and cause a great deal of pain and discomfort, a unsettled nervous system; "hang-over" and sense of exhaustion upon waking, barely mustering the energy to get motivated; loud buzzing in the ears and intense pulses of energy moving up and down the spine causing muscles to spasm; nosebleeds, headaches, eye pain, chest pain, nausea, fatigue, vomiting, tinnitus, dizziness, flu-like symptoms, and cardiac pain and madness. Suicidal thoughts, sleep difficulty, negative behaviors, loss of social bonding and cohesion, collapse of higher functioning.

The new 5G towers and transmitters for wireless technology have major health implications and most people are sitting ducks, as they currently are not aware about much beyond their personal business and self gratification. In 2011, The World Health Organization classified all sources of cell phone and wireless WiFi radiation as a possible carcinogen. Besides neurological damage, memory problems and confusion after being subjected to prolonged periods of radiation exposure from 5G cell towers and antennas, 5G will promote anemia and ultimately cancer, but before that will be depression, brain fog and dementia.

5G microwave technology is yet another eugenics challenge to humans, and an environmental challenge to the continuity of life on earth. Radiating water with 5G from towers and from Satellites WILL make water toxic to life, as it destructures the water in the atmosphere that falls as rain. The anti life-frequencies will also toxify the water within our own bodies and all other living things. 5G is all about hackability, surveillance and full spectrum dominance, so that nothing can be held back from the all seeing Evil Eye of Sauron (Talpiot Program - Israel's push for technological supremacy and total surveillance).

Wireless and microwave (radar range) radiation opens the blood-brain barrier allowing more aluminum, heavy metals and toxins into the brain. Microwave frequencies cause metal amalgams in the mouth to release mercury, and people with metal inside the body could receive internal burns. So all forms of EMF pollution mitigation will reduce the effects of chemtrails on our health. However now with 5G and smart meters it makes it increasingly harder to avoid being cooked by microwaves. More than 65% of the world's population are projected to live in cities by 2050, with major implications resource use, energy, water and sanitation, health, sanity and well-being.

Babies born within the EMF smog will be more basic, with lower complexity and more easily programmable and manipulated. 5G will drop IQ levels faster that most everything else, making whatever countries that adopt it vulnerable to economic collapse, famine and invasion from countries smart enough NOT to adopt 5G. If you don't want to get cancer, and DNA and neurological damage then clean up your electromagnetic environment by eliminating cell phones, wifi, 5G, smart meters and dirty house electricity. 5G millimeter transmitters will be located near every 2 to 10 homes, exposing your family to harmful, carcinogenic, neurotoxic, and genotoxic wireless radiation. See YouTube "5G Wireless Radiation Dangers" www.Bioinitiative.org

Mainstream buildings are generally toxic to living things since they are cut off from contact with the earth's etheric aura and the ground for earthing. Any EMF shielding of houses will have to be compensated for both for grounding, and for connecting to "God." If 5G comes to your town you may need to harden your house against microwaves. Block windows with thin metal camping blankets sold by Walmart. Use EMF blocking paint as underpaint on walls, ceilings and doors. Unplug all electrical devises in your bedroom and most of the house as they are EMF producers. Cover your smart meter with an EMF protective shield. Cover at least three square feet of the wall between your head and the meter with metal screen. You can put a large canvas on the inside wall opposite your smart meter and cover the back of the canvas with a metal screen, as well as painting the entire wall with EMF protective paint.

5G TOXIC SHOCK: If in toxic shock caused by a response to microwaves you can create a paste of baking soda and cover your body until you feel you are out of danger. Microwave toxic shock symptoms include: feeling like you're on fire, water hurt like bullets, your heart stops and your system was down. Keep thin metal camping blankets on hand just in case for EMF toxic shock emergencies. Burying the body in the damp sand at the beach will quickly normalize the body's EMF, as will swimming in the ocean. stopsmartgrid.org

PROTECT MELATONIN PRODUCTION: The pineal gland produces Melatonin during sleep, an extremely powerful antioxidant mopping up potential cell-damaging free radicals in the body. Thus, melatonin plays a major role in cell repair; body rejuvenation and disease prevention. The dark of night and sleep signals the pineal gland to produce melatonin, however when we are bathed in a sea of EMF waves, the pineal gland is unable to detect night time, leading to a lack of melatonin production and impaired immunological function. In the long run this may lead to diseases such as Alzheimer's and cancer. Making your bedroom both EMF protected and as dark as possible, along with grounding your bed will go a long way to preserving your melatonin production while you sleep.

Structured water will help reverse the "frequency dissonance." Negatively charged oxygen or water is an antioxidant—having an extra electron in the oxygen outer shell and offering up electrons to quench unstable positively charged free radicals. Excessive free radicals in your cells can attack the cell membranes, causing cell and tissue damage. Free radicals can also break strands of DNA, which can lead to cancer. Water features and humidifiers that used negatively charged water into our houses may go a long way to counteract the extreme oxidizing effects of the chemtrails. **Tools for creating structured water via vortexing: www.balancedenergystructuredwater.com**

To counter *toxic frequencies* diet should be largely raw and must include high antioxidants and plentiful colorful pigments, along with olive leaf and plentiful greens, microgreens and sprouts. Grounding, magnetite foot baths, grounding shoes, earthen floored houses, negative ion generators, indoor fountains, houseplants and EMF protection will become ever more important. Crystals, orgonite devices, shungite pendants, radionic devices should be employed.

TENSOR RINGS: Radionic Tensor Field Tools in copper and silver for energizing your environment, personal space, water, and all forms of EMF protection. Pendants, dowsing rods and devices for clearing harmful electromagnetic and microwave frequencies. https://twistedsage.com/

CRYSTALS: Psychotronic assaults with frequency weapons and anti-life frequencies like 5G can be reduced with crystals throughout the home, and worn as jewelry. Magnesium containing serpentine & rhodonite offer EMF protection, as does magnetite and shungite. Apparently silicate crystals like quartz, lepidolite, opal, etc... are to be avoided for EMF protection due into their going into resonance with electronics & microwave radiation; as silicates & quartz is an excellent semi-conductor of energy. Crystals are however used in orgonite for EMF protection so more research will need to be undertaken.

MAGNESIUM: Stress from EMF & radiation pollution drains magnesium levels and increases adrenaline so baths with Epsom salt and Baking Soda help to normalize the body and increase serotonin. Magnesium oil (Mg Chloride) sprayed on the skin is also great for frequency normalization and pain.

NATURAL SUNSCREEN: An aloe-astaxanthin lotion would amplify effects of a colloidal silver topical 5G protection. This silver-based sunscreen product shields against harmful x-rays and extreme ultraviolet radiation. https://www.silversafetan.com/

HEART MEDITATION: The heart's electrical field is about 60 times greater in amplitude than the electrical field generated by the brain. Focusing meditative energy on the heart allows the body-mind to come into sync, and by building up your toroidal heart field you can provide some protection from antilife and dissonant frequencies, including those that come from other humans.

THE INNER ARTS: Heart-Tree Meditation, Heart-Wings Meditation or Heart Breathing, the felt-visualization of a 10ft toroidal heart field around you, plus dropping into the heart throughout the day will maintain a strong heart field to deflect negative-energy, or DOR. The Primal Release Pose opens up the "roots" of the heart at the 12th Thorasic. *My spiritual exercise book one "The Inner Arts Practicum"* can be bought from Lulu.com.

FACEMASKS: We need to invent special face masks that include an anti-chemtrail slogan and logo to wear on saturation days. If everyone wears one, it becomes an advertisement, activism and protest as well as protecting our health, and a warning to others. I imagine there will be more street protests, so people could wear them then, but also for getting around town on high spray days. These allergy type masks look great: https://www.vogmask.com; and the Cambridge Mask Company - Anti Pollution Mask Military Grade N99; or Unigear Activated Carbon Dustproof/Dust Mask. You can wet a large cotton handkerchief and fold it in 4, and then putting it over my nose and mouth held in place with a painter's mask. ***However a carbon-filter respirator and goggles will be necessary during a saturation spray attack on your town or city.

SHIELDING HAT: We could wear 5G protective hats, but any headgear will also cut us off from celestial intelligence (God). Make flat shungite buttons to attach on the inside areas of the hat where you want more protection or healing. Shungite attached to headbands will allow it to be positioned over the pineal, temporal lobes or brain stem. Cleopatra used to place a magnet on her forehead to stimulate the pituitary to restore her youth and good looks. We will have to invent a whole range of protective products and methods. For shielding materials for clothing and housing the risk on Esty.com is a good place to start, and here is a shielding hat company shieldheadwear.com.

LADIES FASHION HAT: With Shielded Lining—I found an EMF protection store that sells high tech shielding material that would be good to make hats that protect against EMF. A stylish women's soft hat is perfect for cool weather. 50% Linen, 50% Cotton, with a 100% silver coated mesh lining. Blocks radiofrequency radiation (cell phones, wifi, 5G, TV and radio broadcasts, for example) from EMF Safety Shop, EMF Safety Meters, grounding pad and Shielding. Make wrist guards for use with a Macbook. Hat linings and clothing with Safety Silk from www.etsy.com/shop/EMFSafetyShop

PONGEE SILK CLOTHING: Looks like we could wear Pongee silk Vintage Kimonos, and clothes and hats made from them to protect against radiation/ frequencies. Pongee (Tussah) is an organic wild silk gathered in the jungle from cocoons of wild silk moths.

SHUNGITE: Shungite water has powerful anti-inflammatory/antioxidant/ antihistaminic effects, detoxifies the body and revives the pineal gland as is evidenced by increased dreaming. In my experience shungite shifts the electromagnetic resonance in tissue that is resonating in dis-ease. It is so effective at doing this almost instantaneously, that I got rid of my scenar device. I am not saying it protects against the EMF holocaust itself, but that it re-conjuncts frequency in tissue that has fallen out of healthy synced waves. The fullerenes in Shungite have pronounced anti-inflammatory, antihistamine, analgesic, anti-allergenic, detoxifying, immune-enhancing effects, and can be ingested like activated charcoal. The shungite also cuts any cellular dissonance (inflammation), and the whole body responds to shungite disks put on the surface of the skin. I use them in bed for healing and meditation.

SHUNGITE JEWELRY: Shungite can also be used as a power healing stone to heal EMF damage by placing it directly on the body to head aches, pain, dissonance and spasm and alleviate radiation damage. My shungite pendant moves clockwise when I hold it over my left side of the chest while lying down, and moves anticlockwise on the right side of the chest, while in the middle of the chest it moves backwards and forwards. This is because the heart has a double toroid electric field that represents an infinity symbol or mobius strip, like in the YouTube video: A MODEL OF THE UNIVERSE Proposed by Nassim Haramein.

CARBON 60: One of the best defenses against 5G and other EMFs is Carbon60, either in olive oil, or charging your drinking water with shungite. Also use shungite in jewelry and orgone type protective devices. Shungite buttons can be sown around your shielding hat for extra protection. Putting magnetite or shungite powder in paint to paint on the walls of our houses may also work. Magnetite or shungite in concrete, hempcrete or aircrete may be a good way to shield EMF pollution in dome houses and earth-hobbit houses.

BASALT: If building new housing you need to design towards 100% self-sufficiency, build for winds up to 200mph and use EMF protective technology. Will basalt sand or magnetite sand mixed in with concrete, hempcrete or ceramics help block EMFs and galactic cosmic rays? I thought of the idea of using basalt sand in making ceramic roof tiles, along with basalt siding and basalt floors, as a method of resisting **5G and galactic cosmic rays**. Best to live in a country that respects the sovereignty of its citizens and doesn't mandate compulsory smart meters and such. The free people are those able to break away from the existing industrial extortion matrix. It is a sovereign imperative.

SUPER CERA POWDER: Super Cera powder is used in construction materials and in agriculture is a gray ceramic powder from Japan that is made with EM•1® Microbial Inoculate. The powerful vibrational energy as a result of the high temperature firing process is effective in stopping off-gassing of volatile organic compounds in building materials, increasing tensile strength in concrete, and protecting from EMF waves. We may be able to come up with a cheaper alternative using Hemp fiber fermented with Microbial Inoculate, Diatomaceous Earth, Zeolite, Shungite, powdered lava mixed with structured water.

BIOGEOMETRY: BioGeometry uses specially designed shapes, color, sound, motion and wave configuration, to induce harmony into biological subtle energy systems. It also is a way of 'harmonizing electromagnetic radiation. Dr. Karim has developed a 'science of shape' and the 'physics of quality', or qualitative measurement, which has applications in medicine, architecture, and all other aspects of our lives. *"BioGeometry Back To A Future For Mankind,"* by Dr. Ibrahim Karim.

EMF SHIELDING STORES:

www.emrss.com/ —EMR Shielding Solutions

www.etsy.com/shop/EMFSafetyShop —EMF Safety Meters; Shielding Fabrics, Paints and Other Materials

coolesttechever.com

https://lessemf.com/

NATURE AND THE EMFs OF LIFE: Before buying all kind of supplements and health devises check out YouTube videos by **Dr. Jack Kruse**. His teaching on health and wholeness is the most sophisticated and advanced I have come across. You will learn through him how to tune into cosmic rhythms with sungazing at sunrise, grounding, enhancing mitochondrial numbers and function. By restructuring our lives to tune into Nature we can recover our HUman integrity and natural pleasure in existence, without breaking the bank. By intermittent fasting, getting up at sunrise for sungazing, conscious breathing and running/hiking we can get clear enough to reach escape speed and break out of the wage-slave poverty trap. His book: *"Epi-paleo Rx: The Prescription for Disease Reversal and Optimal Health,"* 2013

FREQUENCY THERAPIES

The depolarization of the electromagnetism of living things leads to sickness, madness, foggy consciousness, cancer, and the acid metabolism of violence, war, competition, disharmony and hyper focus on the material world.

SUN AND EARTH: The sun and the earth are the ultimate frequency medicine. Since the negatively charged earth exists inside the positively charged ionosphere, the tension between the two, gives rise to the Shumann frequency at 7.83 hertz. The resonance of the Earth's magnetic field is extremely close to the frequency of alpha waves emitted from the human brain. Because we are beings of Nature simply being exposed to nature can improve our overall mood and health, and we change out of the beta brain wave patterns that are consistent with high arousal or stress. Our DNA communicates via the invisible 7.83 frequency electromagnetic field that surrounds our living Earth and which we are all connected to…thus the planet essentially creates us and all life. Since our atmosphere is now heavily inundated with man-made radiation and various frequencies Schumann Resonance is being drowned out by wireless technologies which will warp, pervert and degrade the sublime perfection of Nature's creation.

FREQUENCY MEDICINE: Infrared saunas get rid of Morgellons symptoms for at least 24 hours after a 30 min infrared session. A new LED device coming, can load with the same 1400+ frequencies and treat with this rechargeable device. The FIR LEDS penetrate the tissue, and improve microcirculation and cAMP levels (known and proven science, not conjecture). And this is MEDICARE reimbursable, too. Actual medical device, like the other three RADIANT PHI devices. See *"Theraphi and PHI Beam Healing Community"* on Facebook.

ELECTROMAGNETIC THERAPY: Lyme is susceptible to ultraviolet, infrared, gamma radiation especially in pupil and larval stages. Electromagnetic field therapies include Rife Machines, Hulda Clark's Zapper, Denar Devices, Infrared, Acupuncture Pen, Theraphi Machines. Pulsed electromagnetic field therapy PEMF devices with Tesla coils; the VIBE Machine, the Tesla Photon Machine, the Light Beam Generator, Infrared Lamps, the Lakhovsky multiwave oscillator (MWO), and sunlight. Raising body temperature with an infrared sauna powerfully assists the body to kill cancer tumors, bacteria, fungi, yeast, parasites, viruses and other chronic infections.

MICROPULSING BLOOD: Bob Beck's Protocols to kill all infections of the body. Blood electrification, Magnetic pulse, and colloidal silver broadly wipes out bacteria, mycoplasmas, and probably also viruses. Electromedicine is often referred to as blood electrification, blood purifying, magnetic pulse therapy or micropulsing. Basically, they use microcurrents of electricity to create a very small 3.92 Hertz or ½ of the Earth Schumann frequency of 7.83 Hz alternating electric current (i.e.: the cycle of polarity change happens 3.92 times a second). The microcurrents of electricity prevent viruses from infecting human cells which prevents the virus from hijacking the cells' reproductive capacity and multiplying. Drinking ozonated water helps to remove the disabled pathogens and other toxins so that the body safely excretes the disabled viruses. Micropulsing, or blood electrification, also supplies the body with an abundance of antioxidant electrons. Bob Beck Protocol ~ CancerTutor.com

PULSED ELECTROMAGNETIC FREQUENCY THERAPY: PEMF is a physiological modality that increases ATP (energy) production in the cells of your body. In doing so, this dramatically increases the tissue healing rate. The magnetic fields generated by the MR7 are about 60 milligauss. The magnetic field of the Earth is almost 10 times stronger: 250-650 milligauss.

The THERAPHI Device was conceived by Dan Winter and built by Paul Harris, is an extraordinarily powerful Rife-like device. Broad spectrum / centripetal conjugate field effects – rejuvenate and reorganize biologic systems, raise metabolism and eliminate pain. theraphi.net/

A new LED device coming, can load with the same 1400+ frequencies and treat with this rechargeable device. Available soon. The FIR LEDS penetrate the tissue, and improve microcirculation and cAMP levels. See "Theraphi and PHI Beam Healing Community" on Facebook

PLAZMOTRONI DIACOM TECHNOLOGY: Plazmotroni Diacom Technology is a plasma healing devise by Dr. Khachatur Mkrtchyan, a Russian inventor living in Czech Republic. The light wave from PLAZMOTRONIC plasma generator destroys pathogens like borrelia in minutes by "shocking" the pathogens with vibration. Besides being more powerful than any other zapping machines it recharges cells too and eliminates pain! Continuing on from the research of Nikola Tesla, Albert Abrams, Royal Rife, Hilda Clark and Georgy Lakhovsky, the Diacom company created the new Diacom-Plazmotronic device which produces specific radiation via plasma. Diacom-Plazmotronic is used for the destruction of pathogenic microorganisms and other factors that cause chronic and severe diseases, psycho-emotional disorders, as well as metabolic diseases such as multiple sclerosis and Alzheimer's, cancer, skin diseases; it also improves the human or animal's energy field and normalizes sleep.

ULTRASOUND ALZHEIMER'S CURE: Australian researchers have come up with a non-invasive ultrasound technology that clears the brain of neurotoxic amyloid plaques. By oscillating super-fast, these sound waves are able to gently open up the blood-brain barrier, which is a layer that protects the brain against bacteria, and stimulate the brain's microglial cells to activate. As part of the glymphatic system of the brain, Microglial cells are basically waste-removal cells, so they're able to clear out the toxic beta-amyloid clumps that are responsible for the worst symptoms of Alzheimer's. Focused therapeutic ultrasound waves are able to gently open up the blood-brain barrier, and stimulates the brain's microglial waste-removal cells to activate.

Using a particular type of ultrasound called a focused therapeutic ultrasound, fully restoring the memory function of 75 percent of the mice they tested it on, with zero damage to the surrounding brain tissue. The main strategy to eliminate mycoplasma and fungi infections are now centering on the building the immune system, detoxification, raising cellular energy production, remineralizing, enzyme therapy, raw diet and strengthening the terrain of the body. Frequency generators like the Rife machine, Hulda Clark Zapper and the Theraphi Light therapy may be the best way to go for intensive treatment.

INFRARED HEAT: Infrared heat not only helps to detoxify your body of the build up of various toxins, but improves any neurons that have been damaged; helping to stem further deterioration. Infrared heat causes a release of proteins known as **Brain-Derived Neurotrophic Factor (**BDNF), which activates brain stem cells to create new neurons while sustaining existing ones. Supporting your long-term memory, neuron pathways, and firing speed. Infrared saunas support overall mind, body, and soul wellness. During a heavy metal detox, or for removing amyloid plaque you may consider using an Infrared lamp or wand on your brainstem and spine, if you do not have access to an infrared sauna.

Infrared light therapy speeds wound healing, reduces inflammation, increases testosterone production, activates detoxification via the skin, raises the production of Heat Shock Proteins - specialized cellular repairmen that improve cell detoxification and repair malformed proteins, increases blood and lymph circulation & tissue oxygenation, increases tissue growth including Human Growth Hormone production.

Infrared heat causes a release of proteins known as BDNF, Brain-Derived Neurotrophic Factor, which activates brain stem cells to create new neurons while sustaining existing ones and improves any neurons that have been damaged; helping to stem further deterioration. Supporting your long-term memory, neuron pathways, and firing speed. Infrared saunas support overall mind, body, and soul wellness. During a heavy metal detox, or amyloid plaque removal fast you may consider using an Infrared lamp or wand on your brainstem and spine, if you do not have access to an infrared sauna.

INFRARED SAUNAS: Tumors and chronic infections are intolerant to heat and are easily killed with infrared saunas. Near-infrared saunas raise body temperature by 3° F (-16° C), inducing a fever. Infrared penetrates the skin and heats from the inside as well as on the skin, this means the air temperature in the sauna can remain much cooler. Near-infrared saunas kill cancer, parasites, yeast and other infections and assist in eliminating heavy metals and chemicals. Near-infrared is helpful for wound healing and cellular regeneration as well. The near infrared bulbs emit a small amount of red, orange and yellow visible light, which provides stimulating color therapy.

The inexpensive bulbs and lamp housing can be found at most hardware stores as heating lamps for brooding chickens. Three bulbs in a sealed enclosure (a shower or closet) is all you need for an in-home sauna. Do not ever look at the lights when they're turned on. Drink 10 oz of spring water and take some kelp for minerals (Nature's Way brand, or Frontier Herbs) before your sauna. Begin with 20-minutes sessions once a day to avoid massive healing reactions. Wipe the sweat off every few minutes with a towel. Shower with a natural soap like Miracle 11 Soap or Dr. Bronner's, and do 10 minutes of yoga stretches after your sauna. Infrared Saunas and Hydrogen Peroxide or Ozone Foot Baths are a winning combination against Chemtrail Flu and Lyme Disease. Combining negative ions with near-infrared saunas amplifies the benefits. Make sure you get near infrared bulbs, as far-infrared saunas emit electromagnetic fields that can be extremely harmful, especially to those who are sensitive to EMF's.

INFRARED LIGHT WAND: You can also use an affordable option with infrared light wand to eliminate all toxins from the brain and body and ease pain. Infrared light on certain points for 2-3 minutes on prefrontal cortex, ears (+temporal cortex), foramen magnum (brainstem), thymus, celiac plexus, liver, spleen, kidneys and symptomatic areas. The Infrared light turns on the ATP production in cells. I like the Infrared Light Wand (CE0434, ST.302).

ELECTRONIC-ACUPUNCTURE-PEN-MERIDIAN-PEN: The Infrared light turns on the ATP production in cells. An Infrared Light Wand Massager like the CE0434 eliminates toxins from the brain. Infrared light on certain points for 2-3 minutes on prefrontal cortex, ears (+temporal cortex), foramen magnum (brainstem), thymus, celiac plexus, liver, spleen, kidneys and symptomatic areas.

http://www.bwgen.com/ — With the brain wave entrainment programs of the BrainWave Generator take you to the state of mind you want.

TOURMALINE: Free hydrogen is one of the most powerful antioxidants known to man. Free hydrogen has been proven to fight the worst of the free radicals – the Hydroxyl radical, which is known to cause damage to the DNA. Because it's so small, hydrogen can penetrate the smallest reaches of your body – within the cells – fighting the dangerous free radicals. Filtration through Tourmaline activates high levels of free hydrogen, reducing oxidative stress, eliminating inflammation and pain along other changes associated with youth. Tourmaline clay balls can also be added to your shungite water charging system. When milled into fine powders the boron-silicate crystal tourmaline also emits Far Infrared (FIR) and the characteristics of the FIR emission depend on the particle size. I put these tourmaline-clay pellets in my water filter jug, and it greatly softens, charges and purifies the water.

Preparations containing tourmaline powder have been applied to the skin with the aim of enhancing blood flow. In a similar manner discs of Far Infrared emitting tourmaline ceramics have been attached to the skin with the intent of producing a beneficial effect. A blanket containing tourmaline discs reportedly improves quality of sleep, and gloves have been made out of FIR emitting fabrics can be used to treat arthritis of the hands. While socks manufactured from tourmaline-ceramic fiber material in patients with chronic foot pain resulting from diabetic neuropathy or other disorders. And belts made out of fabrics of synthetic fibers embedded with powdered tourmaline-ceramic have been used for weight reduction. Black tourmaline can be used for EMF protection.

USING SHUNGITE DISCS FOR MEDITATION: Shungite is electroconductive, conjuncts or orders energy, is EMF protective, and has an anti-bactericidal effect. You can use flat shungite discs to place anywhere on the body that is inflamed or out of sync. You can make bracelets, anklets, necklaces, earrings, put in pockets, attach to the inside rim of hats, use discs for cellphone protectors and many other uses. You can also use them to put on the forehead or over the eyes while meditating lying down, or use an eye mask, sleeping blindfold to keep the discs over your eyes. My favorite Russian Shungite Store is **boho_cat** on Ebay.

Biophotons and the Biophysics of Light: Royal R. Rife, Wilhelm Reich, Nikola Tesla, Marcel Vogel, Georges Lakhovsy, Albert Abrams, Ruth Drown, Jacques Benveniste, T. Galen Hieronymous, and other pioneers in the psychotronics field. Alexander Gurwitch, Konstantin Korotkov, Alex Kaivarainen and Fritz-Albert Popp for biophotons. Stuart Hameroff for light communication in DNA and Microtubules. Healing is Voltage, Jerry Tennant. www.emergentmind.org/

Sympathetic Vibratory Physics www.svpvril.com/Hier.html

Bioelectromagnetic Healing, its History and a Rationale for its Use, Thomas F. Valone

10

THE WATER OF LIFE

My principle eureka of fortifying the body from the fires of kundalini pointed to "silicon" as being the one element in particular that allowed increased "Light" flow in the body without breaking down nerves and the collagen structure of the body. Again with finding the solutions to the Chemtrail Holocaust it is silicon that is the one element that is indispensable to building tissue that is resistant to pathogens and nanometals, and helps remove heavy metals and aluminum from the body and brain.

It is for this reason that I invented Philosopher's water, so named as a play on the idea of "The Philosopher's Stone." However rather than an object capable of turning base metal into gold and silver, Philosopher's water protects our "ability to philosophize" by preventing the inflammation, mutation and brain damage derived from the aerosol spraying assault.

Chemtrail Syndrome essentially involves the increase and acceleration of the following: aging, dehydration, oxidation, AGEs or Advanced glycation end products, leukoaraiosis or age spots on the brain, accumulation of heavy metals in biofilms and calcium deposits, degradation of DNA and other metabolic molecules, insufficient energy to detoxify the body, leaky tight junctions, inflammation, immune system compromise etc… Basically Chemtrail Syndrome constitutes the rapid breakdown and rotting of the body and destruction of the mind and a loss of soul (separation from Spirit). Drinking deuterium depleted silicon rich water for is the principle cure for Chemtrail Syndrome.

PHILOSOPHER'S WATER

ORTHOSILICIC ACID/COLLOIDAL SILVER/MSM

The principle health countermeasure to the chemtrail holocaust is "silicon, MSM, Colloidal Silver drinking water." This special water helps with both the aluminum poisoning and the infectious agents. The natural antidote to aluminum (Al) toxicity is silicon (Si), as silicic acid, as it has shown to promote the urinary excretion of Al from body stores. If you are silicon deficient the body absorbs aluminum and silicon is one of the only things that removes aluminum from the brain. Besides getting aluminum out of the brain, silicon also strengthens the nerves so the light of life can flow more freely, and helps strength all the collagen structures of the body to guard against infection. For all the structural and water-holding tissue in the body you need silicon as it is the architectural element in collagen. This will strengthen cartilage, joints, connective tissue, skin, bone, teeth, hair, eyes etc…

Philosopher's water uses sodium silicate which is known to decompose quantitatively into bioavailable ortho-silicic acid (H4SiO4) in the acidic gastric juice (HCl), and as such being absorbed in the body. Sodium Silicate (low alkali) mixed into distilled water at minute amounts along with the acid Sodium Bisulfate to balance the alkali has amazing the youthifying effects. Hair, skin, joints and the entire structure of the body regains its youth and integrity. The body is lighter, the mind sharper and teeth and gums heal, and skin and hair are youthified. You will notice your skin gaining more plumpness and strength, nails and hair improving, spine lengthening, breasts becoming perky, eyesight and hearing improving and less pain in the joints etc....Philosopher's water produces great results with increased consciousness, energy, anti-depression, lighter body, weight loss and reduced pathogen load.

In an effort to detoxify aluminum and heavy metals from my brain and body and to deal with the Chembug infection which leaves itchy spots on the back and arms I decided that a mixture of silicon, colloidal silver and MSM or DMSO in drinking water would work—and it does beautifully! While the sulfur rich transporter molecule DMSO drives the colloidal silver into the cells where it can kill harmful bacteria and dissolve biofilms. The Philosopher's water recipe is a lifesaver, it fortifies collagen helping to clear up chembug sores, and reduces the pathogen load of the body. I am drinking around 3/4 gallon of Philosopher's water per day and it is working marvelously for me to strength collagen, bones, hair and nails. I am about to up my game, by water fasting 3 days per week to reset my immune system—to get rid of the irritating Chembug sores. Charging the water with Shungite provides extra benefits such as decreased surface tension, increased hydration. Shungite water is oiler or holy and plants love it. I personally charge the water prior to distilling in order to discourage bacterial growth.

Orthosilicic acid ($Si(OH)_4$) is readily absorbed from the gastrointestinal tract and then readily excreted in urine. Healthy individuals given monosilicic acid as found in beer, excreted 56% of the silicic acid content within 8 hours, along with a significant increase in aluminum excretion. Aluminum and silicon interact to form a metabolite in the kidney lumen that is subject to rapid excretion such that silicon limits the reticulation or reabsorption of aluminum. The silicon moves heavy metals through and out of the body so the elimination organs (kidneys and GI tract) need to be working well to remove the toxins rather than getting restored elsewhere. This is why clay, zeolite, brooms, algae and chelating foods are useful during cleansing heavy metals and remineralizing. Silicon removes calcium from where it shouldn't be and puts it where it belongs. However, if you are prone to gallstones or kidney stones put a little apple cider vinegar in your Philosopher's Water.

My nails used to be bluish due to hypoxia and poor circulation, but after 3 weeks of Philosopher's water—the nails grow stronger and faster, and are no longer blue. So the silicon water repairs the blood vessel walls and helps to recharge the blood so that the red blood cells can carry more oxygen. The silicon is also essential for teeth. The calcium and other minerals for teeth and bones can be taken in a natural multi-mineral such as Puritan Pride's Super Chelated Multi-Mineral and/or kelp pills.

Strength and Protection: Both plants and animals use silica for protection from aluminum toxicity and for structural strength and protective barriers. Silicon was particularly abundant in the mitochondria, in nuclei and chloroplasts, especially so within organelle membranes. Silicon stimulates

DNA polymerase activity and so is needed for DNA synthesis, along with the manufacture of proteins. Silicon adds strength to collagen preventing microbial invasion and skin becomes less "absorbent" to toxic chemtrail aerosols in the air. The chemtrail aerosols are desiccants and EMF microwave frequencies dry out our eyes, sinuses, body, skin and hair, however, silicon rehydrates our tissues due to its special hydrophilic relationship to water.

Silicon is the hydration, strength and barrier element. It is essential to make the body impervious to "invasion" by candida, mycoplasma, viruses, Morgellons, and nanobots...both through increased epidermal strength and enhanced electromagnetic/colloidal environment for a strong immune system. Silica exists predominantly in the connective tissues — skin, blood vessels, cartilage, bone, teeth, tendons and hair. You will notice a rapid reduction in inflammatory joint pain and the lengthening of the spine and youthifying of the skin, hair and nails. Eyesight also improves with the correct hydration of the eyeball...due to the hydrophilic relationship of silicon to water.

After an original detox period you will notice your GI tract and digestion/ elimination improve as the pathogenic strains of bacteria and candida overgrowth are eliminated. Philosopher's water helps to eliminate the biofilms that harbor "bad-actors" in the body. This drinking water starts working immediately. If you spray it on your skin it quickly eliminates the itchy chembug sores within hours. You can spray it on your face and the rest of the body to enhance collagen strength...promoting more of a barrier to toxic chemtrail air and other pollution. If sprayed on your feet it will help to eliminate fungi, and if you wash your teeth with it, the bacterial film doesn't come back between brushings.

You put it in a spray bottle to spray on skin, hair and feet—.hydrating the skin and making you appear much younger. If sprayed on the scalp it will speed hair growth. Apple cider vinegar with six to eight ounces of water and drinking the mixture frequently throughout the day, and especially before meal times to help dissolve kidney stones. Malic acid is derived from food sources such as tart apples, Apple cider vinegar and is used/synthesized in the mitochondria as part of the ATP-producing citric acid or 'Krebs' cycle, to bump up the ATP. I soak schisandra or elderberry in Apple Cider Vinegar which I use to make salad dressings. The Philosopher's water makes great ice as well.

PHILOSOPHER'S WATER WHAT IS IT?

Since this water is to counteract the multiple harmful effects of Chemtrail Syndrome it is intended as an "Elixir of Youth" or a cure all. Thus with reference to the "Philosopher's Stone" we could call this water "Philosopher's Water." Rather than implying a negative such as calling it Anti Chemtrail Drinking Water, it would be best to refer to it in the positive sense. I think the term Philosopher's Water fortifies sovereignty.

Using a home distiller reduces deuterium (H+) by a few parts per million. I first charge the tap water with shungite for 3 or more days. This changes the bonding angles to lower the surface tension and make it more "absorbable." Then I distill it. This removes bacteria that may grow in the water due to contact with the shungite. The shungite enhanced properties survive the distillation process, so this is what I use as my base water.

For aluminum detox ideally you would drink 1 gallon of this water per day. Basically the quantities in that recipe is the daily dose if you drink a whole gallon, since most of us are not going to drink 1 gallon per day, you don't have to worry about OD'ing on Philosopher's water. This water should be taken on an empty stomach, before meals or between from meals. I also put a pinch of Himalayan Salt and 1 drop of Lugol's iodine to the gallon. I added the colloidal silver and MSM or DMSO to deal with pathogens. The DMSO is to transport the colloidal silver into the cells to kill spirochetes and other pathogens. DMSO is a natural solvent that has anti-inflammatory and anti-cancer properties. It is converted in the body to MSM which also kills cancer cells.

This drinking water is used to counteract CHEMTRAIL SYNDROME, the effects of which are aluminum poisoning, dementia/Alzheimer's, compromised immune system, dehydration, increased pathogen and parasite load, candida overgrowth, brain fog, apathy, lack of mental focus, chemtrail delivery of bacteria, fungi, viruses, cancer viruses, mycoplasma, Morgellons fibrous nanomachines, enzymes used in recombinant DNA and toxic chemicals like Ethylene Dibromide. Ethylene dibromide is a known human chemical carcinogen and immune suppressor that was removed from unleaded gasoline because of its cancer-causing effects. Now it has suddenly appeared in the jet fuel that high-altitude military aircraft are emitting!"

PHILOSOPHER'S WATER

RECIPE FOR 1 GALLON OF PHILOSOPHER'S WATER

***You will need to get the **micro measuring spoons** measuring spoons, and make sure you buy only "food grade" Low Alkalinity Sodium Silicate powder. *Sodium Silicate low alkalinity Product Code: SSG from chemicalstore.com

• Low Alkalinity Sodium Silicate powder 1 level Dash spoon (1/8 Tsp) and 2 level smidgens(1/32 tsp).

• Add to 1/2 cup of boiling water and boil stirring for 30 seconds (70% dissolves).

• Add some more water (or Philosopher's ice) to this or cool it so you can run the mixture through a Brita Water Filter. You can also just run it through a coffee filter to remove the undissolved silicon.

• Add this to make up a gallon of distilled or reverse osmosis water (or Shungite charged water).

• Add 1 level Pinch spoon (1/8 tsp) of Sodium Bisulfate dissolve by stirring.

• Add 1/8 cup of colloidal silver and 2 tsp of Methylsulfonylmethane (MSM) an organo-sulfur compound to the gallon of drinking water.

• Add 1 smidgen of Baking Soda and 1 smidgen Himalayan Salt and 1 drop of Lugol's iodine.

***Keep the Brita filter you use to filter the dissolved Sodium Silicate solution in a glass distilled water between uses. You should always store drinking water in glass.

The MSM transports the colloidal silver into the cells, however if you are sensitive to sulfur leave it out of the Philosopher's water. Kyolic Garlic pills and/or Monolaurin may be useful when first taking Philosopher's water to assist eliminating candida and other pathogens, and chelate heavy metals. Garlic prevents red blood cell membrane damage from the effects of various heavy metals. You want the pathogens and toxins to "exit" the body with as little damage to tissue as possible.

For more instructions on to make your own orthosilicic acid $(Si(OH)_4)$ water, starting with a base of distilled, reverse osmosis water or shungite charged water. Dr Dennis Crouse points out the connection between Alzheimer's, autism, and stroke and as being neurotoxic forms of aluminum. For more on how to make Silicade water read the book *Prevent Alzheimer's, Autism and Stroke: With 7-Supplements, 7-Lifestyle Choices, and a Dissolved Mineral,* by Dennis N. Crouse Ph.D. His website is: aluminum-alzheimers-autism.blogspot.com/ If you are a coffee drinker you will need to find a coffee maker that doesn't add aluminum to the coffee, such as BRUNN Speed Brew®. www.bunn.com/Speed-Brew

By using colloidal silver in the silicon drinking water and topical spray, the chembug red spots on the arms, candida and the pathogen load are reduced. Colloidal silver ionically breaks down biofilms. The amount of biofilm and toxic waste from pathogens in the blood reduces, reducing sludgy blood and improving the blood's oxygen carrying capacity. Use Philosopher's Water until you are symptom free, as broad spectrum protection against Chemtrail bugs, other pathogens and dementia.

You start noticing the difference and the sensation of relief from the "pathogen load" of the body after one glass. Its effectiveness has something to do with the increased electrical properties of the water and the geometry of the water in association to the silicon molecule. The water is more "active," that is it has more electrical energy and ionization thus speeds detoxification, metabolism and consciousness. This water can be spraying on the skin and hair, and even at the drinking water strength it is remarkably quick at getting rid of the nasties topically and internally. Use this drinking water in a neti pot or nasal spray for sinus issues also.

Making Colloidal Silver: Colloidal silver is nontoxic to humans and it can destroy 650 different types of germs, fungi and viruses which is incomparable to other antibiotics. Colloidal silver makes vaccination intoxication and antibiotic poisoning unnecessary. Colloidal silver made by using your own battery setup with wires of these pure precious metals. If you want to make your own colloidal silver you will need a water distiller so that the water is not exposed to plastic containers. The 4L-Dental-Medical-Pure-Water-Distiller is inexpensive and efficient. Use vinegar to dissolve the scale off your distiller. See the YouTube video: How To Make COLLOIDAL SILVER The Easy Way.

Heavy Metals are stored in the body in calcium deposits, atherosclerotic plaque, the calcium deposits around tumors and cancer cells, and in the biofilms of bacteria and fungi. The calcium deposit plaques are dissolved through adding apple cider vinegar to the Philosopher's Water. Heavy Metals are also stored in the biofilms produced by pathogens. Colloidal silver ionically breaks down these biofilms so that it can attack the pathogens within. Once the heavy metals and aluminum are liberated from their hiding places you will need to use chelators, methylators, fiber brooms, algae, clays and zeolite to prevent reticulation by removing the toxins from the body.

If you remineralize with kelp and raw greens etc... you replace the "bad" minerals with good. As long as you are not hyper-feeding your pathogen load with bread, sugar, alcohol or other excessive carbohydrates Philosopher's Water does help eliminate the overgrowth of yeast, fungi, and bad bacteria in the mouth and elsewhere. You do notice some loss of intestinal bacteria in the first week, but the overall pathogen load is greatly reduced without a Herx reaction. With the Bravo yogurt healthy intestinal bacteria are fully reinstated.

Spirochetes and other chemtrail bugs get "inside" the red blood cells and other cells, this is why the DMSO/Colloidal Silver Protocol is helpful to amplify the cellular uptake of Colloidal Silver. For those with serious health issues like cancer, DMSO can be substituted with MSM instead, as they both turn into each other in the body. When consuming DMSO orally take a probiotic and fermented foods to replenish your good bacteria, because bacteria cannot survive or thrive in DMSO and will be flushed out of your system. MSM is a superb anti-cancer supplement because it contains two extra oxygen atoms, sulfur and a methyl group. In fact the DMSO/Colloidal Silver Protocol is a gentle, safe and to quickly revert cancer cells back into normal cells.

DMSO specifically targets cancer cells and "opens" the ports on the cancer cells, which in turn allows colloidal silver to get inside the cancer cells to kill the microbes which are causing the cells to become cancerous. With the cancer microbes stealing glucose and excreting mycotoxins the production of aerobic ATP-energy in the cell is greatly reduced. Consequently the cell must revert to anaerobic fermentation to create even a small amount of ATP molecules. Some of the DNA damage inside cancer cells is caused by the DNA of the microbes which cause cancer. When you kill all the microbes inside a cancer cell the cell is able to restore its production of ATP molecules and thus revert back into a normal differentiated, aerobic cell. https://www.cancertutor.com/dmso-cs/

The PHILOSOPHER'S WATER recipe of silicon/colloidal silver/MSM does work to get rid of the Chembugs, but you will need to do a series of 3 day fasts as well to **reboot the immune system** to make it super adaptive. Lyme and other pathogens are constantly changing to try and outwit the body's defenses. Along with fasting and removing toxins from your diet, the Philosopher's Water will shed 20+ years off your body-mind. There is a rapid reduction in body-pain due to quenching inflammation, clearing up the pathogen load, and heavy metal detoxification. Silicon helps to transport minerals and removes heavy metals, especially in association with fulvic acid…this combo fights the fungi that complexes and stores heavy metals in the tissues.

See Dennis N Crouse's YouTube video "Brain Fitness in the Aluminum Age - Eliminating Aluminum."

Another excellent book on silicon is *"Silica, The Amazing Gel,"* by Klaus Kaufmann

ID=26-414454457&id=SSG —Sodium Silicate low alkalinity Product Code: SSG from chemicalstore.com

www.balancedenergystructuredwater.com —Tools for creating structured water via vortexing.

SILICON – THE ELIXIR OF YOUTH

Silicon is the "hero" in the fight against the chemtrail holocaust.

Silicon is the second most abundant element in nature after oxygen. It is not surprising therefore that silicon represents the third most abundant trace element in the human body, with the serum silicon levels being similar to other trace elements, i.e. of iron, copper, and zinc. Dietary intake of Si is between 20-50 mg Si/day for most Western populations. Higher intakes (140-204 mg/day) have been reported in China and India where plant-based foods form a more predominant part of the diet.

Drinking water and other fluids provides the most readily bioavailable source of $Si(OH)_4$ in the diet. Silicon concentrations in drinking water is higher in "newer" rocks and soil minerals that are less weathered, thus the amount of Si in water is dependent upon the surrounding geology. High levels (30-40 mg/L) have been reported in Spritzer and Fiji mineral waters, from natural sources in Malaysia and Fiji respectively.

All living metabolism and structure depends on the bioelectro-geometric relationship of silicon to water. Cell membrane integrity, cellular hydration and cytoplasm zeta potential, cell oxygenation and ATP generation, plus the morphogenic "light" blueprint, or the "supra-intelligence" that organizes life. Silicon is essential for growth and development, as it orchestrates all the other minerals in growth and development. Silicon is an important part of building bone matter. Without it, calcium goes elsewhere to potentially calcify in the soft tissue of inner artery walls and the heart.

Corentin Louis Kervran (1901 –1983) who worked on **Biological Transmutation** proved that fourteen atoms of silicon and six atoms of carbon makes 20 atoms of calcium. Professor Kervran discovered that silica from young horsetail sprouts in the springtime make it more available to the body. He found when the horsetail tissue is gentle and soft the silica is in a different state, and makes an effective water extract. Mean bioavailability of silicon in horsetail is ~41%. Cereals, grains & products: 49±34%; Fruits & vegetables: 21±29% (bananas: 2.1%). Seafood is also high in Silicon with mussels having the highest levels.

Silicon is naturally present in food as a silicon dioxide (SiO2), free ortho-silicic acid (H4SiO4), silicic acids bonded to certain nutrients, and in the silicate form. Generally, silicon is abundantly present in foods derived from plants such as: cereals, oats, barley, white wheat flour, and rice. As a general rule I agree that plant-chelated minerals are the best. However, to overcome aluminum toxicity, and reduce the hypoxic terrain that supports both candida and chemtrail spirochetes, Philosopher's water was the only thing that made a dent, because it breaks down the biofilms, allowing the heavy metals to be removed and the pathogens to be seen and eliminated by the immune system. You start noticing a reduction joint inflammation within 2 days, and within 2 weeks you notice your spine strengthening and elongating. Both foot fungi disappears and oral health improves markedly after about 1 month on the Philosopher's water.

The highest silicon concentration in the body is found in the collagen rich connective tissues, especially in the aorta, the windpipe, bone, cartilage, tendons, ligaments and skin. It is silicon that is largely responsible for improving the quality of the whole lymphatic and immune system. It improves the cardiovascular system including the flexibility of the arteries and the ease of blood circulation. It strengthens all the connective tissue, it thickens and hydrates the skin, improves the hair.

It is really important in the brain and in the nervous system. Silicon improves mitochondrial function and stimulates metabolism for higher energy levels. Silicon deficiency has been found to be connected with bone defects. Silicon effectively fights ulceration and the decay of bones and teeth and also lessens inflammation. Silicon hardens tooth enamel, prevents cavities and protects teeth against oral bacteria, and also prevents gum atrophy, bleeding and recession of gums that could ultimately lead to tooth loss. It's known that silicon is an important part of building bone matter. Without sufficient silicon, magnesium, and vitamin K2, calcium doesn't become part of bone matter and remains in the blood with the potential to calcify the soft tissue of inner artery walls and the heart. Zinc, copper and manganese are essential cofactors for enzymes involved in the synthesis of the constituents of bone matrix.

Silicon metabolism is controlled by steroid and thyroid hormones, and as we age the reduced hormone or thyroid activity decreases silica absorption. The epidemic of osteoporosis, or low bone mass, is a leading cause of morbidity and mortality in the elderly. As we age, we burn out the reserves of our silicon and thus the minerals are not orchestrated, and so calcium becomes depleted from the bones and is deposited everywhere we don't want it (sclerosis); and we're aging or becoming a living fossil. Age reduced gastric acid output, as occurs with aging, is suggested to reduce the ability to metabolize dietary silica. The body is more injury prone when we are silicon deficient and there has to be a silicon deficiency in the body for a period of time before the problem of degenerative or infectious disease arises. Typical sign of aging skin is fall off of silicon and hyaluronic acid levels in connective tissues. This results in loss of moisture and elasticity in the skin.

It was shown that orthosilicic acid (OSA) stimulates fibroblasts to secrete collagen, suggesting that silicon is important for optimal synthesis of collagen and for activating the hydroxylation enzymes, improving skin strength and elasticity. Thus ortho-silicic acid may stimulate collagen production and connective tissue function and repair. Skin, hair, nails and eyesight improves and the overall youthifying effect is profound. If bad habits are overcome and a raw diet and considerable detoxification is undertaken there is the potential to look, feel and act 20-30 years younger.

The bioavailability of silicon is to a great extent dependent on the specific chemical form of the compound. The mixture of ortho-silicic acid (OSA) and choline chloride (ch-OSA) significantly increased silicon levels in both the blood and in urine excretion. The choline present in the compound may have a synergistic effect with ortho-silicic acid, since choline is a precursor of phospholipids, which are essential for the formation of cell membranes, as well as being involved in processes such as cell signaling, lipid metabolism and protection against the collagen breakdown.

Choline is found in lecithin and you can find the substance in vegetables and legumes like Brussels sprouts, cabbage, cauliflower, beans and most leafy veggies. Eggs, cheese, yogurt, milk and other dairy products are also healthy sources of lecithin and Sulfur. The silanol group, present on ortho-silicic acid, is known to form complexes with amino acids and peptides. Appearance of hair and nails can also be affected by lower silicon levels, since they are basically composed of keratin proteins. Keratin is distinct from other proteins in that it is rich in cysteine (a sulfur-containing amino acid) giving keratin a unique strength and protective quality. A diet rich in silicon, sulfur and lecithin (phospholipids and choline), will ensure strong cell membranes and collagen in order to resist the invasion of pathogens, which breakdown and consume cellular structures.

Aluminum (Al) is passed out through the urine when silicon is consumed in sufficient quantity. It seems there's little danger of taking too much silicon as long as adequate water is consumed and vitamin B1 and potassium levels are maintained. Silicon helps ensure collagen elasticity of all connecting tissues in the body, including tendons and cartilage. This reduces aches and pains and maintains your body's flexibility. It has also been determined that high levels of blood serum silicon keep arterial plaque from building and clogging blood vessels. A major culprit for arterial plaque has recently shifted from cholesterol buildup to arterial calcification from serum calcium that is not absorbed as bone matter.

DEUTERIUM DEPLETED WATER

Deuterium is hydrogen with a neutron added to the nucleus, which doubles the mass of the hydrogen atom. About one in every 10,000 hydrogen atoms is deuterium, or "heavy hydrogen." Whereas ice normally floats on the surface of water, ice made with heavy water actually sinks. Water is actually a mixture of H_2O and a little D_2O. In North America, typical drinking water has a deuterium concentration of about 150 ppm, roughly equivalent to a few drops per every quart.

Deuterium-depleted water (DDW), or light water, has a lower concentration of deuterium than occurs naturally, usually about 145 ppm-125 ppm or less. This lighter deuterium-depleted water more readily penetrates cell membranes, carrying nutrients and electrons that destroy free radicals, plus improving cell, hydration, nutrition and detoxification! Water with hardly any D_2O, or "light water," can boost the immune system and benefit plant and animal health. Deuterium-depleted water is more supportive of living cells because the heavy hydrogen (H+) has a neutron in the atom making it too large or "heavy" to fit through the ATP generating protein nano-motors in the mitochondria.

Experiments showed that bacteria can live in 98% heavy water. Whereas EUKARYOTES or life with nucleated cells that comprises all life except bacteria, makes strenuous efforts to avoid and excrete deuterium. Organisms have a preference for deuterium-depleted water. In fact our cells and mitochondria do everything they can to filter out deuterium so that it doesn't enter the nano-motors of the mitochondria. Thus deuterium is the most abundant inorganic ion in our blood plasma due to it being constantly rejected from the tissues. 1500 Hydrogens per second pass through the nano-motor machines, while deuterium is too large to pass through the nano-motors, and in fact it breaks them, reducing the cell's ability to respire aerobically.

Mitochondria dysfunction (due to being damaged from the presence of deuterium (Heavy hydrogen, H+) is what kicks start cancer and genetic dysfunctions. When mitochondria become dysfunction due to deuterium damage the cells turn cancerous; that is they change to metabolize glucose anaerobically via fermentation in order to attain energy. This shift to the inefficient anaerobic ATP production is the main reason why those with cancer have low energy. Deuterium is higher in non-organic and GMO industrial-foods. Only by aligning with Nature using permacultural-style agriculture can food be produced with low deuterium levels. Plant photosynthesis increased with the use of light water. Plants grown in nature or organic –permaculture produce food that is already deuterium depleted, as photosynthesis breaks down water, thus fracturing deuterium. If deuterium depleted water is used, the germination percentage and the root and shoot length are higher .

Carbohydrates/glucose can act as a Trojan horse to convey heavy hydrogen all the way to our mitochondrias where it can incapacitate the ATP nano-motors. This is why a low carbohydrate/Keto diet is healing to many illnesses including cancer, by avoiding deuterium damage to the mitochondria. Fat in nature has less deuterium in it so offers relief to those with mitochondrial dysfunction. The more photon energy we get from sunlight, the more metabolic water we produce, the cleaner our ATP-atase nano-motors can spin without creating inflammatory free radicals. One of the main functions of the mitochondria is to produce water. The water produced by the body, referred to as metabolic water, IS deuterium depleted. Healthy mitochondria act to filter out deuterium.

The more oxygen, food, exercise, grounding and sunshine you get the more metabolic water your body produces. Dr. Jack Kruse recommends what he calls an Epi-Paleo diet that includes plenty of seafood for the DHA-Omega 3 in order to enhance mitochondrial function. Dr. Kruse says that sunlight and grounding, ie: Nature's frequencies, are more important to health than food and supplements. We have been unnecessarily complicating things, while missing the fundamentals…circadian compliance. Man-made, non-natural EMF causes Calcium Efflux in all cells and in the mitochondria, reducing the control of the Ca gated phenomena. Ca influx/efflux determines how much free radicals the mitochondria make, therefore it is critical for longevity….re: the Mitochondrial Theory of Aging.

The efflux of protons from the mitochondrial matrix creates an electrochemical gradient (proton gradient). This gradient is used by the ATP synthase complex to make ATP via oxidative phosphorylation. At the inner mitochondrial membrane, a high-energy electron is passed along an electron transport chain. The energy released pumps hydrogen out of the matrix space. The gradient created by this drives hydrogen back through the membrane, through ATP synthase.

Inflammation involves excess protons, or positive charges ie: acidity, which induces a breakdown of the electrochemical gradient and lowers the REDOX potential (antioxidant/anti-inflammatory potential). The more protons and the less negative charge cells have the less REDOX potential. Protons must be removed from the mitochondria to spin the ATP-atase nano-motor which induces a magnetic field. This magnetic field created by the spinning of the ATP-atase nano-motors is the "lifeforce" or Spirit.

The hydrogen bonds in the bound-water surrounding the DNA molecule plays a major role in the structure and function of the helical shape of DNA. The enzymes and proteins involved in DNA replication and repair make extensive use of hydrogen bonds. The neutron in the hydrogen atom of Deuterium (H+) destabilizes DNA thereby causing mutation damage and cancer through the mechanism of hydrogen bonding. Deuterium content of water increases depression susceptibility via a serotonin-related mechanism.

Due to the neutron the bonds created by deuterium are stronger than normal hydrogen bonds...up to 80 times stronger than those associated with hydrogen. This tighter bonding by deuterium stiffens proteins and requires more energy to break during metabolic reactions. As you can imagine, deuterium affects the shape of molecules, including the shape of enzymes—many of which are involved in DNA synthesis and repair. The presence of deuterium in these enzymes slows DNA replication, it causes errors in transcription, and it hinders DNA repair. Deuterium-depleted water can reverse this DNA damage, stabilizing DNA and protect DNA from radiation damage. Deuterium depleted water delays tumor progression in mice, dogs, cats and humans.

Deuterium-depleted water could be a significant method to guard against DNA damage and protect our mitochondria from breaking down under the onslaught of nanometal poisoning, radiation and 5G frequencies. Mitochondrial DNA is more susceptible to damage by ionizing radiation, UV, electro-smog, nanometals, deuterium and free radical oxidation than nuclear DNA. Damage in mitochondrial DNA leads to the generation of toxic reactive oxygen species (ROS), which precipitate further damage in mitochondrial DNA setting up a vicious cycle of mitochondrial dysfunction. The accumulation of mutations in mitochondrial DNA leads to progressive lack of ATP energy production, cellular damage, degeneration and eventually death. Light water significantly lengthened the lifespan of terminal cancer patients.

We can only imagine what damage the frequency wars...with HAARP, 5G, Direct Energy Weapons, Super Dual Auroral Radar Network, infra-sonics, laser/maser/scalar technology and cell phones is doing to human DNA and the energetic basis to the foundation of all life on earth. The good news is that structured water in plants, deuterium-depleted water, ORMUS Trap water and octagonal water can help us preserve our genetic integrity and protect mitochondrial ATP production. The secret to anti-aging and chemtrail thrival is to protect, preserve and enhance our mitochondrial DNA.

https://www.torustech.com — Nassim Haramein's Torus Tech is delivering proof of concept prototypes in the field of vacuum energy and related resonance technologies. Water treated with PGQmem demonstrated increased conductivity theorized from greater proton mobility (self-ionization): a change in the water that may increase its ability to facilitate the transfer of energy, charge, and signals in the biological system.

www.waterconf.org/

See the YouTube video: *"Resonance, Beings of Frequency"* documentary.

DEUTERIUM DEPLETION SOURCES IN NATURE

Natural water has tiny amounts of D2O molecules, deuterium and oxygen, mixed in with the dihydrogen monoxide. Since evaporation favors hydrogen over the heavier deuterium, water vapor is lower in deuterium. Because it is heavier Deuterium evaporates last and condenses first. Thus in areas where there is a greater degree of evaporation (equator and deserts) the deuterium content of the surface water is high. On the other hand, where there is less evaporation (polar regions and mountains) the deuterium concentration of the surface water is lower. Nearly all deuterium found in nature was produced in the Big Bang 13.8 billion years ago.

The deuterium ratio on earth has been constant ever since the planet got its water, and there is no effect from the solar wind either. Water molecules in liquid state exchange hydrogen ions constantly; thus, a mixture of heavy water and light water quickly becomes a fairly well-mixed mixture of light water, semi-heavy water, and heavy water. The abundance of deuterium in the water on Earth is approximately one deuterium atom to 6.400 hydrogen atoms. 'Aqua Forte' that is a deuterium depleted potable water (60 ppm deuterium) with beneficial effects in animal's health maintaining.

DEUTERIUM % IN NATURE IS DETERMINED BY:

Temperature/Season—In colder climates water contains less deuterium than water in warmer climates. Winter precipitation has less deuterium than does summer rain. Higher humidity increases deuterium levels.

Ocean Water vs. Fresh Water—Oceans comprise more deuterium than fresh water. The Atlantic and Pacific Oceans are 156 ppm, while polar oceans have a much lower concentration eg: 90 ppm deuterium Antarctic ice.

Altitude—Heavy water doesn't rise as high as H_2O, so at higher altitudes have less deuterium. Water from the Rocky Mountains in Colorado is around 136 ppm deuterium. Deuterium-depleted water is even lower in Lake Titicaca in Andes.

Distance from Coastline—Heavy water precipitates (falls) first so the surface water along coastlines contains more deuterium than inland areas.

Distance from the Equator—There is more deuterium in water at the equator than water at the poles. Water from Antarctic ice contains a very low 90 ppm deuterium, while water beneath the Sahara desert is at the high concentration of 180 ppm deuterium.

I can't find the deuterium depletion levels of Lake Titicaca water, however Titicaca is inland, high elevation and cold...all factors that lead to low deuterium levels. Colder inner regions receive isotopically depleted precipitation, with increasing in-land distance from coast. At higher altitude, the isotopic composition of precipitation gets depleted compared to that at lower altitude. The decrease in dD values with increasing altitudes reflects a decrease in condensation temperature as air masses are uplifted by topography over high mountains. Isotopic depletion of deuterium is from -1 to -4 per mil per 100m rise in altitude. The deuterium depletion levels of Lake Titicaca must be similar to water from Antarctic ice which contains a very low 90 ppm deuterium.

HOW TO MAKE DDW

Methods for making Deuterium-Depleted Water take into account the following properties—Normal water boils at 100° C while Heavy water boils at 101.4 °C. Normal water freezes at 0° C while Heavy water freezes faster at 3.8° C.

FREEZING METHOD: By holding the temperature at around 1°C, you can get some ice that contains D_2O or DHO in a higher concentration than in liquid because the freezing point for H_2O is lower. This way you can reduce the D-concentration of the water with 8-10 ppm in one step. If you wish to achieve further decrease you have to freeze this water in further steps.

DISTILLATION: Fractional distillation is the best way to produce DDW in large scale. Since evaporation favors hydrogen over the heavier deuterium, water vapor is lower in deuterium. Home water distillers can at best reduce deuterium concentration by 1 or 2 PPM per pass, which is much less efficient than commercial evaporative methods. But can then be further reduced via freezing method at 8 to 10 drop in PPM per pass.

THE JOHN ELLIS ELECTRON 4 & 5 DISTILLERS: The John Ellis' Living Water Distillers produce deuterium-depleted water (DDW "Light Water") by repeated distilling and cooling water. www.johnellis.com

MAGNETIC TRAP WATER: The vortical ORMUS trap water machines may be "spinning off" via centrifugal vortex the heavier deuterium water molecules, resulting in the collection of deuterium depleted water that has a lower surface tension and life-promoting properties. A sign that Magnetic Trap water IS Deuterium-Depleted Water is that when sprayed on the skin it very easily penetrates the skin and significantly enhances mitochondria activity and ATP production, as is evidenced by the "heating effect" of Trap water on the skin. The fact that ORMUS trap water immediately enhances the mitochondrial activity of the skin, points to the fact that it must provide the correct hydrogen bonding matrix for mtDNA repair. www.cherokeegold.net

PLATINUM CATALYST: The Chinese have invented a machine to create deuterium-depleted water that involves a platinum catalyst that quickly and efficiently removes deuterium from water using a combination of cold and hot temperatures. The resulting water has a deuterium concentration of roughly 125 ppm. "Method for the Production of Deuterium-Depleted Potable Water" Industrial & Engineering Chemistry Research

For more on DEUTERIUM DEPLETION: See multiple YouTube videos on Deuterium in Disease and Mitochondria Function, by Dr. László Boros. He shows how Heavy hydrogen (deuterium) depleted water is THE key to preventing and eliminating cancer etc.... by rectifying aerobic respiration in the mitochondrias. Center for Deuterium Depletion, in Los Angeles.

NATURE ADHERENCE: The core teaching for health (and enlightenment) is how to become a mitochondriac with Dr. Jack Kruse. I love Dr. Jack Kruse's youtubes, and he is so information dense it would be helpful to get his book. He emphasizes the importance of circadian integrity and nature adherence... getting morning sun in the eyes, avoiding blue light at night, grounding and sunlight to defrag manmade EMF toxicity, geo-location and seasonal eating, avoiding vegan DHA-Omega 3 supplements, Depleted Deuterium water for excellent mitochondrial ATP production and so much more.

HYDROGENATED WATER: Hydrogen-rich water is antioxidant, anti-aging, boosts metabolism, reduces fatigue and improves mood. As hydrogen is the smallest element in the universe, it easily penetrates the entire body, including the neurons and the cell nuclei. Hydrogen increases the pH of water by half a point to 7 or 7.5, combating the acidity that results from toxicity, inflammation and oxidation in the body. To purchase a **Hydrogenizer Bottle** with Titanium electrodes to avoid heavy metal poisoning email **H2@wingscoaching.com**

11

GENERAL LIST OF
THRIVAL ALLIES AND DIET

To overcoming Chemtrail Syndrome we need to create a lifestyle that is alkalizing, antioxidant, anti-inflammatory, increases bile flow, detoxifies, removes biofilms and calcium deposits, decalcifies the pineal gland, increases oxygenation and is blood building. Using herbs like Indian Madder root that remove kidney and gallstones is one way to eliminate calcium deposits from the body. And when sclerotic calcium deposits dissolve this releases heavy metals, toxic chemicals, and viruses from their "hiding places" so eat agents that escort (chelate) the toxins safely out of your body (like activated charcoal, MSM, clay and zeolites) so they won't be reabsorbed. To kill fungi, viruses and nano-bacteria that may be released incorporate foods that reduce pathogens like garlic, cat's claw, Reishi mushroom, Pau d'arco etc…

When you start moving heavy metals out of the tissues, you need to simultaneously eat chelating foods like apples, cilantro, onions, garlic, cabbage family, kelp/seaweeds, blue green algae, and fibers like flaxseed, psyllium, chia. Along with Food-Grade Activated Charcoal, clay, zeolite and diatomaceous earth. One of the main points to consider is that if you do not have enough glutathione and assistance to get the heavy metals and toxins out of your system they will be reticulated and restored elsewhere in the body. Liposomal Vitamin C is the best form for high dose protection from Heavy Metals. Increasing the colorful plant pigments like Zeaxanthin from marigold flowers and goji berries are necessary because increased Aluminum concentrations decreases carotene and zeaxanthin. Liposomal glutathione (GSH), Liposomal Vitamin C, Liposomal B complex, Nascent Iodine or Lugol's, R-Alpha Lipoic Acid, NAC, Molybdenum, MSM, magnesium citrate, Transdermal Magnesium, Chitosan, Ortho-silicic acid, Chlorella, Cilantro, Apple and Citrus Pectin and organic pasture fed eggs. You should also take a multivitamin/mineral formula during the treatment for Heavy Metal poisoning to support your body the entire time you do this.

The ultimate colon cleanse should include fiber, aloe, magnesium, anti parasite herbs, Triphala, Fulvic/Humic Acids, Activated charcoal, Zeolite and clay. Probiotics help keep the detox pathways open and will help you maintain 2 bowel movements per day, they also kill yeast. Probiotics and fermented foods are a potential adjunct agent for reducing metal toxicity, pesticides and carcinogens as they can bind and sequester heavy metals and toxins to their cell surfaces, thus removing them through subsequent defecation, and because on probiotics prevent and heal intestinal permeability. Eat sulfur-containing foods such as broccoli, collards, kale, daikon radish, garlic, onions, garlic mustard and mustard sprouts. Use cilantro in your juicing, pesto and cooking, or drink a daily cup of cilantro tea. Asparagus is perhaps the superstar diuretic, detoxifying vegetable for overcoming the negative effects of chemtrail toxicity. Asparagus is the highest dietary source of glutathione, a potent anticancer antioxidant, and many other vitamins and minerals necessary for optimal health.

GO FOR THE REDS: Dark red and deep purple pigments protect against the high radiation conditions of the chemtrail holocaust and Grand Solar Minimum! You will notice plants in your neighborhood increasingly expressing more purple in their leaves. 650 million years ago cyanobacteria, bacteria likely dominated Earth's ancient oceans for hundreds of millions of years, the fossilized chlorophyll in the cyanobacteria samples was dark red and deep purple in its concentrated form.. It was a few hundred million years before blue-green chlorophyll algae would begin to multiply, ultimately forming the base of a food web that eventually led to the evolution of the rest of the biosphere.

Cyanobacteria produce carotenoids such as canthaxanthin, myxoxanthophyll, synechoxanthin, and echinenone. During the evolution of life on earth the dark red and deep purple pigments protected life against the high UV and cosmic ray conditions prior to the blue-green chlorophyll algae producing an oxygen atmosphere and ozone layer. Red pigments include astaxanthin, carotenoids, lycopene, and betalain found in beets, which is made from the amino acid tyrosine. Plants rich in anthocyanins are acai berry, aronia berry, maqui berry, goji berry, blueberry, cranberry, bilberry, mulberry, black raspberry, red raspberry, blackberry; blackcurrant, cherry, eggplant peel, black rice, purple yam, Okinawan sweet potato, Concord grape, muscadine grape, red cabbage, and violet petals.

RED PIGMENTS: Anthocyanin Flavonoids present in tea, fruit juice, red wine, and dark chocolate are already known to reduce the risk of cardiovascular disease. This pigment gives red vegetables their color. It is present in red cabbage, purple peppers, beets, beet greens, purple tomatillos, purple potatoes, radishes, and eggplant skins. Also found in Astaxanthin (Algae), blueberries, blackberries, blackcurrants, elderberries, raspberries, red dragon fruit, pomegranate, goji berries, acai, amla, muscadine grapes. Maqui or Chilean Wineberry have the highest level of high levels of the antioxidant anthocyanin.

ASTAXANTHIN: BioAstin Hawaiian Astaxanthin is a red carotenoid pigment from algae that is one of the world's strongest antioxidants; it's 5,000 times stronger than vitamin C (found in lemons) and much stronger than other well known antioxidants like green tea and CoQ10. Astaxanthin is notable for its anti-inflammatory properties, reduced joint and muscle pain, a fading of brown age spots and sunspots, improved skin tone and color, improved vision, increased energy, reduced fatigue, sunscreen properties, lower pulse rate, improved mood orientation, improved urination, and heightened libido, cardiovascular protection and healing.

ARONIA BERRIES OR CHOKEBERRIES: belongs to the family Rosaceae, native to eastern North America. Aronia berries highest antioxidant capacity among berries and other fruits, such as vitamin C and polymeric proanthocyanidins and anthocyanins are deep purple, almost black pigmentation. These phenolic compound groups in aronia berries are antiviral and have chemopreventive activity against colon cancer. Pre-diabetic rats whose diets were supplemented with chokeberry juice for six weeks experienced less weight gain, lower levels of body fat, and lower blood glucose, plasma triglycerides, and cholesterol levels than the non-supplemented animals. Aronia has greater antioxidant activity than cranberry, blueberry, strawberry, cherry, pomegranate, goji and mangosteen.

BLUEBERRIES: Blueberries are often touted as a rich source of antioxidants. These antioxidants include anthocyanins, a class of compounds purported to reduce inflammation and protect against heart disease and cancer, and increase weight loss. Blueberry extract greatly improved the effectiveness of radiation therapy on cancer cells. Compared to other berries and fruits, blueberries are said to have a high ORAC score, which means they have higher antioxidant activity, protecting the body from damage caused by unstable free radical molecules. Some of the potential uses for blueberries include food poisoning, reducing the symptoms of multiple sclerosis (MS), chronic fatigue, urinary tract infections and hemorrhoids. Blueberries could help prevent the onset of Alzheimer's dementia symptoms, studies found increased brain activity and improved memory and cognitive function in those who ingested the blueberry powder.

BEET JUICE: The raw oxalic acid in beet juice is known to be a good solvent of inorganic (bad) calcium deposits in the body. Beet Juice may be one of the principal methods for removing calcium deposits in the pineal gland and elsewhere in the body. Raw beet greens contain two carotenoids: lutein and zeaxanthin. Support the liver and gallbladder with beetroot. Beets are a valuable source of iron, magnesium, zinc and calcium which all support healthy detoxification and better elimination. Folate, also known as vitamin B-9, is present in high quantities in beet juice, along with manganese, thiamin, Vitamin B3 (niacin), B6 (pyridoxamine), C, and beta carotene, important nutrients for supporting the liver and gallbladder in making bile acids which support detox. The red pigment betalain is a powerful antioxidant, anti-inflammatory, fungicidal, anticancer agent that aids in detoxification. Betalains also occur in some higher order fungi, such as the mushroom *Amanita muscaria*. By dissolving the bad calcium beet juice may be extremely effective in the prevention and possibly reversal of many types of cancer. Beets are widely known to help create red blood cells.

A Basic Juice: 1 large beet; 2 large carrots; 3 stalks celery, 1 green apple, 1-inch piece fresh ginger. (Remember to slow heat a stock made from your juicing fiber for soups and sauces; use it as a base for dehydrated seed crackers or put the fiber on the compost heap.)

CHLOROPHYLL: Super antioxidants, chlorophyll and colorful plant pigments (phytochemicals) and olive leaf will protect the Omega-3 and allow its healthy incorporation into cells. Highest chlorophyll sources are: Dark, leafy greens especially spinach, kale, chard & collards, lambsquarter, nettle, fresh herbs like parsley, dill & cilantro, moringa leaf, wheatgrass and sprouts, duckweed, watercress, asparagus, broccoli, grape leaves, celery, peas and green beans, blue-green algae and seaweed,

WHEATGRASS: Wheatgrass is 70% chlorophyll, contains 17 amino acids; helps your body to build red blood cells which carry oxygen to every cell. Wheatgrass has more vitamin C than oranges and twice the vitamin A as carrots. It is exceptionally rich in vitamins E, K, and B-complex. It is also a natural source of laetrile (B-17). Wheatgrass retains 92 of the 102 minerals found in the soil. These minerals include calcium, phosphorus, iron magnesium and potassium. Wheatgrass produces an immunization effect against many dietary carcinogens. It purifies the blood and organs and counteracts acids and toxins in the body. It helps to increase the enzyme level in our cells, aiding in the rejuvenation of the body and the metabolism of nutrients. These enzymes help to dissolve tumors.

PATANJALI WHEAT GRASS: The Eurasian forage grass called Kernza (*Thinopyrum intermedium*) is a perennial wheatgrass that is actually a distant relative of wheat. A Kernza patch in the garden may be a useful way to generate wheatgrass for juicing, since it is perennial it will require little maintenance, requiring the occasional watering and fertilizing.

CITRUS PECTINS: Pectins in citrus are a very powerful detoxifying substance. Citrus naturally removes heavy metals without depleting the body of important trace minerals. Eat more grapefruit containing naringenin, a special flavonoid that helps the liver burn fat instead of storing toxins in our fat cells.

FRUIT SKINS: The cortex peel wastes of various fruit including apple, banana, kiwi, orange, and tangerine peels act as natural biosorbents for removing pollutants and heavy metals from water. Organic skins and peels could be dehydrated or freeze dried and then powdered to be used as an extra food-chelator during a heavy metal detox. The powders could be added to smoothies of herb mixes for capsulating. Spray peels with Sodium Bisulfate to prevent oxidative browning while dehydrating the peels.

IODINE FOR THYROID: The thyroid is the most negatively charged of all the organs and so needs to be recharged from the earth and the sun. Iodine intake immediately increases the excretion of bromide, fluoride, and some heavy metals including mercury and lead. Bromide and fluoride are not removed by any other chelator or detoxifying technique. Iodide, which acts as a primitive electron-donor through peroxidase enzymes, seems to have an ancestral antioxidant function in all iodide-concentrating cells. Iodine was used by Nature as one of her main strategies of antioxidant defense in plants and animals. A newly discovered oxidant defense system is found in the free radical scavenging capacity of thyroid hormones Thyroxine, reverse-T3 and iodothyronines seem to be important as antioxidants and inhibitors of lipid peroxidation and is more effective than vitamin E, glutathione and ascorbic acid. Seaweed is noted for its ability to bind heavy metals and radioactive pollutants.

The most important nutrient provided by kelp is iodine. Most of us are deficient in iodine, needed for metabolism, cardiolipin, hormones, antioxidant, antibacterial, antifungal, anti-radiation. Iodide, which acts as a primitive electron-donor through peroxidase enzymes, seems to have an ancestral antioxidant function in all iodide-concentrating cells. Iodine was used by Nature as one of her main strategies of antioxidant defense in plants and animals. 2% Lugol's Solution X 2 drops a day to increase iodine, reduce candida, and cancer prevention. Iodine intake immediately increases the excretion of bromide, fluoride, and some heavy metals including mercury and lead. Bromide and fluoride are not removed by any other chelator or detoxifying technique.

A newly discovered oxidant defense system is found in the free radical scavenging capacity of thyroid hormones. Thyroxine, reverse-T3 and iodothyronines seem to be important as antioxidants and inhibitors of lipid peroxidation and is more effective than vitamin E, glutathione and ascorbic acid. The most important nutrient provided by kelp is iodine. Seaweed is noted for its ability to bind heavy metals and radioactive pollutants. Seaweeds (iodine) have exceptional value in the treatment of candida overgrowth. Tyrosine and the precursor phenylalanine with papaya enzymes in water aids in sustaining thyroid hormones.

Small bumps on the skin are often a sign of candida, the small itchy red spots on arms and back are a sign of a mycoplasma or bacteria from chemtrails. Both are symptoms of a compromised immune system. High dose iodine has been used to cure syphilis, skin lesions, and chronic lung disease. Both Lugol's and Colloidal Silver can be used in a steamer along with a few drops of DMSO for sinus and lung conditions. Lugol's solution helps eliminate candida and possibly viruses and other microbes from the bloodstream. Take 3 drops in a shot glass of water twice daily, but not together with antioxidants as Iodine is an oxidant and it is best to reduce the intake of antioxidants while using it. A drop of DMSO in the shot glass amplifies the Lugol's effect.

Classic symptoms of low thyroid activity (hypothyroidism) are evident with persistent internal dysbiosis, candidiasis, and prolonged cortisol elevations, caused by chronic stress. Fluoride and aluminum affects the parathyroid, which works hand in hand with the thyroid gland, resulting in a hyperthyroid condition leading to stress, anxiety, insomnia etc... Hyper/hypo thyroid regulating herbs include: Holy basil, Ashwagandha, Astragalus, Bladderwrack, Ho Shou Wu, Deer Antler, Rhodiola, Ginseng and Guggulu. In Ayurveda, Guggulu means "protects from disease" in Sanskrit.

SEAWEED - MINERALS: To remove radioactive elements, inorganic minerals and heavy metals we must flood the body with good organic minerals complexed in the living protoplasm of plants. The essential elements and trace minerals found in sea vegetables are important to our endocrine system and the regulation of the body's metabolism. Sea vegetables help cleanse the intestinal tract and lymph system, stabilize blood sugar levels, purify and alkalize the blood, and inhibit cancer cell growth. They also promote healthy thyroid functioning, reduce cardiovascular problems, and have been shown to be anti-inflammatory. Kelp cleans and nourishes the glandular system including the pineal and pituitary thus affecting the entire body.

KELP: Kelp contains almost every mineral and trace mineral necessary for human existence. It also contains amino acids and vitamins. The primary known constituents of Kelp include algin, carrageenan, iodine, potassium, bromine, mucopolysaccharides, mannitol, alginic acid, kainic acid, laminine, histamine, zeaxanthin, protein, and Vitamins B-2 & C. Brown kelp seaweed makes up more than 10 percent of the Japanese diet, lowering the incidence of estrogen dependent cancers. 4 kelp tablets/day or 1 Tbsp of kelp a day to provide 500 mcg iodine per day. On average, 20 grams of kelp contain 415 mcg of iodine. Nascent iodine contains approximately 400 mcg per drop. Dulse sprinkle; nori roll ups; seaweeds in soups and salads. I bought a 5lb bag of pet kelp powder just after FUKU, as I knew the northern hemisphere was compromised. *We need some southern hemisphere kelp companies to send product to the northern hemisphere.*
Sea-Crop — Dr. Maynard Murray's Full Spectrum Sea Solids — Sea-90 or Sea-Crop can be used as mineral fertilizer for growing wheatgrass and food and as an electrolyte for drinking water.

HAI ZAO WAN SEAWEED EXTRACT: Sargassum Seaweed, Kombu, Sichuan Fritillary bulb, Tangerine, Forsythia root, Dong quai, Pubescent angelica root, Ligusticum wallichii rhizome, Chinese licorice, Pinellia rhizome. A traditional herbal supplement that promotes healthy lymphatic tissue and helps disperse phlegm, reduces swelling, and softens and reduces masses, tumors and lumps. Drink Sargassum Seaweed broth for lungs and anticancer.

MODIFILAN: Concentrated extract of Laminaria Japonica brown seaweed helps remove radiation, heavy metals, and toxic chemicals from the body. Originally developed as a remedy for heavy metal and radiation poisoning as well as for the rehabilitation of the thyroid, Modifilan is also used for general immune system upkeep and heavy metal detox. Modifilan was first researched and developed in the USSR as treatment for radiation poisoning resulting from the nuclear fallout from Chernobyl.

SODIUM ALGINATE: Sodium alginate is a flavorless gum manufactured from brown seaweed. Alginate is a powerful chelator and detoxing agent, which can assist in pulling radioactive substances from the body, and a surefire way of assisting your body in ridding itself of toxins. It has also been shown to have anti-tumor properties, enabling the body's cells to reproduce at a healthy rate. Alginate also captures Mercury, ensuring your body does not reabsorb is as it normally would, and allows you to simply excrete it instead. Sodium alginate can be used as a thickener in cooking, especially for gel-like foods.

MAGNESIUM: Magnesium is a key protection against the chemtrails, pesticides, poisons, dietary toxins and metabolic wastes, while alternatively is depleted in the presence of their toxicity. Magnesium is a crucial factor in the natural self-cleansing and detoxification responses of the body. It stimulates the sodium potassium pump on the cell wall and this initiates the cleansing process in part because the sodium-potassium-ATPase pump regulates intracellular and extracellular potassium levels. Magnesium protects cells from aluminum, mercury, lead, cadmium, beryllium and nickel. Magnesium protects the cell against oxyradical damage and assists in the absorption and metabolism of B vitamins, vitamin C and E, which are antioxidants important in cell protection. According to Dr. Russell Blaylock, low magnesium is associated with dramatic increases in free radical generation as well as glutathione depletion. Taking magnesium citrate and magnesium ascorbate (Vit C) aids in the removal of aluminum from the brain.

Magnesium deficiency impairs the cell's sodium-potassium pump from working correctly and so the cell's cannot properly detox cellular waste. When too little Magnesium is present, this allows excess Calcium to get inside our cells, literally turning us to stone. Calcium accumulates in your cells, leading to cell dysfunction and even cell death. Magnesium chloride hexahydrate topically applied through the skin is most absorbable, assimilate-able, natural form. Magnesium is absolutely critical for healthy detoxification and moving toxins out of the body and Magnesium thus protects the brain from toxic effects of chemicals.

Magnesium stimulates the sodium potassium pump on the cell wall and this initiates the cleansing process in part because the sodium-potassium-ATPase pump regulates intracellular and extracellular potassium levels. Magnesium protects cells from aluminum, mercury, lead, cadmium, beryllium and nickel. Magnesium protects the cell against oxyradical damage and assists in the absorption and metabolism of B vitamins, vitamin C and E, which are antioxidants important in cell protection. According to Dr. Russell Blaylock, low magnesium is associated with dramatic increases in free radical generation as well as glutathione depletion. Taking Magnesium citrate and ascorbate (Vit C) aids in the removal of aluminum from the brain.

MAGNESIUM MALATE: Malic Acid is a compound of magnesium and malic acid. Both substances help produce energy in the form of adenosine triphosphate (ATP). The body uses Malic acid in the aerobic (oxygenated) KREBS energy cycle, but the tartaric acid produced by yeast infection interferes with the production and use of malic acid for energy production. With insufficient malic acid, your body will be forced into the anaerobic energy production and the glucose is oxidized into lactic acid. Both pancreatic insufficiency and malic acid insufficiency create fatigue, inflammation and discomfort.

Magnesium malate helps to reduce the toxicity of aluminum in the brain. Malic Acid one of several Alpha-Hydroxy-Acids naturally occurring and found in fruits and vegetables. Malic acid is derived from food sources such as tart apples and is used/synthesized in the mitochondria as part of the ATP-producing citric acid or 'Krebs' cycle. **DL Malic**—Malic Acid is a specific and very effective chelator for Aluminum. The DL form is preferred for detox because the L isomer is quickly metabolized as it is part of the Citric Acid cycle. The D isomer hangs around longer to do its chelation work. Both forms can cross the blood-brain barrier to get at aluminum in the brain and nervous system.

MAGNESIUM CHLORIDE: Topical Magnesium Sol absorbed through the skin is great for sore muscles and joints, headaches, constipation, toxicity and fatigue. You can also make a sole solution with quality water and Magnesium Chloride powder and put it in a spray bottle. DMSO or MSM can be added to increase the absorption of the Magnesium deeper into the tissues. Epsom Salts can be used in the same way if you have sore muscles or headache and don't have any Magnesium Chloride on hand, however this mix tends to leave salt residue on the skin. Magnesium is also absorbed systemically via foot baths and baths.

POTASSIUM: Excessive blood levels of barium result in decreased blood potassium (hypokalemia), which may cause adverse cardiovascular and muscular effects such as tachycardia, increased or decreased blood pressure, muscle weakness, and paralysis. Insufficient potassium may lead to chronic tiredness, muscular cramps, and fatigue. Potassium keeps the skin healthy and sends oxygen to the brain. It decreases the risks of kidney stones and stroke. It also stimulates the kidneys to eliminate waste, thereby maintaining balanced water levels in the body. Besides these benefits, supplementing with Potassium restores alkaline salts to the bloodstream by neutralizing acids.

SELENIUM: Shown to be effective in shielding the body from dangerous lead and mercury contamination and poisoning along with other metals. Selenium has been shown to lower cancer incidence by 37% and even decreasing cancer deaths by 50%. The levels of Selenium in our blood are consistently negatively correlated with our adaptive behavior, motor performance, brain function, depression and even social behaviors. All these can be affected by inadequate levels of Selenium in our blood. Brazil nuts Chia Seeds, Sunflower, Sesame, and Flax are the best sources of selenium! Shiitake/White Button Mushroom, Lima/Pinto Beans, Broccoli, Cabbage, Spinach. Fish, grass-fed and pasture-raised meats, whole grains, and nuts and seeds are either good food sources of selenium.

SILICON: (collagen/hydration) found in Horsetail, Oatstraw, Nettles, Hemp leaves, Eyebright, Cornsilk, Comfrey, Lemongrass, Ginger, alfalfa, Blue cohosh, chickweed, dandelion, red raspberry. Other sources include the stalks, peels and cores of fruit and vegetables like celery, spinach and broccoli stalks, cucumber peels. Silicon is the architectural keystone of the collagen molecule and its vital to the electrical and structural integrity of the body. Silicon is also a transporter molecule for other minerals so is essential for removing inorganic minerals and heavy metals safely from the body.

SULFUR: Grow mustard and broccoli sprouts for your salads to ingest sulforaphane, indole-3-carbinol and D-glucarate that help with detoxification. Sprouts also contain up to 20 times more sulforaphane than regular, full grown broccoli plants. Sulforaphane has been shown to prevent the growth of many cancers including breast, prostate, colon, skin, lung, stomach, and bladder cancer. The risk of common diseases like diabetes, heart disease, gastric disease, neurodegenerative disease, ocular disease, and respiratory diseases are reduced with the consumption of sulforaphane as well. Even behavioral disorders like autism have been helped with sulforaphane supplementation. And if that isn't enough, sulforaphane has been shown to decrease fat gain.

GARLIC MUSTARD: (*Alliaria officinalis*) A weed from the cabbage family is the most nutritious plant on the planet, especially for methylation of toxins in liver and brain, DNA methylation, anti inflammation and regeneration. Garlic mustard is delicious and great for salads, or blended in smoothies with oranges and berries. You will notice an immediate boost in mental clarity, well being and vitality from the extra methylation, liver-detoxification and soothing GI tract inflammation. Perhaps one of the most important anticancer and anti-radiation herbs.

MUSTARD SPROUTS: For inexpensive cancer prevention and liver methylation grow your own sprouted mustard seeds, similar in action to the more expensive Broccoli sprouts. The Sprout People sell mustard seed they call "Oriental Mustard," which tastes like horseradish for micro-greens and sprouts

BLACK SPANISH RADISH: Black radish triggers the liver to make vital digestive juices to help break down food and fats in your stomach. Black radish has potential liver-detoxifying and cancer prevention properties, but also the leaves have similar liver-detoxifying effect. Excellent for weight loss and detox regimes, to relieve Gas, Constipation, Intestinal pains/cramps, Heartburn, acid reflux, Bloating, Diarrhea, Nausea, Vomiting. Black radish can be eaten raw, in which case it is usually grated or sliced, and added to salads, plus the young leaves can be consumed. When used for its health benefits, black Spanish radish can also be juiced or ingested in supplemental form eg: Swanson's full-spectrum Spanish black radish supplements.

GLUTATHIONE: Glutathione (GSH) is the most important antioxidant inside the cells, just as vitamin C is the most important antioxidant everywhere else in the body. Glutathione is the mother of all antioxidants because it helps to recharge other antioxidants. Infections can bring down the glutathione levels, along with poor diet, mitochondrial dysfunction, and stress. The greater the toxic burden on the body the more depleted are the supplies of glutathione. Having a deficiency of glutathione is a precursor for one's inability to effectively excrete mercury, aluminum, and pesticides from the body. GSH is an antioxidant, immune booster and detoxifier. Without it, your cells would disintegrate from unrestrained oxidation, your body would have little resistance to bacteria, viruses and cancer and your liver would literally shrivel up from eventual accumulation of toxins. Glutathione recycling is the vital factor in avoiding Alzheimer's disease and dementia.

Glutathione, most important antioxidant produced in the body is synthesized by most cells in the body, particularly those in the liver. Glutathione is a natural, sulfur-containing peptide formed by linking three amino acids together; glutamic acid, cysteine and glycine. Glutathione teams with a selenium to create glutathione peroxidase - an enzyme in the body that is a powerful scavenger of free radicals. Glutathione is so important that up to 6% of the ATP of the body may be used to optimize its antioxidant, chelating, detoxifying functions. Glutathione (especially in the liver) binds with toxic chemicals in order to detoxify them.

The Glutathione levels in aged cells are 20-30 percent lower than young cells. Glutathione has the unique ability to make certain areas of the brain more sensitive to dopamine and helps to preserve brain tissue. Glutathione is the major protector of mitochondrial DNA thereby protecting energy generation and preventing aging. Glutathione is needed both to make T3 and move it into the mitochondria. Glutathione is required to maintain normal function of your immune system.

Glutathione assists in the breakdown of fats and prevents build up of fat in the arteries by deactivating free radicals, especially of the lipid peroxide type. Propolis, Alpha Lipoic Acid, Jiaogulan and Milk Thistle extract stimulate glutathione production in the body. Also cofactors include Vitamin C, D3, B6, B12 and Vitamin E. Schisandra berries taken together with 50mcg of the mineral selenium enhances glutathione production in the liver. Glutathione could be made into the liposomal glutathione by coating it with sunflower lecithin in an ultrasonic device. To increase Glutathione, using a sublingual and a suppository of 500mg glutathione seem the best way to match the advantages of IV.

You can also take the component amino acids of Glutathione: glutamine, glycine and NAC in smoothies. Selenium (selenomethionine) binds with mercury and parks it in the liver in an insoluble form, as well as aiding the manufacture of glutathione which is a mercury detox pathway.

Bilirubin is an orange-yellow pigment that occurs normally when part of your red blood cells break down. Glutathione S-transferase, binds bilirubin and its glucuronides so that they can be eliminated from the liver cells. Whatever you can do to improve the function of the liver will improve methylation and restore glutathione levels, for it is through methylation that the body produces glutathione. Vitamin D3 or spending time in the sun catalyzes production of glutathione, and basking the belly and liver area in the sun will speed the detoxification processes 20X. Dr Jack Kruse mentioned that intestinal bacteria produce light which produces Vitamin D in the intestinal tract!

Asparagus contains large amounts of glutathione. Vegetables rich in sulfur such as the cabbage (Brassicaceae) and onion family enhance methylation and glutathione supply in the body. Prickly Pear Cactus increases GSH and Alpha Lipoic regenerates it.

PAROTID GLANDULAR EXTRACT: Due to the onslaught of heavy metals and chemicals the body's **salivary glands** get exhausted, as it is their job to produce enzymes like Parotid that breakdown and remove heavy metals from the body. Cells die off and regenerate quickly on the skin, but not so quickly in bone matter, heart tissue and the brain and so these are most prone to accumulating and storing Al. The incredible increase in neurological disorders during this "Age of Aluminum" demonstrates the need for eliminating it from our bodies. High silica content mineral waters remove aluminum from the tissues.

RATFISH OIL: Highest form of Omega 3, mega-antioxidant, cleans arteries, pineal gland, removes calcium plaques. This deep sea shark liver oil contains Omega 3, 4, 6, 7, 9 and 11 in an advantageous distribution to the body. Of all the omega-3 sources the synergistic effects of Ratfish oil may be the fastest route to reestablishing mitochondria energy production through the normalization of Ca2+ concentrations, building of cardiolipin concentrations in the mitochondrial membrane, and as a powerful antioxidant to prevent disruption of the electron transport chain. Ratfish oil heals the effects of the toxic halogens on the pineal and thyroid—thyroxin being needed for cardiolipin production.

Ratfish oil is such a powerful antioxidant that it helps to revive the thyroid from the destructive effects of the halides chlorine, fluorine and bromine…thereby raising Thyroxin enough to maintain cardiolipin levels in the mitochondrial membranes. The introduction of chlorine and fluoride into our lives since the WW2 is one of the greatest factors in the destabilization our immune system and instigated conditions ripe for cancer, fungi, tooth decay and candida, by further reducing iodine level our bodies that are already iodine deficient. Combination of Krill oil, K2, Astaxanthin and Spirulina may approximate ratfish oil. http://ratfishoil.com/

BLACK CUMIN SEED OIL: (*Nigella sativa*) for overcoming Insulin Resistance. There is growing evidence that an increased release of proinflammatory cytokines is associated with the development of insulin resistance. In insulin resistance and diabetes addition, the elevation of free radicals and the reduction of antioxidants is associated with stimulation of inflammatory agents. The administration of black cumin oil significantly induced the gene expression of insulin receptors, significantly reduced blood glucose level, improved the lipid profile, oxidative stress parameters, serum insulin/insulin receptor ratio, and the tumor necrosis factor-α, confirming that blackseed oil has significant antidiabetic activity.

MEGAHYDRATE: The hydrogen anion, H⁻, is a negative ion of hydrogen, that is, a hydrogen atom that has captured an extra electron. Negative ions draw out radiation and hydrate cells to flush toxins, hence the need for grounding and nature. Hydrogen has an advantage over other antioxidants because it is so tiny it is able to penetrate cell membranes, and can easily enter deep into cell components, such as mitochondria and the nucleus, where other antioxidants are not able to reach. One of the most powerful antioxidants Megahydrate (hydrogenated silicon) invented by Patrick Flanagan sops up free radicals and radiation, take 3-6 capsules/day in combo with your Omega-3s. http://www.whyhydrogen.info/

MILK THISTLE: Milk Thistle (*Silybum marianum*) is a great support for the liver. Long with helping the body detox, this herb has been linked to reduction in certain cancers, reduced diabetes and even reduction digestive disorder.

MILK THISTLE PORRIDGE: For the beatification of the liver—Grind in a coffee grinder ½ cup Milk Thistle Seeds, ¼ cup Flax Seed, then soak in 1 cup water overnight in the fridge with 6 prunes, dried figs or apricots. Eat with fruit, nuts and yogurt or cottage cheese…and add pinch of sea salt and cinnamon.

LONG PEPPER AND DANDELION ROOT: Long pepper (*Piper longum*) and dandelion root extracts kill cancer cells while leaving healthy cells alone. Long Pepper extract kills cancer cells by stopping the growth and metastasis of cancer cells resulting in cancer cell death. Dandelion root targets cancer cell mitochondria and through the activation of multiple death pathways it turns on the expression of genes implicated in programmed cell death, ripping apart the cancer cells while having no significant negative effect on non-cancerous cells.

GINGER ROOT: Has been shown to inhibit cancer growth, be anti-inflammatory, anti-arthritic, effective against asthma and allergies. One of the best supplements you can take for all health ailments. Ginger Root Supplement administered to volunteer participants reduced inflammation markers in the colon and nausea from chemotherapy within weeks. Ginger contains a chemical that is used as an ingredient in antacid, laxative and anti-gas medications. Daily ginger supplementation reduces muscle pain in scientific studies.

OREGANO EXTRACT: Carvacrol and thymol, two phytochemicals in oregano, are powerful antimicrobials. Research has shown essential oils from oregano may kill the food-borne pathogen Listeria and the superbug MRSA (making it a useful addition to hand soaps and disinfectants). Oregano contains beta-caryophyllene, a substance that inhibits inflammation and may also be beneficial for conditions including osteoporosis and arteriosclerosis as well as metabolic syndrome. Oregano extract has been found to significantly relieve symptoms "immediately" in those with upper respiratory infections. It even encourages sweat production as a mode of detox, and ingesting it may help your body to get rid of unwanted phlegm in your lungs.

GINKGO BILOBA: Been used for 1000's of years as a homeopathic medicinal herb to treat a wide variety of health concerns. Well known for its treatment of immune disorders and longevity properties. Studies have shown that Ginkgo Biloba supplementation is more effective at treating Alzheimer's disease than the drug Donepezil. Ginkgo reduces oxidative stress and enhances mitochondrial respiration, and has been shown as a powerful agent against Dementia, Gout, Glaucoma, Memory Enhancement, and Macular Degeneration.

PAU D' ARCO: Used for generations to treat infections, reduce inflammation, promote digestion, strengthen the immune system, flush toxins from the body, protect against cardiovascular disease and high blood pressure. Pau D'Arco contains compounds which inhibit pathogenic bacteria while at the same time having no adverse effects on beneficial probiotic strains. Long promoted as treatment for dozens of illnesses ranging from arthritis, ulcers, diabetes, and cancer due to its 20 different chemical compounds.

FRANKINCENSE: Boswellia works by blocking the release of 5-LOX an enzyme that causes pain and inflammation. It is anti-arthritic, anti-hyperlipidemic, anti-atherosclerotic, analgesic, anti-asthmatic, anti-colitis, inflammatory bowel disease, and protects the liver and from various cancers.

271

A water extraction can be used for making frankincense tea, and the oleoresin can be mixed with manuka honey, or coconut oil for healing the GI tract and thus the rest of the body. Get rid of stubborn headaches by placing 1 drop of Frankincense on pad of thumb, pressing the essential oil on the roof of mouth and holding for several seconds.

ASHITABA: Ashitaba outperforms all other herbs tested for their antioxidant potential based on the ORAC guide (Oxygen Radical Absorbance Capacity). Ashitaba is a superfood containing eleven vitamins including, Vitamins: β-carotene, vitamin C, vitamin B12, thirteen minerals, chlorophyll, enzymes, carotene, germanium, saponins, proteins, plant fibers, glycosides, coumarins, and a rare class of flavonoids called chalcones, which are unique flavonoid compounds that give the juice its yellow color.

The many potential effects of flavonoids include defending cells against carcinogens, curbing the oxidation of LDL cholesterol and preventing blood clotting, helping to protect the organs from destructive free radicals and slow the aging process on a cellular level and the inhibition of general inflammatory processes. The germanium, in Ashitaba promotes production of Interferons (IFNs), which are natural proteins produced by the cells of the immune system to prevent viruses and bacteria from penetrating into our cells.

ANDROGRAPHIS: Andrographis Paniculata is a medicinal bitters plant from Sri Lanka traditionally used in a wide variety of conditions including fever, gastrointestinal diseases like dysentery, hepatitis, stomach ulcers and colitis, respiratory diseases (influenza), allergies, venomous snake and scorpion bites, malaria, ear and skin infections, and yeast infection. Andrographis is anti-inflammatory, antiviral, antimalarial, liver-protective, and anti-cancer. It is also protective against heavy metal accumulation.

TURMERIC: Curcumin is antibacterial and antifungal. It inhibits leukotriene, which is an inflammatory compound associated with different types of arthritis. It prevents autoimmunity and protects the nervous system. Turmeric also increases the production of glutathione, an important antioxidant made by the liver. With regard to cancer, turmeric induces cell-death in cancer cells, while leaving healthy cells undamaged. According to Dr. Dennis Liotta, an American biochemist, curcumin inhibits the release of a transcription factor that is made by cancer cells.

FO-TI: (*Polygonum multiflorum*) or Fo-Ti is a member of the buckwheat family that has powerful rejuvenating, anti-aging benefits. It is a Jing herb, sedative, anti-tumour, antipyretic, sedative, anti-progestational, anti-inflammatory, decreases blood coagulability, cardiotonic, hypotensive, vasodilatory. The longevity effects of Fo-Ti are greatly increased with Shilajit which contains 85 minerals including fulvic acid.

TRIPHALA: Triphala is a powerful antioxidant consisting of three fruits native to India: Amalaki, Bibhitaki and Haritaki. Triphala is the most widely recommended ayurvedic herbal formulation that cleanse and detoxifies while simultaneously nourishes and rejuvenates the tissues. In addition to restoring the GI tract, triphala supports healthy respiratory, cardiovascular, urinary, reproductive, and nervous systems.

ASPARAGUS RACEMOSUS: Shatavari root powder reinstates peristalsis and when combined with Triphala makes an effective tonifying blood cleanser and gentle laxative, that is gentle but highly effective, without being depleting and is not cramping. Shatavari root increases levels of antioxidant enzymes such as superoxide dismutase, glutathione and catalase.

SPECIAL ATTENTION FOR HYSSOP: Rotate the intense colon cleansers such as Cascara Sagrada, Rhubarb Root and Senna so that the intestinal lining doesn't get habituated and inflamed. Rhubarb is better than laxative herbs such as cascara sagrada or senna which are more purgative. Hyssopus officinalis or Hyssop is an ideal alternative cathartic and colon cleanser. Hyssop is known as the "holy herb," because it was used for cleaning and purifying temples. As a purifier, anti-inflammatory, antiseptic, anti-parasite that relieves anxiety, soothes the nerves, enhances mental clarity and heals respiratory ailments.

Hyssop is one of the most important plants we should be growing in our gardens, adorning our houses with, slathering our bodies with hyssop essential oil and taking internally. The laxative properties of Hyssop leaf help to clear the body of toxins in the intestinal tract and clearing mucus from the intestines, soothing the mucous lining. Hyssop has also been used to expel worms. As an antiviral, Hyssop combats herpes simplex virus and treats Lyme and HIV. Sun Tea made of hyssop flowers is particularly holy.

COENZYME Q10: Essential component of the mitochondria. Our cells simply cannot function properly without enough CoQ10. Low levels of this nutrient are linked to cardiovascular disease, Parkinson's, muscular dystrophy, breast cancer, diabetes, infertility, asthma, thyroid disorders, depression, fatigue and periodontal disease. CoQ10 is one of the strongest antioxidants available. Patients with cancer often exhibit low levels of CoQ10, and researchers have shown that CoQ10 can increase immune response in humans. In one study, supplemental CoQ10 reduced migraine frequency by 27% alone!

VITAMIN E: Powerful antioxidant like vitamin c but works in different pathways to prevent the development of such things as cardiovascular disease and cancers. The right dose of Vitamin E has also been shown to protect the brain from long term oxidation caused by much higher levels of Mercury present all around us than ever before. Vitamin E is also a powerful anti-inflammatory. The antioxidant properties of Vitamin E are also important to cell membranes. For example, vitamin E protects lung cells that are in constant contact with oxygen and white blood cells that help fight disease. Another widely known health benefit of vitamin E is in skincare and hair care. Owing to its antioxidant properties, vitamin E promotes the circulation of blood to the scalp. Vitamin E helps alleviate fatigue and strengthen capillary walls while nourishing the cells.

ESSENTIAL OILS: For counteracting the effects of chemtrails and radiation the following essential oils can be used Juniper berry, helichrysum, lemon (citrus limonum), grapefruit (citrus paradise), lavender, tea tree, neroli, laurel, black cumin oil, Cassia Leaf Essential Oil, cardamom, Dragon's Blood, Sweet Osmanthus or Fragrant Tea Olive. **The top antioxidant essential oils are:** Clove, Myrrh, Clary sage, Savory, Cedarwood, Marjoram, Geranium, Douglas fir, Basil, Peppermint, Celery seed, Lime, Hyssop, Oregano, Wild Massoia, and Helichrysum. *ORAC stands for Oxygen Radical Absorbance Capacity or the antioxidant capacity of a food item. Clove oil = 1,078,700. Oranges = 750

STABILIZED RICE BRAN: Rice bran contains several thousand beneficial enzymes including glutathione peroxidase, methionine reductase, polyphenol oxidase, CoQ10, catalase, and the powerful antioxidant superoxide dismutase (SOD). Stabilized rice bran is a good source of selenium, a trace mineral that is needed by the body in small amounts to make proteins and enzymes. That means if your diet is selenium deficient, your body is not going to be able to manufacture enough enzymes for either digestion or metabolic purposes. Hepatitis and herpes viruses thrive as the human body begins to store extra iron with advancing age. Removal of iron from the liver by periodic consumption of IP6 rice bran extract may be advantageous.

COCONUT OIL: Coconut oil is a perfect fat to use when making the body get its energy from burning fat. MCT oil is refined medium chain triglycerides from coconut oil that can be used in making Bulletproof ™ coffee. 100% organic, virgin coconut oil contains fuel substances called ketones, also helps to rebuild the lining of the nerves so that brain communication is increased and healthy nerve function is enhanced. The primary source of energy for the brain is glucose. In Alzheimer's disease, it's believed that brain cells have difficulty metabolizing glucose. But the theory is that ketones that are produced in our bodies when digesting coconut oil may provide an alternative fuel source to keep the brain nourished.

High amounts of coconut oil can create rampant inflammation, nerve damage and worsen an autoimmune disease. The Short Chain Fatty Acid propionic acid (C3) which is biosynthesized in the large intestine of humans by bacterial fermentation of dietary fiber both prevented the onset and alleviated symptoms of MS by inducing anti-inflammatory, regulatory T cells. So this means don't overdo coconut oil without balancing it with vegetables.

Imbalanced T cell subsets drive numerous autoimmune diseases, and an abundance Th17 cells can result in inflammatory autoimmune disease, including intestinal bowel disorder (IBD) and multiple sclerosis (MS). The immune Th17 cells are meant to attack parasites and pathogenic bacteria, but having too many of them in your body can increase the chances of their attacking your own tissues, such as myelin sheaths in the case of MS.

CAPRYLIC ACID: Well known for its power to kill yeast, fungi and other pathogens. Caprylic acid is a Medium Chain Fatty Acid which is responsible for the benefits founded in coconut oil. Has also been shown to increase energy expenditure thus promoting weight loss. Known to be anti-microbial, anti-viral and to protect against Candida yeast. Applications include anti-cancer, anti-aging, and shown to improve circulatory function. The capric/caprylic and lauric acid found in coconut oil is effective in killing candida yeast by disrupting its plasma membrane.

Increasing the oxygen carrying capacity (VO2 max) of the body is needed to eliminate anaerobic pathogens like candida, but eliminating acid-toxin producing pathogens and parasites is also necessary in order to increase our oxygen carrying capacity. Besides eliminating heavy metals, overcoming insulin resistance and increasing ATP we can incorporate an Anti-Candida diet by slowly working up to a daily intake of 3 tablespoons Coconut Oil, adding fermented foods like live yogurt, Coconut milk kefir, sauerkraut, kimchi and kombucha and eliminating sugars and simple carbohydrates.

APPLE CIDER VINEGAR: Apple cider vinegar is a miracle health tonic that has shown promise in helping fight cancer, improve heart health, lower cholesterol, lower blood sugar and reduce diabetes. 1 Tbsp Apple Cider Vinegar in a glass of water morning and evening will assist digestion, calm a queasy stomach, relieve food poisoning, eliminate candida overgrowth, remove bloat and abdominal fat, overcome obesity and improve weight loss. Anti-fungal and anti-bacterial properties of Apple cider vinegar make it useful used straight on cuts, toenail fungus and for cracked feet, eczema, chemtrail lesions, insect bites, and is helpful for fighting acne.

CONSTIPATION: Arginine, Vitamin C, Magnesium citrate and B5 will cure constipation within a few hours. Diet changes (more rawfood and fiber), hydration and exercise should be employed to avoid constipation in future. Grated cabbage fermented with probiotics in the fridge and used in salads is a surefire way to avoid constipation and bloating.

BLOATING: Try drinking Bay Leaf tea, peppermint tea and ginger tea throughout the day to deal with the bloat. You may also need to take enzymes with meals. Bitters tincture 1/2 hour prior to meals may also help. You can learn to create your own with local trees and herbs. Lemon water, apple cider vinegar, probiotics, papain and bromelain enzymes, potassium-rich foods, watermelon, celery, cucumber, green tea, pepperment tea, ginger tea, cardamom, cinnamon, clove, fennel seed, rosemary, yucca root, fermented foods such as sauerkraut, kimchi, miso, natto and homemade kefirs, triphala, Baobab Powder. Before sleep take activated charcoal in a glass of water after fiber/clay brooms like the PM CLEANSER.

PM CLEANSER: To make a broom cleanser use equal parts Psyllium powder, organic Rice Bran, Bentonite Clay, Yucca root powder, Magnesium citrate powder, papain and/or bromelain enzyme powers. Mix this together and keep in a jar in the fridge. 1 heap tsp in a glass of water before bed; or if cleansing take 3 times a day alternating with cleansing herbs every 3 hours or so. If you want your PM Cleanser to be fizzy add ¼ tsp of Potassium bicarbonate and ½ tsp of Vitamin C powder to your glass. Buy ingredients by the pound at herbalcom. com.

YUCCA ROOT: The Steroidal saponins in Yucca root could be considered as an intestinal soap or cleanser and a wetting agent for intestinal flora. Yucca helps form a protective coating on the intestinal walls. Yucca helps eliminate pathogenic organisms including viruses and encourages growth of friendly bacteria and eliminates intestinal mucus and the wastes on the intestinal lining. Saponins have long been known to have strong antibiotic activity and stimulate the immune system and reduce pains of all kinds.

HUMIC/FULVIC ACIDS: Humic and Fulvic acid is a powerful bi-directional super antioxidant that can eradicate any form of free-radical. That is it can act as an electron acceptor or as a donor if it encounters free radicals in the creation of electrochemical balance. Along with selenium, fulvic acid also increases the activity of the body's main antioxidant glutathione peroxidase. Leonardite or Humalite contains at least 85 minerals as well as Humic/Fulvic acids that are major chelators of heavy metals and radioisotopes.

Humic/Fulvic acids assists the removal of radionucleotides and heavy metals out of the body, especially when used in association with micronized zeolite and structured water! Fulvic acid is just leonardite or humalite watered down, so it is best to just buy the fertilizer by the pound and add it to herb formulas, water, irrigation water, soil mixes etc... You can also mix it in with clay for body masques and detox formulas.

Leonardite and humate are other such carboniferous material that provide fulvic/humic acids and amino acids. Carbon-based redox molecules from ancient fossilized soil help restore the communication network between bacteria in the gut, mitochondria, and shown to help improve tight junction function. Fulvic acid and other humates help increase, strengthen and protect the tight junctions in the gastrointestinal tract against substances that increase intestinal permeability, such as agricultural herbicides, antibiotics, GMOs, gluten and food-borne toxins, thereby impacting the immune system, as much of the body's immune system is in the gut lining. Instead of introducing new bacteria like probiotics, humic acids create an environment where existing bacteria can flourish. The bacterial metabolites can help promote biodiversity in the gut ecosystem and support normal immune function. Our gut health is intimately related to the health of the soil we get our food from. Leonardite/shale/humate powder acts a natural soil and plant growth stimulant of soil microorganisms and promoting Humus formation.

CLAY: Bathe in Kaolin clay or use a calcium montmorillonite clay as they are considered the best for removing heavy metals and pesticides from the body. Zeolite helps to repair the serotonin system. Activated Clays (such as Zeolite and Fulvic acid), bentonite clay, apple pectin and charcoal. You can mix leonardite or humalite into clays to provide the catalysis of fulvic acid, which gets molecules inside and outside the cell membrane and binds toxins in order to escort them out of the body.

• Wheatgrass juice and bentonite clay powder face/body packs

• Clay and humalite face pack with a touch of clove or peppermint oil.

ACTIVATED CHARCOAL: Activated charcoal binds to pesticides and other environmental toxins and then ushers them through the intestines to be purged from the body. It is estimated to reduce absorption of poisonous substances by up to 60% by attracting and trapping thousands of times its own weight in gases, toxins, food additives and other chemicals. Like zeolite the porous surface of activated charcoal has a negative electric charge that causes positive charged toxins and gas to bond with it. Activated charcoal has the ability to help whiten teeth naturally by adsorbing plaque and toxins from the mouth, killing bad bacteria and removing stains. In addition, activated charcoal flushes out all the toxic heavy metals (such as arsenic, copper, mercury, and lead) that are stored in your body. Bamboo charcoal may provide more silicon than wood charcoal. **Whenever you take activated charcoal, it's imperative to drink 12-16 glasses of water per day. It alleviates uncomfortable gas and bloating, by binding the gas-causing byproducts in foods that cause discomfort.**

GI SPRING CLEAN: Combine yucca root, and powders of Vitamin C, Potassium bicarbonate, Magnesium Malate and Papaya Enzymes and keep in an airtight jar in the fridge. In a large glass of water mix 1-2 tsp at the beginning and end of your day.

GI IRRITATION: Aloe, slippery elm, mullein, mallow, yucca root, flaxseed, chia seed, chamomile, horsetail and ginger will help to reduce inflammation in the GI tract. Salba is a variety of Chia and has white flowers and light colored seeds. Salba has 30% more omega-3 than Chia and 35% more protein. Salba scores 8400 on the ORAC scale versus 7000 for Chia, and has 22% more calcium and potassium also.

QUALITY ORGANIC FLAXSEED: Can be ground and combined with cinnamon and used to sprinkle over fruit and breakfasts etc…Ground flaxseed can be used to thickening soups and sauces and in baking. Ginger and flaxseed tea will cut GI inflammation, increase fat burning and speed waste elimination. It provides fiber, which balanced blood sugar helps you lose weight because any excess sugar is stored as fat. Ground chia seed or flax seed can be added to the fiber leftover from juicing when slow cooking a soup stock base.

PERILLA SEED: (*Perilla Frutescens*)—Korean Wild Sesame or Perilla leaves and seeds belong to the mint family and have a minty licorice kind of a taste to them and a nutty flavor. Perilla is probably one of the most commonly used herbs in Korean cooking. Perilla seeds have twice the Omega-3 fatty acids as chia seeds, and better taste than chia. Taking perilla seed oil, which is loaded with ALA, significantly increases lung capacity, enhanced air-flow capabilities, fights inflammation, and reduces allergy symptoms.

PERILLA PESTO: Use of perilla leaves instead of basil leaves, perilla oil and avocado or pumpkin seed blended along with the usual lemon juice, garlic, seasonings and spices. One of the greatest characteristics of perilla leaves is rosmarinic acid, which not only has antiviral properties, but it also has antibacterial, anti-inflammatory, and antioxidant capabilities as well.

SUPERFOOD SPRINKLE: Factors that are usually "removed" from our food sources (fiber, Omega 3, beta glucan) can be added to the diet. Sources should be as fresh and high integrity as possible. Used as a tasty addition to breakfast-style meal of chopped fruit, raw nuts, sprouted buckwheat groats (hulled buckwheat), yogurt. Rice Bran, Oat Bran, Wheat Germ, Lecithin, Bee Pollen, Hemp Seed and a tablespoon of papaya enzymes (Papain); Cinnamon, Sunflower and Pumpkin seeds are optional. Mix these together and store in the fridge. Every week grind up some Flaxseed and Chia seed and add to enough of the base mix to last the week…this way the ground seeds remain fresher. You can also grind the seeds each day, but it is easier to do a weeks supply. You can buy inexpensive bee pollen, chia, flaxseed and papain powder at herbalcom.com

See YouTube: *Chemtrails and Their Effects on the Brain* ~ Dr. Russell Blaylock

CELL MEMBRANES: The key to good cellular nutrition, hydration and oxygenation is healthy cell membranes. The **Budwig Anticancer Protocol** is a recipe by Dr. Johanna Budwig designed to restore the cell membranes: Blend 16 oz cottage cheese with 2 Tbsp Flaxseed Oil. (ie: the amino acid Methionine and Omega 3). As an alternative to cottage cheese you could possibly get by with a seed cheese made from a mix of ground organic soaked sesame, sunflower, hemp, pumpkin seeds, along with moringa leaf and mesquite bean powder. Sesame seeds contain the highest levels of Methionine. Hemp seed oil is rich in Omega 3 & 6 essential fatty acids (EFAs) in an ideal 1:3 ratio. In addition, hemp seed oil contains antioxidants like Vitamin E, carotene, and chlorophyll.

TEAS

ESSIAC TEA

Essiac Tea has traditionally been used for anti-cancer and cancer prevention, and it also cleanses the body. This tea can help the body rid itself of pesticides and chemtrail toxins, and acts as a gentle "releaser" of the colon while undergoing heavy metal detoxification.

Sheep sorrel — (Rumex acetosella), also known simply as sorrel or dock, is the main cancer killing herb in Essiac, especially the root.

Slippery Elm — The inner bark of Slippery Elm is rich in calcium, magnesium and vitamins A, B. C, & K, which soothes organs, tissues and mucus membranes, especially the lungs.

Indian Rhubarb Root — Rhein, a substance present in the root, inhibits disease-causing bacteria and candida albicans in the intestines, reducing fever and inflammation.

Burdock Root — Burdock root contains polyacetylenes, a chemical that kills disease-causing bacteria and fungi.

Additional Herbs — I replaced slippery elm with the cheaper herbs Mullen and Marshmallow; along with licorice root for taste and adrenals. Dandelion root and Red Clover are blood cleansers that improve oxygen supply and upgrades immunity.

Essiac Tea Recipe

6.5 cups of burdock root (cut)

1 pound of sheep sorrel herb (powdered)

1/4 pound of slippery elm bark (powdered)

1 ounce of Turkish rhubarb root (powdered)

Mix these ingredients thoroughly and store in a dark glass jar in dark place.

Bring 3 cups (1 quart) of filtered or distilled water to boil in a saucepan and add ¼ cup of the herb mix. Cover the saucepan. Then turn off the heat, and leave the pot sitting on the warm plate overnight. Or alternatively use a crock pot on low! The next morning, heat the tea again until it is steaming, but do not boil. Let it stand for a few minutes, then strain it into warm, sterilized, glass bottles and refrigerate. To consume it, pour ¼ cup of the concentrated mixture into a coffee mug and fill the cup up with hot water. Start with 2 cups daily and increase slowly as desired.

PINENEEDLE SUN TEA

The Immortal Sisters, the Taoist female sages main diet was pine needles and pine nuts. Pineneedle Sun Tea can be made from 6 branch tips are harvested in the morning from the growing tips of the branches and are pulled off with some of the wood intact. Put these needles in glass containers of rain/snow water in a sunny window and leave all day to steep. Drink that evening if possible or keep in the fridge. This will give you flavonoids similar to those in pycnogenol...its an antioxidant cocktail that tastes absolutely delicious.

SOOTHING TEA

This tea will help, you can get most of the ingredients from herbalcom.com. Licorice, Chamomile, Mullein, Marshmallow, Flax, Chia, Ginger, Galangal, Cinnamon, Fennel. Drink this energizing tea by the gallon during your cleanse to support elimination and fortify the adrenal glands. It is great made in a French Press.

GINGER, FLAXSEED TEA

When heavy metal cleansing you need to significantly increase your water consumption, so drinking detox teas is a good way to go. My latest lifesaving invention is ginger and flaxseed tea. This will make one squeaky clean during a heavy metal detox. First grind the ginger in a bullet or grate it. Then add ground flaxseed. Make up enough for making a day's tea, and keep the mix in the fridge. It works great to make this tea in a French press. If you put the leftover herbs from teas in a watering can, they will slowly build up the garden soil to hold more water. Just don't water houseplants with it or you are likely to get fungi growth. And if you sprout buckwheat for salads and cereal, you can use the goop it produces to build up the water holding capacity of the soil also. The hulled buckwheat gives off significant mucilaginous goo when sprouting, which is a great hydrator for the skin, or for hair gel, as a thickener in raw cooking and it is very good for healing the GI lining. Ground chia seed or flax seed can be added to the juicing fiber when slow cooking a soup stock base.

CHAGA-CHICORY COFFEE

Brewing Chaga Powder + roasted Chicory instead of coffee, would be a great start to significant detoxification. Chaga is rich in beta-glucans, which are immune enhancing and can even shrink tumors. Chaga is a natural source of B vitamins and its mineral content includes copper, potassium, manganese, iron, zinc, calcium and selenium. Chaga is known to provide a variety of antioxidants and it is also one of the world's richest sources of pantothenic acid (vitamin B5), which is an essential nutrient needed by the adrenal glands and digestive organs. Chaga mushrooms contain extremely high oxalate concentrations, so excess consumption can cause kidney stones. Chaga Powder + roasted Chicory can be brewed in a crockpot

SEAWEED TEA

Seaweed is packed with vitamins, antioxidants, omega-3s, essential amino acids, and minerals, including iodine, potassium, zinc and magnesium. In fact seaweed contains 10-100X the minerals found in plants on land. Not only is seaweed full of vitamins and minerals, but it could promote weight loss and helps chelate radiation and heavy metals. Seaweed and Matcha green tea are a powerhouse of micro-nutrients. The seaweeds suitable for making teas include Bladderwrack, Hai Zao – Sargassum – Black tangly seaweed, or dried purple dulse, kelp, Irish Moss. Kombu Cha, (Konbocha) which can be literally translated to "kombu kelp tea" is made from the kombu seaweed. Sea Lettuce seaweed contains 27% protein, which is comprised of all 9 essential amino acids including Lysine which is the amino acid that is typically deficient in most vegetarians. Drinking this tea on a regular basis will help to regulate your hormone production and keep your skin and hair beautiful. Lemon, ginger, basil leaves and miso are a great addition to seaweed tea.

KETOGENIC DIET

In order to break self-destructive habits like alcohol, bread and cooked food, we need a metabolic-cognitive shift that will win-out over the compulsive power of chronic sugar- addiction fueled by candida infection. The chemtrail toxins coupled with the breakdown of the environment's immune system means that we have to rise above the self-destructive habits of Borg culture, in order to save ourselves and create a metamorphic legacy for collective survival and thrival. Consider a Keto diet in along with water fasting as a reset protocol for breaking addictions, overcoming emotional dis-ease, reducing kundalini symptoms, detoxing from pharmaceuticals, and recovering one's shamanic soul. Water fasting, and/or the ketogenic diet would help to reset your neurons to a new plane of existence.

To deal with the chemtrail bioweapons a comprehensive program that needs to be undertaken that includes going on a ketogenic fast, by eating 1 tsp of organic virgin coconut oil every 2 hours, is the fastest way to remedy the situation.

Fat burning, ketogenic metabolism or the ketogenic diet can be useful for treating viral and bacterial infections, because viruses and bacteria have no mitochondria, which means that the ketogenic diet starves them of their ideal food source, "glucose". Intriguingly, evidence from brain disorders in people suggests that abandoning glucose also helps our neurons when they are stressed.

A ketogenic diet protects the brain cells in those who have epilepsy, and is also used as way to fight brain cancer. Since cancer cells get their energy from the fermentation of sugar, eliminating sugar from the diet starves cancer cells. The low-carb, high-fat ketogenic diet can replace chemotherapy and radiation for even the deadliest of cancers, said Dr. Thomas Seyfried, a leading cancer researcher and professor at Boston College. See YouTube. The ketogenic diet has been effective in controlling symptoms of diabetes such as insulin resistance and elevated glucose and triglycerides. The regular Keto diet is suitable as a lifetime diet for those with epilepsy, seizures, cancer, autism or other ailments that positively respond to ketogenic metabolism. For those who want to lean in this direction the Paleo Diet may be a good option. https://peterattiamd.com/

The human primate body is not designed for eating cereals and these days bread is lethal due to Monsanto's *abominable practice* of spraying Roundup on fields to kill-dry wheat prior to harvesting. Rye is a little easier on the GI tract but still takes energy away from the body-mind and is difficult for the body to detoxify. However you will find Quinoa easy on the GI tract and the brain (moods). It is gluten-free, high in protein and one of the few plant foods that contain all nine essential amino acids, including lysine, which promotes healthy tissue growth throughout the body. It is also high in fiber, magnesium, B-vitamins, iron, potassium, calcium, phosphorus, vitamin E and various beneficial antioxidants.

For Toppings Make: Seed cheeses, pumpkin seed pesto, olive miso spread, guacamole, tofu Pâté, Red Pepper and Sun-Dried Tomato pâté, Parsley pine nut pesto, perilla leaf cashew spread, Walnut + Roasted Garlic and Chickpea pâté, Porcini and Pecan Pâté, Zucchini Spread etc... Load your crackers high with tomatoes, peppers, avocado, onion, pineapple and other goodies.

RAW DIET RECOMMENDATIONS

Cooked, industrial Borg culture is not conducive to kundalini awakening or the conductivity of consciousness. Since the end of the Paleolithic age we have reduced levels of Omega-3 and an excess of Omega-6 from cereals. This makes the body's nerve insulation, brain fat, cell membranes and mitochondrial membranes less able to generate and conduct electrical charge. This is one of the main reasons why human society at present is mainly operating on the basic default mechanical level of the consensus reality nightmare.

In order to liberate ourselves the machinations of the Flatland Hindbrain world, and to be free of our own wounding and inner self-sabotage we have to repair our Omega-3 ratio and rebuild our cardiolipin levels. We also have to change our lifestyle so that it is steeped in Nature, fully grounded, adopt a live-food diet, and realign with the circadian rhythms of the sun, moon, seasons and connect to Source. Then kundalini awakening can proceed without burning through the sugar-body and frying us to a crisp, making us even more vulnerable to the ubiquitous toxicity of Borg civilization.

Industrialization has changed our relationship to food and agriculture through commodification of the food supply. Without regard to the best practices of regenerative agriculture, Natural Hygiene philosophy and "raw food science" commercial food has actually become life-taking rather than life-giving. Choice by choice, those in know slowly increase their **food integrity** over the course of their lives. It is the lifeforce in the food itself that informs us whether a food will either give us life or take it away. Thus as a general rule don't buy anything in a package or bottle as it is all fake food—and the agricultural processes are so bad that industrial food has almost NO food value, and is in fact toxic to the body. If our food is anti-life, then Borg civilization itself is anti-life.

Integrity must stand on solid cosmic ground to be valid and true, and only cosmic integrity can create happy outcomes and positive futures. The ultimate diet for health would be picking food directly from your own permaculture food forest and veggie garden. The closer to harvest the more life-giving the food. The complexity achieved through the diverse interspecies planting of permaculture design systems is healthiest for the plants and animals and healthiest for humans. By using Nature's design, we can realize the perfection of our own design.

An anti-chemtrail diet is one that is varied, raw diet with the food grown in remineralized regenerated soil. Nutrient density and high enzymes is essential to detoxing and rebuilding the body exposed to eugenic agents we experience in our current environment. Chimps forage from over 360 food sources. Try and count how few food types we eat, and consider how they are all largely demineralized and devitalized.

Dr. Edward Howell, author of the classic book "Enzyme Nutrition," explains how the digestive system is designed to break down approximately half of the food we eat. The rest of the digestion is "supposed" to be undertaken by 40 to 60 % of enzymes found in the living food itself. Since cooking destroys enzymes, cooked and processed foods are "enzymatically dead" leaving no live food enzymes to help with digestion. These dead foods place a lot of stress on the digestive system, the pancreas, the immune system, the whole body. The faster your enzyme supply depletes, the faster you age and the more likely you will get disease. When fat is cooked or processed, it no longer has the 40/60 ratio and quite often gets stored in the body as excess weight. If fat is not properly digested, it can cause many cardiovascular problems among other things. Poor digestion and consequent low energy, leads to excessive eating to try to satisfy that hunger. Dr. Howell found through his work in a sanitarium that...”It is impossible to get people fat on raw foods — regardless of the caloric intake.”

To assist the digestive process use Papain and Bromelain enzyme powder sprinkled on meals via a salt shaker. A high enzyme diet means maximizing ATP production with a minimum of exhausting the body’s resources for digestion, maintenance and repair. It is obvious when sprinkling or eating papaya enzymes with meals that the food is more fully digested and processed, and the proof is in the toilet bowl. The highest enzyme counts are in the “young” parts of plants — the sprouts and shoots, and the fruiting bodies.

A general anti-candida (antifungal) diet with a marked absence of sugars limited to around 2 pieces of fruit or sweet vege per day and NO cooked carbos, hence AVOID cereals. Sprouted Essene breads made in a dehydrator from a variety of grains including amaranth, quinoa, rye, buckwheat, millet, oat and barley, mesquite flour is OK if you don’t overdo it. Use alternative grains such as sprouted Kaniwa, Amaranth, Quinoa, Sorghum for making raw tabbouleh or pilaf, or dehydrated seed crackers, an ideal bread substitute. I make dehydrated seed crackers with — chia, flax, sesame, sunflower, pumpkin, caraway, poppy etc... which are good for your brain fat.

Any sugar including processed fruit will increase your inflammatory pain level, feed candida and the chembugs and increase your pathogen load. Fresh raw vege juices are a great start — but ultimately for “full health” food must be grown via green alchemy, high biogenic principles to be of maximally regenerative. One super nutrient smoothie in the morning and one raw meal mid afternoon is ideal for a detox-lifestyle and maximum creative energy.

Mega-greens in the form of salads, green drinks, wheat/barley/oat grass juice to provide minerals, iron, oxygen and chlorophyll. Lots of sprouts for salads, fermented vegetables, probiotic salads, seed cheeses/pates are necessary for a high enzyme diet. Virgin olive oil and coconut oil and fermented foods like: Miso, Tempeh, Natto, Kimchi, Kefir, Sauerkraut, and Korean Fermented Brown Rice vinegar. Since 70% of our immune system is in our gut, when we eat remineralized raw food, we provide for the health of our intestinal bacteria thereby preserving our own health and optimizing our mood.

Yet another example of the upside down nature of our current cultural paradigm — “death by medicine” is a twenty-first century epidemic, in that prescription drugs kill over 100,000 people each year. While a raw plant-based diet can prevent pretty much all chronic degenerative disease deaths. It is your choice do you want to live the death-culture, cooked, GMO, criminal medicine, obese, Metabolic X and mentally deranged world, or in the enlightened, intelligent, progressive, vital, raw, permacultural, regenerative, remineralized and reforested world? Perhaps we should shine our rear lights on the dying regime, and our head lights on our enlightened future.

• ONLY RAW IS REAL: Check out on YouTube David Wolfe, Gabriel Cousens, Dan MacDonald (the Life Regenerator), Markus Rothkranz, Tony Wright, Brian Clement, Vaughn Lawrence and Dr. Mercola on YouTube.

Don’t think “treatment,” think LIFE FORCE!

REANIMATION WITH CHELATED MINERALS

The heavy metals and the nanometals in chemtrails interferes with the enzyme metabolism in the biosphere and in our body.

Minerals which have been so altered by heat as to come out of their organic, chelated bonds change to corrosive insoluble salts. In such a water repelling form they are useless to the body, disrupting our chemistry and electromagnetism and the flow of substances to and from the cells. These inorganic-mineral ions bind with cholesterol to form plaque on the blood vessel linings and cell membranes. This cement plaque hardens cell membranes leading to cell suffocation, arteriosclerosis, arthritis and cell insensitivity, such as in diabetes. Unchelated metallic minerals disrupt enzyme systems, thereby reducing the efficiency of all metabolism.

The work of *Dr. Paul Kouchakoff* with leukocytosis proved that even the minerals in spring water evoke an immune response when heated above 191°F. According to Dr. Paul Kouchakoff (Suisse), M.D. Nobel Prize Nominee who wrote "The Influence of Food Cooking on the Blood Formula of Man," the activation of the immune system occurs in response to all cooked food or boiled water. Leukocytosis or the increase in leukocyte white blood cell numbers in response to abnormal conditions, involves the activation of flight/fight response of the sympathetic nervous system and the liberation of adrenaline.

These conditions are directly counter to what should happen during digestion under the normal activating influence of the parasympathetic nervous system. The body essentially goes into toxic shock after the consumption of cooked-denatured food and beverage. This means that even herb tea made with boiled water affects the body adversely. This also means that practically everything that comes in a container or that has been processed by heat does more harm to the body than good. Thus we have to rethink the hundreds of dollars we spend on vitamin and mineral supplements, for these factors are only viable in the context of vital-plant-protoplasm and cannot be stored in a bottle.

Returning to a raw-remineralized diet will save us thousands of dollars on doctor and dentist bills. The money that we used to spend on supporting and repairing the consequences of our cooked food regime, we can then spend on the true nourishment of raw-remineralized-organic fruits and vegetables. If we get it right the first time we save ourselves a lot of suffering and unnecessary expense. Remineralized food increases function at every stage of digestion as well as improving assimilation, cell metabolism and elimination.

The only viable Life-giving way to take in the full quota of chelated minerals and trace elements that we need is if they are in raw plant protoplasm. When the soil is remineralized with rock dust or seaweed then all the life-giving attributes of the plant life are synergistically increased. Remineralized food has more enzymes, vitamins, hormone's, phytochemicals, antioxidants, water, oxygen and thousands of other mysterious vital organic factors. To incorporate these allies into our bodies when they are at peak performance, in their raw-alive state, is the only way to maximize our life force and the only sane way to eat. For in order for food to be fully assimilated, used and eliminated, the nutrients need to be in their electrically alive colloidal state.

If we eat remineralized food then we can be sure of getting the powerful nutrition necessary to restructure our raw-body and avoid the unnecessary repercussions from our "past sins." The higher the enzyme content of the new raw diet the less radical the healing crisis and the easier the cleansing symptoms, for enzymes provide the means to cleansing, protecting and healing — they do all the work. Organic minerals are needed for the production of our enzymes. Minerals are also needed to grow healthy populations of intestinal and soil bacteria.

Microbes in the soil are the agents that make minerals available to plants by decaying rock and vegetable matter. Life which has been grown on demineralized soil lacks minerals and hence is deficient in enzymes, and this lack of enzymes reduces the initial food-enzyme digestion. Thus if we eat a lot of fruit and vegetables grown on such weak soil we will have a hard time breaking the food down, poor intestinal bacteria will result and we will have gas and bloating. Hence when we start eating more raw-food it is important to obtain remineralized organic foods and to always incorporate some high enzyme foods with each meal or to take enzyme supplements. If you can't find or grow remineralized food then take kelp capsules with your meals, sprinkle your food with dulse or supplement with wheat grass and algae.

The communities that historically had uninterrupted perfect nutrition are the Hunzas in Afghanistan and some tribes in the Andes mountains of South America. The longevity of these tribes is attributed to the fact that they use glacial milk containing mineral rich ground rock in their drinking and agriculture water. Thus we might look to them as an example of what is possible. The Hunzas are said to be a very happy, peaceful people who live disease free till 120 years old. And if you have tasted food remineralized by growing with rockdust, as I have done in Hawaii, you would not believe the difference on the senses — the food literally explodes in one's mouth with God-force, an electric bomb of consciousness, and sensory fulfillment, orgastic homecoming of oral gratification — radically waking up body, mind and soul.

The ultimate diet for health would be picking food directly from your own permaculture food forest and veggie garden, or indoor growing system to avoid chemtrail contamination. The closer to harvest the more life-giving the food. The complexity achieved through the diverse interspecies planting of permaculture design systems is healthiest for the plants and animals and healthiest for humans. That which supports lifeforce is pleasurable. Stuart Hameroff proposes that the quantum drive for pleasure is the evolutionary force!

ZEOLITE AND DIATOMACEOUS EARTH

Silicon accelerates the rate of bone mineralization and calcification in association with molybdenum, Vitamin D and vitamin K as such cofactor, which is important in bone mineralisation. Even though plant food contains high levels of silicon, its bioavailability from these sources is questionable, due to poor solubility of actual silicon forms present in these foods. Orthosilicic acid is readily and rapidly absorbed and excreted in urine, and uptake occurs predominantly in the proximal small intestine. Absorption studies indicate that the ortho-silicic acid is a main readily bioavailable source of silicon for humans. Orthosilicic acid is the major silica species present in drinking water and other fluids/beverages, including beer, so these provide the most available source of silicon to man. It is readily absorbed and excreted; at least 50% of intake.

CLINOPTIOLITE ZEOLITE (foodgrade) is non-toxic and completely safe for use in human and in veterinary medicine. Clinoptilolite influences cell viability, cell division, and cellular stress response that results in anti-proliferative effect and apoptosis induction. Although silicon compounds like clinoptiolite zeolite and diatomaceous earth are substantially insoluble in water, they release small, but significant concentration of ortho-silicic acid (H_4SiO_4) in contact with water and physiological fluids. Cancer cannot survive in cells that have the correct levels of silicon, so Zeolite shows positive results on tumor cell suppression and potential in antiviral therapy.

Zeolites are detoxifying when added to animal diets, reducing levels of heavy metals (e.g. lead, mercury, and cadmium) and various organic pollutants, i.e. radionuclides and antibiotics. Zeolite is hydrolyzed at low pH (stomach hydrochloric acid) into ortho-silicic acid (H_4SiO_4) and aluminum ions($Al3+$), so zeolite in feed does increase aluminum deposition in bone. Zeolites are particularly useful for removing heavy metals and radioactive species from water, you can also take a radiation detox zeolite clay bath. I think there is potential for using zeolite in homemade filter systems along with diatomaceous earth. on an empty stomach, 1-2 hours away from food, minerals, supplements or prescription drugs.

DIATOMACEOUS EARTH (DE) is another great source of silicon since it is made up mostly of the substance. Diatomaceous earth is actually millions of tiny, fossilized aquatic microorganism called "diatoms" that are ground up into a fine, white powder. Besides aluminum detoxification, DE also chelates other heavy metals, helps with GI health, and can give you more energy. Some say that food grade D.E. is far superior than bentonite clay because most bentonite clays have an aluminum content of anywhere from 15 to 75 percent. Diatomaceous Earth is 84% Silicon Dioxide (Silicon). Food Grade Diatomaceous Earth is worth considering during the deworming periods of internal cleansing, and can be included in the general PM Cleanser (Bentonite clay, psyllium, yucca root, magnesium citrate).

The presence of sufficient silicon in the intestines will reduce inflammation of the intestinal tract. As Diatomaceous Earth moves through the stomach and digestive tract, it attracts and absorbs positively-charged pathogens throughout the body, including bacteria, fungi, protozoa, viruses, along with endotoxins, pesticide and drug residues, E-Coli, and heavy metals. These pathogens and toxins are trapped and passed out of the body.

After only a few months of taking DE, the intestine wall is no longer coated with mucus and molds but SCRUBBED CLEAN and disinfected. Silicon can prevent or clear up both diarrhea and constipation. Because of the beneficial effectiveness on the lymphatic system, silicon can be used for swelling of the lymph nodes in the throat, and acts as a supportive treatment for inflammation of the middle ear.

Silicon is more essential in some plants, namely rice, oats, barley, maize, cucumber, hemp and tomatoes, as silicon deficiency reduces their growth and vice versa, addition of silicon improves growth and guards against attack by pathogens. Consumption of moderately high amounts of beer in humans and ortho-silicic acid in animals has shown to reduce aluminum uptake from the digestive tract and slow down the accumulation of this metal in the brain tissue.

SHUNGITE C60

THE RECYCLABLE SUPER-ANTIOXIDANT

A rare black stone known as Karelian Shungite found in the Karelia area of Russia. This lustrous black stone consists of over 98% carbon by weight and is claimed to contain "fullerenes." Shungite is a fossilized organic carbon material of Precambrian ocean sediments comprising of amorphous carbon and the graphite crystal containing carbon (30%), silica (45%), and silicate mica (about 20%). The Shungite deposit is composed of nearly all the elements of the Periodic Table. It is believed to be more than two billion years old and exhibits an amorphous or non-crystalline habit, an opaque transparency, a matte or metallic luster, a Mohs scale hardness of 3.5-4 and electric conductivity properties that are palpably "felt" by the body.

The Buckminsterfullerene (C60 Buckyballs) carbon that occurs naturally in the geological deposit of Shungite gives it catalytic abilities, electro-conductivity and chemical resistance. "Buckyballs" or spherical carbon fullerenes form a large spheroidal molecule consisting of a hollow cage of carbon atoms resembling soccer balls, which take the forms of hollow tubes, ellipsoids, spheres or other shapes. Charging water with shungite magnifies and catalyzes all components and it is super hydrating. Charging distilled water with shungite makes the texture of the water oily like Trap Water, showing that it has a low surface tension and super hydrating capacity.

LONGEVITY ANTIOXIDANT: The C60 molecule is not damaged when it accepts or donates electrons from/to free radicals and goes on to work as an antioxidant in the body indefinitely, for when a mitochondrion dies, the lipofullerene C60 can be reused by other cells. It extends lifespan by inhibiting telomere shrinkage, and also enhances DNA-demethylation (which would rejuvenate an individual on the genetic-molecular level). When old mice take C60 their brains get rejuvenated and suddenly perform as well as the brains of three months old mice. It appears that C60 prevents oxidative stress and protects against the liver against highly toxic chemicals. We age mainly because we can not regenerate cells. C60 promotes the disappearance of scars, the regrowth of hair, and the apparent re-stimulation of stem cells. It is reported that by the age of 50 we lose about 50% of our adult stem cells and 90% by age 65. Complementary supplements that promote stem cell proliferation are astragalus, fucoidan, l-theanine, and blue-green algae.

EMF PROTECTION: Fullerenes normalize the nerve processes, influencing the exchange of neurotransmitters and neurotrophic factors, reducing stress, suppressing the development of many allergic diseases and improving immunity. The Fullerenes shield from the electromagnetic radiation given off by electrical equipment, including computers, mobile phones, wifi, microwaves and televisions. Worn as a pendent it heals those who have developed a sensitivity to man-made electrical devices. Pyramids of Shungite along with clay balls or Tourmaline crystal can be used in water storage and water filter jugs to charge and purify the water. Shungite pyramids guard against harmful radiation from computers, microwaves, TVs, mobile phones, power lines, etc...

Shungite began being used in cast iron production - for coating blast furnaces, as well as for water purification sand. It is now being used in paints, concrete, brick, and finishing solutions for building material to shield against electromagnetic radiation. The electromagnetic (EMF) shielding qualities of building material made from Shungite is being used not only in schools, hospitals and rest homes, but also in enterprises electronic, radio, nuclear industry, communication centers, residential homes, buildings on tectonic faults, near high-voltage lines or cell towers. In fact, Shungite is at the forefront of a new class of building materials to protect the public from electromagnetic radiation without metal screens.

HEALING: Shungite has amazing properties unlike any other stone. It is so powerful is that it is said to be the "miracle stone" or "the stone of life." Shungite is truly an amazing electrically alive healing stone - when placed on painful or blocked areas of the body the tissue instantly responds and normalizes. Provides healing on all levels: mental, emotional, physical, and spiritual, leading to considerable growth and transformation to occur in every area of our life. Shungite is so electromagnetically alive it helps to normalize electrically spastic tissue and pain within minutes. Shungite efficiently carries an electric current, so can be used in electronic vibratory healing and meditation devices. You can hook a large piece to your colloidal silver maker clips and hold the shungite round in your palm. (Esp. good for kundalini actives.)

PALM WORRY STONES: There is the nervous system which is supposed to cross over to feed the opposite side of the body to the brain. There is also multiple layers of energy frequency fields from scalar down to the visible light spectrum that constitute the EMF egg of the aura or electro magnetosphere of the body. A shungite egg can be clenched in the hand while walking to massage the side of the brain most damaged by vaccines, trauma, bumps, strokes and kundalini awakenings. Heat the stone in the sun before using. Wearing Shungite pendants and jewelry also helps to calm and defrag the body's energy and protect from toxic EMF frequencies. Wear a shungite pendant over the Thymus gland to improve the body's immune system.

SPIRITUALIZING: By wearing shungite jewelry this increases personal power, clears and balances energy, raises vibration, increases earthing, promotes positivity, enhances psychic and spiritual abilities and a feeling of "light and space" is created by rebuilding the integrity of the body's electromagnetic field. It is believed to bring both physical and psychic protection, as it grounds spiritual energy and brings light into one's auric energy field Shungite also protects against social toxicity, warding off negative energy and the evil eye. It can be used to help remove negative people or bad luck from your life, and helps in easing anxiety, insomnia, inflammation or even acne. Wearing shungite, meditating with it and/or keeping it near seems to calm and relax everyone in its vicinity, making it a beneficial stone to keep around the house.

DETOXIFYING: Wood charcoal and shungite increased biomass of plants and reduced the concentration of pesticides in rhizosphere up to 57%. Shungite and zeolite – the minerals refer to new generation of natural mineral sorbents (NMS). Zeolite and shungite work better at purifying water than activated carbon. Shungite removes free radicals out of water in 30 times more effective than activated carbon, thus reversing the negative effect of free radicals that formed during water treatment with chlorine and its derivatives. Shungite cleans water and removes fluoride, chlorine, pesticides, volatile organics, pharmaceuticals, and eliminates sour taste. Shungite adsorbs on its surface up to 95% of contaminants, including organochlorine compounds, phenols, dioxins, heavy metals, and radionuclides removes turbidity and color of water and gives the good sensory properties and saturates water with micro-and macro-elements. Boil and charge shungite in the sun to purify and charge it.

ANTIMUTAGENIC: Ignatov and Mosin show that a water solution of shungite or zeolite on a molecular level inhibits the development of tumor cells, slowing both the growth of cancer cells and the development of the AIDS virus. Shungite initiates cell rejuvenation and enhances cell and DNA / RNA repair, eases headaches, stomach aches, back aches, rheumatism, nerve pain, nervousness and skin spots.

ANTIBACTERIAL: Shungite water has strong antibacterial, antiviral ability, and helps lessen the symptoms of the common cold, chemtrail flu, vaccines and other diseases. During the experiments, water was contaminated with various types of streptococcus bacteria groups. The experiment showed that only after half an hour in Shungite water the concentration of streptococcus bacteria groups decreased by a factor of 100%, and other groups of bacteria was reduced by a factor of 900%!

ANTI-ALZHEIMER'S: Russian Academy of Sciences (RAS) confirms Ukrainian breakthrough in Alzheimer's treatment with Hydrated Fullerenes or C60-HYFNs or Water Soluble Buckyballs. A study suggests that C60 may also enhance autophagy or could elicit cytoprotective and help to eliminate the accumulation of Beta-amyloid through autophagy. There have been several rodent studies that suggest that hydrated C60 derivatives are neuroprotective and may enter into the brain through the bloodstream. Another study found that the neuroprotective properties possessed by these water-soluble carbon fullerenes depend on activity that mimics superoxide dismutase (SOD). SOD mimetic activity is caused by the presence of an enzyme named superoxide dismutase (SOD), which is not present in unhydrated C60 molecules. In contrast to these synthetic derivatives of C60, unhydrated C60 dissolved in olive oil has no published scientific studies human or animal studies have been conducted to determine whether C60 treatments may benefit patients with dementia or mild cognitive impairment.

SHUNGITE IN OLIVE OIL (Lipofullerene): Ultra Fine Carbon 60 Fullerene Nano in extra virgin olive oil. The product Lipofullerene C60 is composed of olive oil and fullerene-C60 through an extensive amalgamating and filtering process. The product Carbon 60 Olive Oil (GoodAndCheapC60oo.com) is made by grinding the C60, then use a magnetic stirrer to mix it into the olive oil for 2 weeks in the dark, and then put it through a vacuum 0.22um filter. Lipofullerene is reputed to embed semi-permanently in the lipid bilayers of the cells and mitochondria, where it acts as a reusable, recyclable antioxidant. Since the cell walls are lipids Lipofullerene is therefore readily absorbed by the cells and ends up where it is most needed – that is in the mitochondrial bilayer membranes, where it will neutralizes free radicals like no other molecule.

Lipofullerene acts as a recyclable super-antioxidant that is 270 times more potent than vitamin C. In fact C60 may be tens of thousands of times more effective as a long-acting antioxidant than Vitamin C because Vitamin C is not lipid-soluble nor recyclable. Shungite water and/or Shungite Fullerene in sunflower or olive oil can be used topically for joint pain, injuries, cancer, infections, inflammation and as an antihistamine. Longecity.org is a forum for people interested in life extension and dozens of people have been pioneers in taking C60 in extra virgin olive oil.

HOW TO MAKE SHUNGITE WATER: Shungite C60 imparts its structure and healing properties to water. The C60 molecule contains fragments with five-fold symmetry (pentagons). I charge water for 3 days, after which the water is very much softer, oiler, purer, smoother, silky, tastier, and absorbs additives like lemon slices or teas much more profoundly, meaning the water is more highly active. Plants love to have their leaves sprayed with Shungite water, as does your face and hair. You need to make and store the water only in glass containers as it is highly activated and will absorb toxins from plastic. Wash a cup of it in water, use the black rinse water to water the plants.

Put the stones in a large jar or gallon bottle and fill up with filtered water. Leave for 3 days and then start drinking. If you have 3 large glass jars/bottles going at once you will never run out. Imagine the stones last for about 3 months, after which you can charge the stones in the sunshine and use them again, or use them for charging irrigation water for the garden. I charge my water with shungite chips prior to distilling so that I eliminate bacteria. It still seems to transform the water.

Horsetail, cucumbers, and diatomaceous earth powder lack the ionic suspension of Orthosilicic ($H4SiO4$) or ionic silicic acid found in the mineral waters to penetrate the blood-brain and reduce aluminum toxicity in the brain to help ward off Alzheimer's Disease. Since I charge my distilled water with shungite prior to making Philosopher's water, the water has exceptional "drinkability." It is also a lot easier than making tons of horsetail-nettle tea, cucumber-spinach juice, eating expensive bamboo sap and other forms of plant-chelated silicon.

***To make sure it is Shungite you are buying it might be best to buy only from Russia. I use a cup of shungite in the bottom of a gallon jar and have 2 jars charging at once.

https://shungit-store.com/shungite-water/view-all-products —Powdered and rough stone for oils and water treatment.

See the YouTube video: *Side Effects of Living Silica - What You Don't Know!* by **Dr. Robert Cassar**.

Dr. Robert Cassar on YouTube is a super advanced healer/alchemist. He is very helpful and outstanding—the perfect Doctor for fortifying our knowledge to survive the chemtrail holocaust. YouTube.com > EarthshiftProject

Stimulating Hair Growth Removing Scalp Toxicity, Fungus & Hair Mites Part 1 by Dr. Robert Cassar.

12

THE GLOBAL EUGENIC DEEP STATE

Oligarch: a ruler in an oligarchy. ORIGIN late 19th cent.: from Greek oligarkhes, from oligoi *'few'* + arkhein *'to rule.'* An "Oilogarchy" is government against the people and for big oil. There are going to be countless energy generating alternatives which will allow people to unplug from the entropic established cancerous matrix. Then with communities of soul-soul communion and mutual self-sufficiency and permaculture based urban centers we will be well on our way to liberated advanced human existence. The biodiversity of Life is infinitely more precious than gold or black gold!

The so called ĒLites are at war with the world for their own ends. The central impetus of this war is depopulation coupled with resource gathering and territory acquisition for themselves. Without any pushback, blowback or reprisal they can use the entire mechanism of State and international organizations like the UN, WHO, NATO against the people and the planet because THEY (tyrannical, hegemonic, evil yahoos) rule the world. The arch enemy has co-opted the US government and all other governments except for those not in the central banking system—it is a global cabal of money changers—and other dark figures hiding behind their expensive facades.

The head of the leviathan is the so called ĒLites, which are comprised largely of the Rothschilds, Rockefellers, UK Royals, Vatican, Illuminati, Council on Foreign Relations, Trilateral Commission, Club of Rome, Tavistock Institute (Rockefellers), and the Bilderberg Group. War is about rich people stealing stuff. All around the world there is war and genocide for body parts, drugs, antiquities and natural resources (oil, gold, diamonds, silver, lithium) and all of it goes back to the Rothschilds, the Vatican and the Royals as the head of the Fourth Reich. The neo-feudal czar, the "Rothschild syndicate," is the force behind the UN and the paramilitary intelligence army, the CIA.

The "secret government" or the "deep state" of the US has been a law unto itself over the past seven decades. America is the 4th Reich – meaning successor to the Nazi Third Reich. With its raving puppets. Its draconian laws. Its mendacious medicine forever pushing vaccines and drugs. Its eugenic poisoning. Its mutagenic GMO experiments and the 5G euthanasia grid. Its global "defense"empire. Its blatant, deceitful propaganda. Its mind control and the frenzied fanning of fear and stranger danger—and its Agenda 21. Those who have profited the most from industrial capitalism, now seek to impose socialists austerity measures on the serfs with Agenda 21 "sustainability." Read "Agenda 21: Earth Summit: The United Nations Program of Action from Rio, United Nations."

We live in a hologram of lies. All authorities are compromised, so we cannot rely on them for information, protection, inquiries or answers. The hierarchical authoritarian power system is presently working AGAINST the people and the planet. Power grabs by systems—political, governmental, religious—using fear tactics, are a desperate effort to maintain control. The inescapable truth is that you cannot bomb, kill, invade, occupy, steal and torture, and then expect no pushback, no retaliation and no blowback. Blowback is the unintended consequences of a covert operation that are suffered by the civil population of the aggressor government. So as people wake up, THEY have to increase the stressors, the economic hardships, the taxes, the poisons, the environmental disasters and weather disruption to prevent an outright global revolution. Sovereignty and freedom are best acquired when they are challenged. The attempt of authorities to control our freedoms are out of alignment with our true nature and will naturally fall apart. When we allow others to control us we give up responsibility to our mature, divine selves.

"Total Dominance Global Weather Control" — this is the overriding ambition behind the global chemtrail assault, to both euthanize and sicken the population, and asphyxiate them into a compliant stupor, so the NWO psychos can carry out their plans of a Total Dominance World Government managed by absolute surveillance. An incarcerated world that is not fit for humans to live in. With everything that is happening in the world, and from the gleam in their psychopathic eyes, it is easy to see that this is what they are aiming for. THEY are building a Hindbrain world and closing all the exits to the Matrix so that no one can escape the asylum. Hindbrain dominance occurs when the older brain regions hijack the prefrontal lobes, and so we become cunning, devious and manipulative, and our world reflects fear rather than love.

Our leadership model is currently built around a disconnected, chaotic mode of fear, scarcity, profit-first and self-gain. While the heart-driven approach to social organization is centered around love, abundance, growth and connection. Operating from this more evolved modality not only paves a clearer pathway to success, it also expands human consciousness into making the prefrontal lobes the manager of human affairs, rather than being dictated to from the reptilian brain. Do we want a dark, dying world run by dinosaurs? Or do we want a world run by those who are the most evolved, altruistic, humanitarian, public-spirited, philanthropic, kind, magnanimous and unselfish, resulting in a beneficent isocracy and a garden planet? **Isocracy**, is a government in which all individuals have equal political power. A philosophy of Isocracy expands from the legal right of isonomia to political and economic systems, from equality of law, to equality in governance.

The Death Machine is a progressive deadening of all life on earth. As an individual living within the death machine of a fallen civilization it is terrifying to look into the hopelessly **dystopian future** that is inevitable if we follow this present trajectory. We must turn our backs on Sodom and Gomorrah and lose our morbid fascination with the mental illness of the predator class and tragedies of the collapse. Civilization has been molded and hoodwinked by predatory capitalists, and both science, observation and natural law are being ignored. It is ill advised for the lamb to ask the wolf how best to survive. It can only end badly. Those living in underground cities might protect themselves for a few years more than surface dwellers, but they are likely to be already "mad" in order to obtain citizenry to these Ark cities. https://deepstatemappingproject.com/

"Monopoly capitalism, Communism, National Socialism (Nazism), and Fascism all came out of the Rothschild offices in Frankfurt, Germany." ~ Eustace Mullins.

HOW IS IT POSSIBLE?

How is it possible for there to be a global campaign of spraying chemical weapons when such military operations have been outlawed by the Geneva Protocol?

Geneva Protocol: Signed in Geneva on 17 June 1925, the Geneva Protocol prohibits the use of "asphyxiating, poisonous or other gases, and of all analogous liquids, materials or devices" and "bacteriological methods of warfare". How is it then that there is a worldwide campaign of blanketing the globe with asphyxiating, poisonous, omnicidal and genocidal aerosols? We are under daily attack by the most diabolical biological-chemical warfare ever devised. https://en.wikipedia.org/wiki/Geneva_Protocol

The Convention On Biological Diversity: Geoengineering is banned already via the multilaterial treaty — "The Convention on Biological Diversity," which recognized for the first time in international law that the conservation of biodiversity is "a common concern of humankind," and is an integral part of the development process. The agreement covers all ecosystems, species, and genetic resources. The UN Convention on Biological Diversity states that no climate-related activities that may affect biodiversity take place, until there is an adequate scientific basis on which to justify such activity and appropriate consideration of the associated risks for the environment and biodiversity and associated social, economic and cultural impacts with the exception of small scale scientific research studies that would be conducted in a controlled setting in accordance with Article 3 of the convention and only if they are justified by the need to gather scientific data and are subject to thorough prior assessment of the potential impacts on the environment. Signed in Rio de Janeiro, effective 29 December 1993. Out of the 168 signatories the United States was the only country to not ratify the agreement. www.cbd.int

Presently this stage of the global cull appears to be to destroy the immune system of the environment with chemtrails and to eliminate forests with fire and to kill off wild food sources. Next stage will be 5G microwaving of the population, and the spreading of pandemic superbugs along with the collapse of agriculture. The climate and geological extremes brought about by the Grand Solar Minimum are assisting the psychopath's weather warfare campaign. THEY seem all-powerful, but evil is ultimately stupid and weak. The existence of those who are anti-life is doomed, but we don›t have to go down with them.

Virtually the entire dominant cultural matrix is off kilter and needs to be overhauled to get it back onto cosmic alignment. In order to transcend the Matrix we must disembed, and see beyond the Matrix and move as far away from the pharmaceutical hypothesis of medicating sickness — it doesn't work and it never will. Health or wholeness is only achieved when we live in congruence with nature. Regardless of what THEY are doing, regardless of the encroaching night, it is up to us to use these constraints, stressors and negatives as the rungs of a ladder on which to climb. Let us never feel alone in this struggle, but together support each other in the breakthrough to the regenerative culture. Keeping the faith is our main spiritual practice these days as we move towards the great renewal. But we need to redefine faith as being the connection to the free, sovereign, liberated and actualized sense of self. Keeping the faith, means opening this portal into the enlightened, sane and transcendent future!

"And in the contemporary warfare arena, where experts in biological chemical warfare convene and discuss the ways that are ideal to conduct warfare today, to really take an enemy out, you don't want to kill the people. You want to produce people who are chronically ill and become dependent on the state and totally sap the resources of the country. And then you can move in with your military-medical-industrial complex and your international medical-pharmaceutical cartel. Then you sell these defeated countries all of the pharmaceuticals and chemicals that they need to maintain any semblance of healthy function. Once they're completely depleted, they can't put together a military. You create a dependence and thereby you weaken the population, and weakened populations are easy to control. So you've got population control, and you make vast fortunes doing it, versus just blowing up a nuclear weapon and devastating the infrastructure that you own. You and your colleagues own that infrastructure. You want to get rid of the people. You don't want to get rid of infrastructure."
~John P. Holdren, President Obama's Science Advisor and Director of the White House Office of Science and Technology Policy. His books written with Paul R. Ehrlich outline his global eugenics plan.

"The war is not meant to be won. It is meant to be continuous." ~ George Orwell, 1984

Headlines read: "Scientists to Spray the Skies with 'Reflective Particles' to Cool Down Plant Earth." But they are anything but "scientists" – for this an't science it is genocide!

http://eradicatingecocide.com/ — **Eradicating Ecocide** – Criminalizing ecosystem destruction; pollyhiggins.com/
https://www.YouTube.com/embed/8EuxYzQ65H4 —Ecocide, the 5th Crime Against Peace: Polly Higgins at TEDxExeter

https://www.facebook.com/ —The Farming Gardening Bill Of Rights

THE FOURTH REICH?

The Fallout of the Baron Rothschild's Caspian and Black Sea Oil Company—Israel was created by the Khazarian Rothschild banksters who funded both sides of WW1 and WW2 in order to set up a military state in the Middle East to oversee Rothschild-Rockefeller oil interests in the region. The Rothschilds "bankrolled" the holocaust in order to bring about the supreme dominance of their global financial empire. The Khazars, are a Tatar people from the south of Russia who converted to Judaism in mass at the time of Charlemagne... c. 812–814. See: The Protocols of the Elders of Zion, 1903. Now, they practically own the planet and are undertaking the slow holocaust of the entire earth, via chemtrail poisoning, ecocide and weather warfare. Now having made their money, they stand to lose more than they gained from conflict.

Israel was created by the Illuminati banking families and they essentially interned the Palestinians in concentration camps. By extrapolation, the fate of the Palestinians is the same fate for the rest of the world's citizens under the zionist's imperial global enterprise. Although the methods of global cull are more clandestine - via the slow gassing by chemtrails from the sky. As an illegitimate nation, Israel won't survive the ice age as it is focused on war, not survival. As we go into the trials of the Grand Solar Minimum the USA will stop supporting Israel when it will need to focus entirely on its own survival. Israel's guilt drives their homicidal mania and rapid slide into despotism, and since she is not likely to reconcile with her neighbors, she will be consumed. Israel must know this and is bent on technological global conquest.

The global eugenics program is obviously immoral and unethical, however it is legal because it is the industrial pirates make the laws. The forerunner to United Nations, the League of Nations was created and funded by the Rockefeller Family in 1919. The Rockefeller and Rothschild families both created the United Nations in 1945, without them the development of this global organization would not be possible. Thus the UN cannot save us from the global eugenics program because they are the ones that are conducting it. The CIA is also controlled by the Rothschild syndicate.

The Rockefeller and Rothschild families that comprise the global government have decided there are too many people on the planet and so they are asphyxiating and slow poisoning everyone. However these fossil dynasties will collapse when humanity breaks away to hydrocarbon fuels and establishes a new money system. When hydrocarbon fuels are outlawed as an energy source, this pact with the devil between Israel and the U.S. will fold, and other countries will be released from the threat of constant bullying, subterfuge and trickery.

Chemtrail spraying operations are now active in all 50 states of the US and all NATO countries. Who is chemtrailing? It is all governments complying with UN and WHO directives given to them by the 1% who want to poisoning the planet to reduce population. Whoever "owns" the planet, is who is instigating the chemtrail spraying. The Rothschild dynasty ($500 trillion), British Royal family, Vatican, Bill Gates etc... Global Empire is not war, it is cancer! It kills its host and dies of excess.

The conspiracy theory of the UN-New World Order (NWO) is claimed to be an emerging clandestine totalitarian world government masterminded by the Rothschild syndicate. We are told that the United Nations (UN) is headed and funded by the Rothschild and Rockefeller families. The European Union was also created by the Rothschilds (Schumann, a Khazar). Rothschilds created the corrupt money system + FED, Council on Foreign Relations and United Nations. See the YouTube video Myron Fagan Exposes UN As Tool Of Rothschild Luciferian ĒLite.

Banking is the mechanism of control over humanity by the Luciferian Illuminati. These "money changers" are the puppet masters behind the Deep State and the world eugenics program presently underway. This means that the we cannot appeal to the United Nations to stop the chemtrail gassing of all living creatures, because it is the United Nations that has ordered the attack on the planet. It appears that the foxes are guarding the hen house.

In the year 2000 there were only seven countries without a Rothschild-owned central bank: they were Afghanistan, Iraq, Sudan, Libya, Cuba, North Korea and Iran! It is the international Ashkenazi banking cabal who are the dogs wagging the American tail, and have been since the creation of the Reserve Banking system. A quarter of Israel's operating budget funded by America. Just like Germany was used for the Third Reich, America is being used as the beast of the Fourth Reich.

The oil-banker barons are destabilizing, raping and pillaging the Middle East and other oil rich countries, killing millions in the process. The only way to stop them is to get the global community off of the use of fossil fuels and to outlaw their use. It is possible to save the Titanic if the truth gets out and the people reboot and revolutionize society. Eliminating oil for energy, central banks, international banking cartels, debt currency, disaster capitalism and war profiteering for all time. Ironically the US debt is $21,823,094,510,705 and the missing/stolen public money is over $21 Trillion. Looks like a balanced budget. No one should be profiting from disease, death and destruction period, and anyone who does needs to locked up.

The world does not need US-corporations to meddle in rebuilding what the US military destroys. Structures in the USA are breaking down under the assault of chemtrails and electro-smog and HAARP. Older building methods using stone and traditional craft skills will stand the test of time better. The concrete in the USA is already breaking down and crumbling within 2 years of being laid. The solution is to simply STOP with the destruction and excel in "creation" instead. Disaster capitalism should be outlawed, just as war should be outlawed. Game is up! It is time for humanity to deal with its propensity to organized evil, and to create eternal systems to prevent it.

There is no way we can stop a global cull via legislation "within" the current corrupt judicial and political system for it is complicit with the NWO-Globalist Agenda 21. You can't sue the United Nations in a domestic court or any court because governments have signed the treaty and some countries like the U.S. have even put it in domestic legislation. By virtue of the Convention on the Privileges and Immunities of the United Nations, and the UN Charter, the U.S. Federal Court has ruled that "the UN is immune from suit unless it expressly waives its immunity." Individuals however could be sued for complicity in global genocide and damages to people's health and property. Those pulling strings behind the curtains must be made accountable to their actions.

Since the Rothschild-Rockefeller United Nations is at war with MOST countries of the world except for the most demonic, world citizens must unite and organize to create a One World Court of highest authority that offers protection against defoulement and upholds the integrity, security, and liberty of world citizens against the threat of persecution, violence, chemical genocide and the violation of all human rights. Besides policing against such assaults against health and wellbeing, this High Court must enforce the need for the criminal agents carrying out these acts of ecocide and genocide, to pay full restitution damages, along with life-term imprisonment in high security prisons catering to the psychopathically insane.

All those complicit this is diabolical program should forfeit their own capital to recompense all those who are suffering and to pay for restoration of the planet. We can now plainly see the forces at play, and the question is—how to reverse the regressive trend and reclimb the evolutionary ladder? Work for mere survival "within the entropic system" is futile, might as well be dead. There must be multiple exits off of the hamster wheel. We must each EXIT the entropic culture and create a global syntropic community of planet healers.

Without an enforcement mechanism to curb total dominance, absolute power runs rampant absolutely

Great book for a head's up on the End Game plan. *"Illuminati Covenant and Protocols,"* edited by Zen Garcia. Also *Collusion: How Central Bankers Rigged the World*, by Nomi Prins, 2018

Brendon O'Connell's phenomenal Youtube channel has the finger on the pulse of the globalist regime. His comprehension and dot connecting is unsurpassed.

Dean Henderson is the author of "Big Oil & Their Bankers In The Persian Gulf: Four Horsemen, Eight Families & Their Global Intelligence, Narcotics & Terror Network," (2010). Illuminati Agenda 21: The Luciferian Plan To Destroy Creation (2018), by Dean and Jill Henderson. His blog is at www.deanhenderson.wordpress.com

See on YouTube videos on the big picture of the leviathan, how Rothschilds control the Media, the Banks and the Oil — "Are the Rothschild's More Powerful Than the Monarchy? Are They Really Worth $500 Trillion?" by The Money GPS; and others.

http://illuminatisecretsexposed.com/ — Myron Fagan exposes the Illuminati/ CFR [1967]

https://deepstatemappingproject.com/ — Dylan Louis Monroe mapping the Deep State.

YouTube: "How the Jewish Rothschild Zionists Created Modern Israel" by Jake Morphonios shows how Churchill was involved in establishing the Balfour Agreement allowing Palestine to be used to build the state of Israel; and how the global central bank and oil industry was established by the Rothschilds and their Rockefeller relatives.

Our Global Neighborhood: The Report of the Commission on Global Governance, by The Commission on Global Governance

Food production within genocidal/ecocidal conditions needs to be of primary concern for communities and individuals. The Grand Solar Minimum and weather disruption is already undermining agriculture harvests, consequently food prices will rise and an economic depression will ensue. Farms can remain viable if they are permacultured with contour farming, swales, compost, mulch, remineralization with rockdust and kelp etc, compost tea, mycorrhiza, chicken tractors and drip irrigation — this reduces the water bill and holds water in the soil. Sucken greenhouses and earth heating and cooling may be necessary in temperate and unstable growing conditions. Follow Adapt 2030, Ice Age Farmer and Oppenheimer Ranch Project on YouTube.

The faster each of us propel ourselves into harmonious right relationship with the planet, the less inertia and lag we will feel as the old confining skin is discarded.

THE SCORCHED EARTH

Twenty plus years of massive chemtrailing with nanometal fire accelerants over California and other states...has produced a nation poised on the verge of an inferno.

California is one of the areas experiencing historic fire losses in the last few years. For the large part, the California energy company Pacific Gas and Electric (PG&E) is owned and operated by the Rothschilds; and Rothschilds owns Weather Central as well as being involved in weather modification globally. Rothschild's PG&E lies at the heart of the Agenda 21 United Nations Development plan, who have adopted 'MAPS', a common approach to help countries implement the 2030 Agenda and achieve the Sustainable Development Goals (SDGs), promising to leave no country behind. www.undp.org/.../sustainable-development-goals.htm

We must look into The PG&E SmartMeter™ program. Note that laser or other Directed Energy Weapons (DEW) directed at Smart Meters can turn houses into instant fireballs, but also the SmartMeter™ gas module attaches to your traditional gas meter, thus the gas supply to the houses can be targeted simultaneously from drone, orbital drone or satellite by homing in on their radio frequency. Even the RFID chips in your credit cards can be used to locate and identify you by satellite. Intercepted Pacific Gas & Electric (PG&E) documents profess the fact that they were going to use Directed Energy Weapons on northern California's Sonoma County. For 100% DEW evidence watch out for wood burning fiercely when in contact with metals under DEW attack, because the metal conducts the electrons from the DEW electromagnetic frequencies.

 What happens when you put a metal wire in a microwave? Microwaves cause electrons in metals to become excited move. This build-up of electrons creates a strong electric field in the surrounding air. When the electric field becomes strong enough, it causes free electrons in the air to accelerate creating an electrical charge in the air, which shows itself as sparks. Microwaving wires can create "sparks, and the electrical wiring of buildings is covered in inflammable plastic, in close contact with wood.

Guidance and Policies on 2030 Agenda is the United Nation's sustainable development and resilient cities cultural renewal program. With the burning of outlying subdivisions they are condensing population into denser housing, opening up land to rewilding and taking people's property via eminent domain. Sonoma was chosen to locate the **rectanna** for the solar-satellite. A rectenna is a rectifying antenna—a special type of receiving antenna that is used for converting electromagnetic energy into direct current electricity. The answer is to pull the rug out from the oil-war machine with New energy systems—which will quickly change power and wealth to a distribution model.

The Fukushima hot blob in the ocean and rising desert temperatures are creating a high pressure dome which is keeping moisture out in the Pacific hundreds of miles away from the west coast of the US. They have been heavily ship chemtrailing 500+ miles out to sea for over a year now, so when this air does reach the California coast, it makes people sick! It appears they are intentionally making California hell on earth. I assume it is for depopulation in order to create another Israel-like military state for the Zionists.

THE ELECTROMAGNETIC KILLING DOME

Chemtrails are part of Star Wars. It involves the combination of creating an "atmosphere" that will support electromagnetic waves, ground-based, electromagnetic field oscillators called gyrotrons, and space based ionospheric heaters. Chemtrail particulates and ionization of air molecules make directed energy weapons, Space Based Lasers and HAARP technology work better.

Having both gas and electrics on Smart Meters means that entire houses can be targeted with lasers to instantly explode in an inferno. This is the perfect method of clearing out sprawling subdivisions that are in the road of Agenda 21 resilient cities and the Wildland's Project brought forth by the UN BioDiversity Plan. California is ahead of the curve for Agenda 21 of the United Nations Development. I suppose THEY feel that if they can break California, they can break any state or nation.

The aluminum oxide and other metals in the chemtrails act as radical desiccants, drying out the trees, houses, fences and even the rocks and concrete, such that everything is becoming oxidized and decomposing. This provides **extremely volatile fuel** for burning, in association with the fact that the Aluminum oxide and other chemicals in the chemtrail ARE fire accelerants.

Flammable metals like aluminum oxide produce fires that cannot be extinguished with water. They produce very hot fires known as a Class D fire. Even the desiccation and ionization of the air by the chemtrails would contribute to the severity of wildfires, and the microwaving by HAARP technology would create an electrical inferno—a fact of which must be the intended strategic goal and the real purpose of the chemtrail program, for how could the military and scientific community be so stupid?

I assume that if they are going to torch an area then they would add more iron to the chemtrail mix, as nano aluminum from chemtrails mixing with iron in the trees basically becomes **thermite**. Aluminum, barium, strontium and fluoride are fire accelerants. All trees that have been heavily chemtrailed for years are basically dead, as the phloem is so compromised that it is only a matter of time before the tree is completely dead.

The chemtrails also are desiccants and oxidizers—both processes make trees, houses and everything else more highly combustible. When tree stumps rot on the inside in an enclosed space, the fungi and bacteria produce ammonia, which on a hot day can spontaneously combust—the ammonia enhancing the "thermite" like effect. Microwaves from communications and military amplify this pyrotechnic effect.

Most of California is a fire waiting to happen. California is moving and volcanically coming alive (as per Dutchsinse), one would assume that this ground movement would create leaks in the gas pipes—hence fires to the houses. California is insolvent—it does not have sufficient assets to pay all of its present liabilities! California is drowning in 'irretrievable' debt - more than $428 billion, so chances are it has already been sold out to the highest bidder.

The Feds cut them off. The only way to get Federal assistance is to create a state of emergency through a "natural disaster" to bring in more federal money. Numbers of homeless have tripled since the fires in 2017-18. These people made homeless are victims of DEW weather warfare, rent hiking and economic warfare on the sovereignty of the individual.

The most heavily geoengineered region has been California. One motivation could be that they are trying to shut down the onshore flow to keep the air born radiation from Fukushima from ruining the farming lands of CA. It appears that they ship chemtrail 500-1000 miles out into the Pacific to overseed and dry out the ocean air, so that the marine layer doesn't reach the coast like it is supposed to, this leaves a 1000 mile hole of cloudless sky off the coast. This was noticeable before fires in Sonoma 2017, and as far back as December 2011 when the state of California experienced one of the worst droughts to occur in the region on record. Apparently it has been happening since 2012—theoretically as a response to the Fukushima disaster, to create a weather wall to keep the radiation off of the west coast.

A contrary or conjunctive possibility is that this is a weather-warfare strategy to use the summer heat in the Californian desert and HAARP to create a high pressure heat dome, which keeps the moisture and precipitation from coming onto the West Coast. This phase of the UN Agenda involves chemtrailing, shiptrailing, HAARPing, jet stream manipulation, weather warfare, disaster capitalism and anomalous Directed Energy Weapons land clearing fires is a global phenomena. This is easily observable from NASA Worldview, all you need to do is to look at old satellite images of the earth from prior to 1990's and compare them with today's sad looking earth.

They don't usually chemtrail the heat dome, they ship trail in the North Pacific to the west of the heat dome itself in order to stall the weather and dry out the air to prevent rain onto the West Coast. This is an act of war against California, and part of the SPRAY, ZAP AND BURN attack on the state in the name of Agenda 21.

Spraying millions of tons of highly conductive metals into the atmosphere and then microwaving it with HAARPs and Scalar Radar will undoubtedly increase lightning storms frequency and strength, with destructive consequences to human electrical installations, buildings and increase in wildfires. The Alaska HAARP array pumps out 3.5 *million* watts of radio frequency energy. There are also HAARP capabilities from ships, planes and satellite. HAARP technology can move weather around, create earthquakes, tsunamis, atomic-like bomb blasts, create drought or flood, hurricanes, cyclones, lightning-fire storms etc... Since none of these behave normally (seismically etc....) it is easy to tell what is geophysical warfare and what is nature.

The atmosphere has been ionized to become the "ideal medium for scalar energy weapons." When you cross two strong beams, you can create scalar energies. Such powerful god-like technology was used to bring down the towers on 911. These energies can be used as untraceable weapons for nuclear size explosions or for defense. You need lead, ceramics, and a deep underground facility to avoid the effects of scalar weapons. If we watch the Solar Radiation Managers behavior on satellite maps such as NASA-Worldview and follow the sequence of the consequences, we can understand their climate warfare methods and their goals. In this way we can protect ourselves from the catastrophic consequences of their war games. I am not sure what we can do about the geospatial war against the people via EMF-firestorms, earthquakes, tsunami, hurricanes, tornados, floods and drought.

See the YouTube video by The Haarp Report - *"BEST SCIENCE - REAL Purpose of Chemtrails, Ozone Layer Destroyed."*

MARINE CLOUD BRIGHTENING

Geoengineers have been stopping moisture from entering the western US since Fukushima 2011. The hotspot in the ocean off the coast is causing a heat dome off of California and Baja — which even prevents the marine fog layer from reaching the coast. This is caused by the build up of a FUKU radiation hot spot, increased oceanic volcanic activity, El Niño, the north magnetic pole moving into Siberia, and Grand Solar Minimum disruption of the jetstream patterns. The hot spot and heat dome is also caused by the MASSIVE ship chemtrailing thousands of miles into the Pacific. These are sulfur rich bunker fuel burning ships on irregular courses and meandering shipping patterns, whose job it is to overseed and dry out the air before it reaches the west coast.

Marine cloud-brightening (MCB) is geoengineering technique that involves seeding marine stratocumulus clouds with copious quantities of sea water particles to enhance the cloud droplet number concentration, and thereby the cloud albedo and longevity. Marine Cloud Brightening, via spraying seawater and sulphates, to increase the Earth's albedo via spreading massive chemtrails via ships off of the west coast of America is causing widespread severe illness for those in Oregon in particular. The Oregon Illness is no doubt related to the crazy ship trails 500 miles off the coast for months, resulting from sulfur rich bunker fuel.

Multiple ship chemtrails in far out in the Pacific off the coast out from Washington state and Oregon during spring and summer of 2018 are blowing onto the continental US and causing grievous health problems in the citizens of those states. On the Oregon coast the symptoms reported late June'2018 were reported to have been occurring for two weeks: 104°F fever, massive sneezing attacks, stomach upset - diarrhea, even vomiting again, confusion, flushed skin or shivers, WAVES of dizziness, weak legs, barely able to stand up, racing heart - all the symptoms of panic attack, drop in potassium levels, skin tingling and numb spots on the body. Lump in the throat when you try to eat, either you're on the couch flat or doing hyper behavior stuff. Dogs are completely wiped out, cats don't want to move. People are easily angered, and there is lots of wacko driving.

 The massive meandering ship chemtrails appear to be laid out prior to the Agenda 21 Fire Storm events in order to ionize the air moving onto the West Coast so that Direct Energy Weapons can be used to light the anomalous subdivision clearing fires. This electromagnetic technology is so effective that they can create wind and lightning storms on demand, directing air currents with the microwave heating effects of HAARP arrays — with complete disregard for the property, safety and well-being of the citizens.

What is the best a person can do for themselves and their family? Look at the Agenda 21 & Agenda 2030 maps for suburb consolidation and sell your property if you are in the redevelopment zone. Move away from areas with 5G; www.antennasearch.com. Going rural and subterranean for housing seems like a good option. Look for areas with water supply that is unsullied by fracking, mountain spring water if possible. Ideally you want to be in areas that are away from the jet stream coming over from Fukushima. And areas that are not of strategic importance for military, mining, industrial-GMO take over and such. Avoid nuclear power stations, military bases, large cities and earthquake faults. Go where you can find supportive, loving community who are moving ahead. Resist smart meters, get OFF the grid, fire proof your property, create a bugout bag, have your emergency plan in place and go down guns blazing.

SIGNS OF ANOMALOUS DIRECTED ENERGY FIRES

When distinguishing between natural wildfires and the DEW fires look for:

- Prior droughting via generating heat domes to keep maritime air off the coast and deflect the jet streams.
- Heavy Chemtrailing for weeks prior, white powder on the tops of the trees, possibly thermite fire accelerant.
- Signs of the solar satellite moving into position, ie: sunburst in wrong place, or light flash across a continent.
- Aerosols ionized/charged into a plasma-like atmosphere with GWEN or 5G microwave frequencies, increasing static electricity.
- DEW Lasers from drones cause conductive metals to "spark" which kindles wood in its vicinity — ie: houses, telegraph and power poles etc..
- Smart Meters for GPS positioning of buildings, and GPS in cars to laser people on the roads escaping the fires.
- No Alarm, roads congested, cars lose power, sitting ducks for DEW attack.
- Extreme heat of the fire, instantaneous combustion of entire buildings.
- Complete burn-off of buildings down to their foundations.
- Houses neatly burned and dustified leaving surrounding trees intact.
- Look for wood burning around metal nails, bolts, wire fences, railings etc...
- Exploding cars that flip over onto their roofs, melted glass and aluminum.
- Electrical EMP effects and electrified air before the fires start.
- Sudden extreme wind out of nowhere.
- Initial fire bomb explosion rising thousands of feet creating huge blast radius.
- Multiple fires lit in a line or all at once. Multiple areas in a state.
- Blue lasers from the sky at night seen through the smoke.
- Blue circular flashes seen on satellite images before and during the fires.
- The location of the fires in association with UN Agenda 21 Maps.
- What buildings, facilities and areas are left untouched by fire.
- Holding rain back with atmospheric heating (heat dome). using HAARP.
- After the fires allowing maritime air and rain in to deluge the land, creating more damage and eliminating evidence of the anomalous fires.
- Weak fire fighting, too little to late …Fire trucks guarding non-burn areas.
- Firefighting planes can't fly because the sky is filled with drones.
- Citizens lose the financial ability or legal right to rebuild.
- Citizens not allowed to live in RV due to toxic soil layer and may not be able to rebuild due to benzene from the burnt city water pipes.

Video taping these attacks while they are happening is essential to prove culpability, by capturing the laser strikes through the smoke on film. We need more home owners taking video footage of the fires during and after in order to document the anomalies and set them before a group of scientists and engineers. Heavy chemtrail spraying and holding back rain with high pressure systems, sending in the solar satellite or the orbital drone, lighting fires by laser or lightning, then letting the weather go so the deluge washes away the evidence.

SATURNIC ĒLITES AND WORLD DOMINATION

Non participation is the sane response to the villainy of the global tyranny.

Now technology has developed to the point where evil is in our face and in our skies daily. But the dark ones get chemtrail pneumonia same as everyone, so we really have to wonder about the sanity of the perpetrators. It could be, the risk of getting sick themselves is overcome by the joy they receive over making everyone else sick? Our human world always has had its evil side, but we were ignorant and innocent to its machinations. It is truly amazing how at this late hour there are intelligent individuals who cannot see what is occurring, perhaps they live in areas where the chemtrailing is not so bad, or they have not seen the atmospheric mess on NASA-Worldview and have no idea what the earth is "supposed" to look like.

In past years Boulder Colorado has been chemtrailed heavily making us wonder how it is that those working for military industrial machine and geoengineering program are going along with the daily aerial assault to their health and well-being. Boulder after all is *Borg-city*, harboring as it does so many companies that support aerospace and the American "Defense"Industry: IBM, Lockheed Martin, Ball Aerospace, Boeing, ITT Exelis, Lockheed Martin, Northrop Grumman, Raytheon, CASA, LASP, NCA, NIST and NOAA. Both the Colorado Nanotechnology Alliance and Colorado Photonics Industry Association are also headquartered in Boulder. DARPA uses universities University of Colorado (and Carnegie Mellon, Cornell) and giant Tech companies (Siemens, Heron) to build their military technology.

Power-addicted psychopaths are not rational, they feel they can do whatever they want without regard to consequences. THEY revel in the fact that the people know what they are up to, but are helpless to do anything about it. THEY (Tyrannical Hegemonic Elitist Yahoos) also revel in the fact that some people will always be sheep. I wouldn't call people who don't have eyes that see, nor brains that know the reality of nature, or minds that cannot conceive of the demonic nature of the unfolding human folly your friends...they are lemmings. Go find friends you can walk into the transcendent future with.

As is observed by all the shenanigans going on in California it is obvious that the THEY want to turn California into a manufacturing center and military border state for the total dominance Global Empire, as is seen in the predictive programming movie "Elysium" (2013). If you live in a targeted area like California you have to study the videos of Deborah Tavares and look at the Agenda 21 Maps to see what they have in store for your region. (See YouTube: Cooking of Humanity - Invisible Global Warfare.) If your area is slated for "redevelopment" you should sell up ASAP and get out of the region, perhaps to a different state, or country. You also have to keep in mind all the earth changes and weather disaster effects associated with a Grand Solar Minimum with its disrupted magnetic field, wandering jet streams and deluges.

http://agenda21news.com - The Wildlands Project brought forth by the UN Convention on Biological Diversity Plan to Restore Biodiversity in the United States in 1991, by setting aside at least 50% of USA for wildlands to encourage biodiversity.

See Neil Hague's exceptional article Online: *"Elysium – Life after Death in the New World Order."*

THE UN WAR AGAINST SELF-SUFFICIENCY

The war against self-sufficiency, and self-determinancy is the UN Agenda 21 Depopulation Agenda…poisoning crops to quicken the famine, preventing people from growing and sharing their own food and collecting their own rain water. The breakdown of the physical/mental/emotional human radiation, GMOs, chemtrails, vaccination, pharmaceutical drugs and agricultural toxins like Glyphosate (Don Huber) is an accelerating and accumulative decent.

The global cull is a full spectrum weather, chemical and frequency war. This "diabolical" war against the earth and its people is coordinated with HAARP, microwave towers, scalar waves, chemtrails and biological weapons etc. to target specific areas for Agenda 21 redevelopment. Geo and weather warfare, chemtrail weapons of mass destruction, Reality Show Politics and disaster capitalism merges nicely with the deprivatization of land via UN and federal land grabs through Agenda 21's corrupt resilient cities network using branches of the leviathan: Local Governments for Sustainability (ICLEI), Department of Housing and Urban Development (HUD), Bureau of Land Management (BLM), Environmental Protection Agency (EPA) etc… The EPA and other so called regulatory government agencies are in fact mercenaries protecting the criminal behaviors of multinational corporations and enabling ecocide.

FULL SCALE MULTI-PRONGED ATTACK

We are under full scale multi-pronged attack which is breaking down immunity via:
Geoengineering Chemtrails and Pathogens via "sky vaccine"
Chemical pneumonia
Lithium mood modulation
Fukushima Radiation
Smart meters and Directed Energy Weapons
EMF Poisoning, 5G
Fluoride and Chlorine in drinking water
Vaccines-Autism
ADD/ADHD
Endocrine disruptors-Estrogenization
Carcinogenic Glyphosate and GMOs
Fracking-Poisoning of aquifers
Corexit, Pharma, Coca Cola, Junk food, Industrial chemical farming
Demineralization, soil microbiome and soil organic matter depletion
Nature deprivation, ecological devastation
Blocking sunlight and Vitamin D deficiency
Sugar, Candida/Cancer
Biodome GI tract destruction.

It is not going to get any better under these circumstances, it can only get much worse. This is a eugenics war against the land and people that will destroy the soil microbiome, plus poison air and water, and deforest the environment. Land, house and livelihood prices have outpaced wages, and a "service economy" is not self-sustaining. Such a fragile economy is bound to collapse into widespread homelessness and the hopelessness of wasted lives. However by recovery of our magical shamanic soul, our sovereign self—we can turn the big lemon into a truckload of lemonade. By expanding the psychology, spirituality and technology of awakening we need to thrive regardless of what the darkside throws at us. Instead of euthanizing, we will youthenize!

Quit following the **Circus of Satan**, they are not going anywhere, but round in ever maddening circles. The trauma-based mind control via "shockn'awe" keeps the amygdala and the reptilian brain over-stimulated, causing the brain to become inflamed and the body full of stress hormones. This paralyzes the conscious mind from making rational judgments and zeitgeist of intellectual and spiritual darkness gains hold. The hypertonal reptilian brain prevents the higher transcendental brain from kicking in, and so as a species we are trapping in this lower mundane mechanical mode of functioning in which pathological power and false hierarchy can perpetuate throughout the centuries.

Thus we see the **piratearchy** (mal-patriarchy), inequality, rogue governments, criminal military, mafiosa police, and exploitive predatory economics that make human life almost impossible. Evil is out of sync with the lifeforce, so evil is inevitably undone by itself. Evil thoughts and actions breakdown the body, the mind and the genes, so evil is negatively selected against by evolution. Justifiably Nature abhors that which "doesn't" further life's success and abundance. Nature IS the light of life! It is this foundational principle of life that points to human civilization eventually ending up in a good place. You cannot build a stable, substantial life for yourself on a pirate ship run by psychopaths.

"He who controls the weather, will control the world." Lyndon Johnson, 1962.

***Paul A Philips has a great article online on what we can do to help turn things around – *"Now That You've Awakened How Do You Awaken Others? – 8-2-16"* www.newparadigm.ws/

THE SHIRKY PRINCIPLE

"Have you heard of the Shirky Principle? It's that institutions exist to preserve the problem to which they have a solution Sending food to starving countries is this knee-jerk reaction." Charlie Paton, Founder of Seawater Greenhouse

We are living within a cultural mental illness with similar qualities and motives as Nazi Germany. Mass delusion, is a socially contagious frenzy of irrational behavior. The government, military and police societal functions are honorable, but not when directed by a corrupt ÉLite that is bent on reducing global population by 99%. Under such an omnicidal regime all factions of authority right up to the UN, along all judicial bodies cannot be trusted to be operating in the best interests of any human, nor in the interest of the planet. This makes Borg civilization itself highly toxic and obsolete to the entire population of the earth. Since we cannot fight this madness, nor fix it, the only viable option is to refuse to feed it and to somehow get away from it.

The Borg is surface - void depth and authenticity, therefore always seeking outer approval and the stamp of authority. It abhors truth, reality and original thought. The Borg is the anti-HUman. The propensity to blindly cooperate with evil and corruption simply because it is the leading Powerhoe of the day will be the death of humanity. Unless we can rapidly grow beyond being human cattle and corroborating with our own demise. To save our soul we must leave our comforts behind when we seek to escape the madness of the Borg, and step bravely into the new world. You know that fascism is taking over when censorship and propaganda reaches an all time high. Shirking personal responsibility is intrinsic to fascism!

The social disease of fascism can only infect a population when the people are traumatized, threatened and separated from the vitality of nature. The work of **Wilhelm Reich** explained the bio-physics of fascism, a lesson we will have to re-learn in this weird, martial, hypercapitalist era in which we find ourselves. Governments psychologically manipulate public mood through the economics of scarcity and surplus, and as individuals we "contract and armor" our body-mind when we feel our survival or thrival is threatened.

When in this bioenergetic armored condition we forfeit the energy and traits of creative, entrepreneurial, executive and sovereign function. This loss of passion, optimism, motivation, creativity and risk taking allows for the domestication, passivity, obedience and conformity which underlines the submission to fascist domination and political immorality. When people fear for their survival they shut down and become conservative and defer authority to a dubious "higher" power. Sick, low consciousness people more easily follow bad orders as they shirk doing what is right through being in automaton (Borg) mode.

"The biological process of armoring disrupts work function through immobilization, and this impairs the individual's ability to develop and find satisfying work and to earn an adequate wage. This process takes place at the individual level leading to individual poverty, or at the national level leading to national poverty." Charles Konia, M.D., The Emotional Plague, The Root of Human Evil,

We need to study examples of cultural renewal from history, and also tune into the transcendent. We must assume that the pirates at the top of the food chain always were insane, but they are now truly showing their true colors. Reading The Mass Psychology of Fascism by Wilhelm Reich, may give us some answers as to how to proceed. The evolution of consciousness and community has never been more important than it is now. We each must do everything we can to wake up to our sovereign self, and to bring that wealth of brilliance to the party. Need a collective awakening fast—share information far and wide. This is not a fight, this is a celebration of life. When lifeforce rises, that which is anti-lifeforce drops away.

We as a species assign responsibility to those who are tasked with a duty or responsibility to perform an obligation to the common-weal. When those in positions of power shirk their responsibility and evade the performance of their duty, they are remiss or negligent. We have created a culture where to be successful and rise to the top we have to operate in reverse or in the opposite of the highest objectives of the field of human endeavor. We have a civilization that shirks, avoids and neglects the founding tenets and operatives of the civilizing principle itself.

Mass civilization produces food that creates disease, medicine that promotes death, education that prevents creativity and original thought, clothing and housing that cuts us off from the Earth's telluric and magnetic fields, relationships that promote stagnation, music that hurts the senses, entertainment that dulls the mind, sports that distract us, transportation that pollutes the air we breathe, jobs that enslave us, governments that manipulate and prey on their people, and military that creates war to feed its own agendas. No aspect of degenerate society is free from the Shirky Principle.

There is no aspect of human life that is not besieged by the ongoing encroachment of the "Shirky Principle." The term "shirk" perhaps comes

305

from German *"schurke,"* (scoundrel, rogue, knave, villain, or shark.) There is perhaps no greater example in human history of the failure of responsibility of governing body's towards the people and the planet than the colossal screw-up of geoengineering. After the earth is rendered almost "uninhabitable" by this massive failure of science and common sense, the perpetrators of this folly will go down in history as the most extreme imbecilic criminals ever to walk this earth.

Political dementia or "End Times Political Alzheimer's disease" is not a party issue, it is systemic to exploitative capitalist culture. War Hysteria is fomented by a gaggle of old, sclerotic, impotent men invested in expanding or protecting their own economic interests, power and legacy. An immortality project born of the bloated egos of power addicts and the enemies of humanity. Things are corrupt because they are corrupt! We must stop those in positions of power from shirking their responsibility to life. Anything less is planetocide.

Shirking is intrinsically tied to "commodification" and commercialization of all aspects of human action or "work." The collective ego doesn't have a conscience due to "deferred responsibility" — for we have fallen under the authority of man's will, not Thine Will of the creator. The effort to run away from responsibility produces human lives that constitute a long series of addictions, our will having been hijacked by our survival centers. The divine energy to "create" is lost to us when we have given up personal accountability and self-care, to survive in a mad, upside down world of ever diminishing returns. A civilization ruled by rebellion from cosmic union is always heading towards entropic collapse — reacting against the collapse only further amplifies the self-destruct mechanisms.

Authorities complicit in the UN agenda are saying that chemtrails are an "urban myth." Blind obedience to delusion is essential to the continuity of evil empire. In this fashion of "the emperor wears no clothes" the earth is being destroyed by those who refuse to admit the naked truth. The saying, *"The Emperor Wears No Clothes"* is often used in political and social contexts for any obvious truth denied by the majority despite the evidence of their eyes, especially when proclaimed by the government. When people say "The emperor wears no clothes", they mean that other people need to stop being ass kissers to a political leader and see things for what they truly are instead of denying the truth of the situation. It takes a person with guts to speak the truth and blast through the bullshit and lies." www.urbandictionary.com:

The average citizen of contemporary consumer-driven society is focused on instant gratification and pleasure-oriented habits, and is impulsive with a short attention span. The type of irrational human we have become, capable of extreme feats of denial, is not equipped to deal with extreme survival conditions, thereby ensuring the death of billions. Cognitive dissonance or psychic rift, bad observation skills or poor education perhaps? Mytho-religion, and patho-politics have melted the rational faculties to the point where even the animal senses of humans are insane. Hence the remarkable ability of chemtrail denial. **Willful denial** is just as anti-life (evil) as planet killing itself.

In the slow apocalypse we can kid ourselves that we are floating rather than drowning. When the crisis reaches an acute phase people may wake up to their inner leader. We need to organize and inspire leadership in each other "prior" to man-made or cosmic disasters. I think we are perhaps collectively stunned by the realization of the inverted world. My father used to say everything is the opposite of how it appears. The lemmings want to believe that there is no cliff. Let them—they will turn around eventually. Lack of observation, malignant denial, toxic compliance, comfort addiction, hedonism and immediate gratification make the plebs perfect victims to the global genocide, for they will not know what is upon them until it is too late. We cannot "save" those who are still not differentiated from the Borg matrix. Instead of wasting our time and energy it is best to sing to the choir, and join other Thrivalists to create joint homesteads and communities. When leaders have lost their way it is time for the people to lead.

We may be headed towards the limitless of galactic civilization, however we won't get there if we continue to behave without accountability, sanity and goodwill toward planet earth. We should withdraw our attention and support for high jinx nations and rogue empires and find some way to make the planet killers pay for their crimes. Those criminals who are so stupid that think they can spray toxic chemicals to ionize earth's atmosphere should not be allowed any political or cultural influence, nor any bank account to carry out such dastardly deeds. Together we must hold the "shirkers" accountable and rebuilding our lives in ways that ensures greater sovereignty, resilience and sustainability. Just as success as an entrepreneur is all about accountability, so too success as a politician should be all about accountability! Culpability marks the dividing line between good and evil, and is intimately tied to freedom, empowerment, agency, initiative, flexibility and free will.

First Do No Harm, the precautionary principle, has been thrown by the wayside. John Whyte of the "Consciousness Beyond Chemtrails Conference," interviewed retired USDA Biologist Francis Mangels, who pointed out that the aluminum deposited in the soil from chemtrails CANNOT be removed. It just goes on accumulating in the soil and water cycle for as long as they continue to spray. Within the decades that military jets have been chemtrailing over Mount Shasta the soil aluminum in Francis's garden has raised the soil pH from 5.5 to 6.5. With chemtrailing acid soils become 10 x more alkaline. The pH of normal rain is 5.5-5.6, while chemtrail contaminated rain is 6.5-7.6. What this means for humanity is that soils are rapidly becoming too alkaline to grow trees and food. Besides the pH, nano aluminum is extremely effective at killing the root hairs and rapidly killing all plant life exposed to the accumulation of chemtrailed aluminum fallout in the rain and snow. Thus if things continue as they are we are headed with the collapse of the biosphere, mass extinction (including humans) and a desert planet.

"Political reaction lives and operates within the human structure in the thinking and acting of the suppressed masses in the form of character armor, fear of responsibility and incapacity for freedom, and, at last but not least, as an endemic crippling of biological functioning." Wilhelm Reich, The Mass Psychology of Fascism.

Read the *"Culture"* series of science fiction novel by the popular Scottish author **Iain Banks.** The Culture is a fictional interstellar post-scarcity civilization or utopian, post-scarcity space society of humanoids, aliens, and very advanced artificial intelligences living in socialist habitats spread across the galaxy.

SIGNS OF EUGENIC PSYCHOPATHY

• So now we see why the microbiologists scientists and GcMAF doctors were killed off.

• Why the wild animals are being culled and forests are in decline as they serve as for backup food sources for survivalists.

• Why the weather is being manipulated to destroy the food supply.

• Why the abominable Monsanto is aggressively pushing food that genetically mutates and developing seeds that tolerate high aluminum.

• Why there is red blood cells, pathogens and heavy metals in chemtrails, essentially delivering "live vaccines" from the sky.

• Why the desiccating chemtrails, atmospheric microwaving, smart meters and directed energy weapons are being used to fire-bomb strategic areas.

• Apparently they will spray until the population is reduced enough to reach their goal of maintaining the world population under 500 million.

• Why stratospheric geoengineering could continue for the next 100-years non-stop in an effort to thwart alleged "global warming."

• Why Bill Gates has funded millions of dollars on geoengineering, or "chemtrails and Harvard and scientists are now publically admitting to the program.

WHY IS THIS HAPPENING?

We must ask how we arrived at the place where the human race is engaged in a murder/suicide with Nature and planet earth? The chemtrailer's are vaccinating us from the air, using up billions of gallons of fuel, polluting the world, destroying the soil and precipitating mass famine, hardship and illness and killing people, forests and all life.

How in the world could the global geoengineered omnicide be happening? It is happening because the predators at the top of the food chain are certifiably insane and have taken it upon themselves to eliminate the majority of people on the planet. The upcoming Grand Solar Minimum will foil their global warming cover that allegedly justifies chemtrailing and weather manipulation, so they will have to come up with a new raison d'être to fulfill their dastardly plan. To move beyond the state satanic barbarism we must look at how we arrived at this absurdity.

The Global warming scam was a front for geoengineering—a multi-pronged attack to put in place the UN Tyrannical One-World Government and reduce population numbers. So the plan all along with the solar dimming chemtrail program was to break the immune system of the biosphere, weaken the human population and bring about mass genocide. However, they are too late, for the people have already awoken to self-governance and will not tolerate a fascist New World Order.

They are burning, poisoning and otherwise destroying potential food growing areas around the world to prevent people gaining access to free and wild food — so they can speed the level of dumbing down and compliance they need to maintain their power. To ensure famine they destroy crops with fire, freezing, flood, hail, drought, hurricanes, chemicals, and GMOs. With the current Grand Solar Minimum and the following ice age wild animals will be more likely to survive than farmed animals. Thus only wilderness and forested areas will provide food for the few enterprising hunters. The 1080 poisoning of the wildlife, land and water catchment in New Zealand is making human survival questionable in the upcoming climate disruption cycles. Native animal and bird species will be made extinct by the indiscriminate dispersal of this highly toxic and inhumane systemic poison into the environment.

Once you look at the historical graphs you can see that we are on the verge of the Mini Ice Age, followed by the large ice age. The self-serving Governments as they are presently constituted are a GRAVE threat to Homo sapiens' survival. The nuclear power stations need to be dismantled and all nuclear material reburied miles underground, away from potential ice sheets. And the military need to be redirect away from wars over arcane fossil fuels, to re-engineering human habitation in habitable zones of the planet. The alternative energy inventors need to be supported and given all the resources they require — NOT killed off. Thus we see, it is imperative to eradicate the predatory leviathan that is feeding on humanity and the globe, so we can become all we were meant to be as a species.

How is it possible that science, government, religion and the military are all failing us, and have turned against the earth and all her lifeforms? I blame the global omnicide on the "fallen" nature of the incorporated or Borgified human (the Wetiko, see Paul Levy) — not on aliens, gods, spirits, demons, or the Vatican. We must educate the masses and unplug from the psycho Borg, for compliance means a loss of our humanity and Spirit.

The ĒLite globalist eugenics program appears to be playing out via Borgification mechanisms, medical tyranny, gender confusion, fluoride/lithium compliance, toxic food intoxication, life-harming EMF frequency and lighting, chemtrail nano-poisoning, cashless society, the chip, disarming the public, Hollywood predictive programming movies. That is, soft kill by multiple vectors leading to the zombie apocalypse, or "hell" on earth. Basically the "Borg" is a term used to represent socialized retardation to Hindbrain function through fear, intimidation, competition, deprivation, disrespect, usury, harassment, slavery and dependency, that is missing out on the "refuge" of higher HUman qualities via mass psychosis.

The service-to-self cretans have hijacked everything that serves toxic power, leaving the rest of us locked into the given entropic culture, with little capacity to see beyond the fallen world. We need a revolution in human evolution, and we need it fast. This revolution cannot be monetized, or it is simply just more of the old. As the left brain hemisphere gains greater supremacy we fall into a progressive state of delusion fueled by runaway feedback loops of cause and effect as we react to circumstance without the wisdom of holistic thinking, integral wisdom and transcendent gnosis. The chemocide death of the planet is occurring because Homo sapiens is insane. Presently our world is run by the most brain damaged among us and if we follow this track our species will descend into ever greater peril and madness.

Tony Wright exposes the original cause of our species fall from grace when we left the tropical forests and a diet of raw fruit to moving around the world to colder environments and turned to hunting, agriculture and cereal production. Humanity lost its moral compass as its diet descended to meat and cereal grains and the body-mind became dis-eased and discombobulated. This shift in the metabolic makeup of the "human" rendered us increasingly left-brained—with focus on control, **piratearchy** (malpatriarchy), technological mechanization and commodification. This imbalance to left-brain dominance explains the profound mental illness and systemic dementia in our species today, a sickness which is progressing at breakneck speed as the mental illness compounds on itself, and generates ever greater demonic technology and pathological control systems that cause ever greater "self harm" to ourselves and our planet.

The question of the age is, are we to have a Luciferian Deep State Global Dystopia or a Paradise on Earth? Everything the ĒLites do is one organized satanic, sadistic, machiavellian psyops to demoralize and render the global population into a permanent PTSD, learned helpless condition. It is not being Judeo-Christian, that is the problem - it is organized crime—the global religious-military-banker-corporate mafia that is the problem. Why do we keep on projecting our hatred on systems of past tyranny...Socialist/Communist/Republican/Labor/Libertarian? It is the same monster with different heads. Chop the head off the kraken—and the people can live in peace and abundance.

We have 7+ Billion cocreators on the planet, and we can create what we love, if we turn away from the existing dis-eased decivilization. We create a heavenly realm through this realm by focusing on the things we love. We must focus on the solutions, not the problems. Remember or imagine the green full trees, the deep blue sky, the buzzing of the bees and be grateful that we will see that again. The garden planet will manifest as soon as we all intend it and each do our part. We are the most majestic, powerful beings in the Universe, and we have Lifeforce on our side. We can change this whole world to the awe-filled mysterious, scintillating transcendental dream we know in our hearts is true.

""Recognize everything around you as Nirvana; hear all sounds as mantra; see all beings as Buddhas." So John Blofeld was instructed by his Tantrist lama. [That same central teaching is honored in the Hermetic tradition as...] "As above, so below." Find the sacred within the profane, the profane within the sacred; for the two are organically related, hierarchically ordered. Or so they are experienced and taught to be by the visionary Few, whose role is to keep open the bridges of experience that run between the two realms."" 156, The Unfinished Animal, Theodore Roszak

Ice Age Farmer, Adapt 2030 and the Oppenheimer Ranch Project YouTube on the upcoming Grand Solar Minimum, which we are now in. See Youtube: "(MIAC #130) Step by Step What to Expect as the Eddy Grand Solar Minimum Intensifies." Adapt 2030, Oct 29, 2018.

Also on YouTube Robert Felix, "Not by Fire But by Ice."

"Standing up against radical evil even in the face of overwhelming odds gives us meaning, dignity and integrity." Christ Hedges on the scourge of global corporate fascism.

THE ROOTS OF ANCIENT WISDOM

"By the mid to late 2010s, hardly any region on Earth was free of the newly ionized and metalized atmosphere, or by virtue of particle fallout, the ionization of the electromagnetic grid system of the planet." ~ The Silent Invasion of Our Planet Earth, E.M. Nicolay.

The Death Machine has its roots in authentic geomantic and cosmic science, stemming from the Atlantean era and the non-sapiens Master Race. Knowledge of the Sacred Science was passed down to Homo sapiens and was expressed in the worldwide megalithic age, the Persian, Egyptian and Andian civilizations, and on through the classical era to the modern age. Various rulers and secret societies kept the science alive from the Druids to the Templars and the Freemasons.

The ancient megalithic structures were temples used for astronomy and divining—with high quartz rock directing earth telluric currents up to be used to amplify the human biofield and consciousness. Humans were more sensitive in those days and the earth had more energy. In former times the sun, moon and planets (the Gods) were closer to the earthcand so they played on the imagination giving birth to astrotheology or "religion," from the fortunetelling astrologer priests that studied the heavens and could predict events like eclipses and comets.

Such events and myths associated with the heavily bodies were used politically and economically to manipulate the ignorant populous. Governments and religions were established, and thus militaries were concocted to protect the sky-priests, the nobles, kings and the government officials both from competing tribes and the citizens they feed off. Now however the lust for power and total dominance has perverted the sacred science of planetary stewardship, geomancy, telluric and magnetic fields, space weather and climate into a systematic war against the earth and all its living things.

Geoengineering in the hands of the discombobulated and profane, power mad Borg will be the death of us all. Thus we must consider that this is the intended goal of the UN-NWO globalists, as is suggested by the tenets of the Georgia Guidestones. The Illuminati/Freemasonic Georgia Guidestones that calls for the world population to be no more than 500 million people, was translated into various languages by the United Nations (Rothschild Syndicate). The Guidestones are signed by an "R.C. Christian," which is the pseudonym for the founder of modern Rosicrucian mysticism, Christian Rosenkreuz (1378--1484). The predator class need to be eliminated or there is no hope to stabilize society or the environment, and the planet will always be careening out of control.

Sacred Science: The King of Pharaonic Theocracy, R. A. Schwaller de Lubicz

The Spiritual Technology of Ancient Egypt, Edward F. Malkowski

Astrology in Ancient Mesopotamia: The Science of Omens and the Knowledge of the Heavens, **Michael Baigent**

Earthmind, Communicating with the Living World of Gaia, Paul Devereux

Tutankhamun Prophecies, The Sacred Secret of the Maya, Egyptians and Freemansons, Maurice Cotterell

THE MURDER/SUICIDE OF HUMANITY

Chemtrailing or injecting reflective particles into the stratosphere is one of the methods for albedo modification or solar geoengineering, raises a whole host of serious socio-political and ethical issues.

Over and over again, profit trumps life. A Nazi gas chamber raining down on us on a daily basis. From a manical fascist point of view it is economically sensible to try and kill off the elderly, the sick and the poor so they are not a burden on the welfare system. It is a fine trick to play on people who have been paying medicare and Social Security all their lives and have little savings. Raising the pension payout age to 68 years shows exactly what these so called leaders are about. FEMA prison work camps are the ultimate contingency plan in the power game of preventing upward mobility. " Israel/America is heading for a full on fascist regime unless something shifts within the zeitgeist. Remember they have been murdering the microbiologists, and the anti-cancer GcMAF doctors over the last decade trying to eliminate resistance to their harvest.

We must consider that the Lyme, Mycoplasma, Morgellons and Chemtrail Flu coinfections are possibly high-tech bugs they have been dropping on us for decades, and ramped up since Jan 2015 **Indigo Skyfold**. We are under attack by effective soft-kill bio-warfare. A disturbing consequence of "sickness descending on us from the sky" is that it drives more people toward vaccination which ironically further compromises their immunity, weakens their health and burdens the body with heavy metals. Then they go get fluoridated antibiotics that destroy their intestinal microbiome and make them more vulnerable to the next chemtrail attack. We are victims of a silent war of fingerprintless weapons, but we can clearly see the enemy by pointing to lines in the sky.

The people throughout Tornado Alley in the USA are in danger from breathing in bacteria, fungi and viruses drawn up into the air by the vortex. Three men got pulled up into a tornado in Oklahoma. They survived the tornado, but almost immediately came down with Morgellons, flesh-eating bacteria, and various viruses. Like giant vacuum cleaners, tornadoes would also concentrate the heinous chemtrail pathogens, along with all the pathogens drawn up into a tornado from the soil and earth surface. After the Joplin, Missouri, tornado on 22 May 2011 there were several individuals coming down with "flesh eating fungus" caused by the fungus *Apophysomyces trapeziformis*, which is commonly found in soils, decaying vegetation, and water containing organic matter. Those with acid blood, hypoxia and diabetes are more susceptible to catching diseases by tornadoes.

William Thomas is an investigative journalist who wrote the book "*Scorched Earth*," where he examined the "exotic weapons system" and uncovered a direct link between biological warfare experimentation and the aerial spraying of pathogenic material in chemicals (chemtrails) over our cities throughout Canada, the United States, England, Australia, Holland, Italy, Germany, and New Zealand. He and others attribute the main cause of the rise in autoimmune diseases we have seen in the wake of the chemtrail spraying - such as chronic fatigue, multiple sclerosis, lupus, transverse myelitis and meningitis to the new genetically-engineered pathogens - particularly mycoplasma and other fungi which are sprayed on the general population via the chemtrail aerial spraying program. He also finds that there is mental-emotional component to this spray that disorients and makes people lethargic and mentally confused, with short-term memory loss and the inability to concentrate.

312

It would only take one generation to break the pattern of the master-slave game. Tell the kids the big lie of resource wars. Wean them off of slave education through entrepreneur-creator education, and stop feeding them junk food and GMOs. Everything about Borg culture is so corrupt now, that collapse is inevitable. Research, education and establishment of Civilization Next should be the driving force of human existence. *The global cull is forcing us to resuscitate our shaman, warrior, sage, seer and saint.*

The planet murder/suicide front need to grow up and join the progressive edge. Men need to redefine their role on the planet and work passionately towards creating Civilization Next. The husband-provider role no longer works for many, so what then? If you are a soldier or even a scientist then you are probably working for the devil and supporting the corrupt corpromilitary regime. We have no choice but to recreate our lives beyond what this corrupt culture can offer us. Whatever it is we WANT we must CREATE. If good people become cocreative we can manifest a GOOD world. The cure for the tyranny of evil empire is self-determinancy!

IT'S A MAD MADE WORLD

Willful ignorance is perhaps the most obvious sign of a loss of soul or humanity.

Everywhere people are either unconscious in the Borg, active participants of the Borg, or they are rejects and refugees or recluses from the Borg. Other than assimilation you can also be a spiritual sovereign standing up for and reinforcing the free, whole and higher HUman. Take your pick which one you want to be. Those in the Borg call those outside of it mad or underprivileged. Current civilization is mad, and the organizational structures of culture are becoming hostile to the people they are supposed to serve. It is only a matter of time before the madness spins out of control—as anti life technology breaks down the physical matrix necessary for higher-complex consciousness and HUman life.

We must be able to fortify and make resilient the wholism of our own humanity, move to locations that preserve the organism, find community of mutual recognition, create a fertile environment for creativity and bring home our contribution to worthy collaborators. Human companionship is imperative, but impossible to find in the Flatland commercial world. We need to start composing social get-togethers as if they were paintings or symphonies. That is to create "conscious" relationships, where both, or all participants are actively engaged in bringing all they are to mutual communion.

The foundations of civilization is civility! Civility has its roots in *"first do no harm"* and in the Buddhist ethic of non-harming or non-violence (ahimsa) to all living creatures from the lowest insect to humans. This basic principle of not killing and the cherishing the life of living things is not widely expressed in Western culture. Love and appreciation for "all living things" requires that we first give up our fear and worry over our own existence. This extension of the self-sense into the larger world beyond self-concern emerges through a felt-appreciation and gratitude for one's own existence and the miracle of life in the universe—hence is deeply related to our concepts of God. However, our knowledge of God is deeply warped by our retarded level of spiritual development within an exploitative civilization where everything including God is bought and sold. Civility or attunement to the mystery via cosmic consciousness is pretty much the opposite of the operating mode we are presently in as a species. Thus the need to atone and attune to rise beyond the psychotic, defeatist regime we are presently a party to.

The headless chicken society differs responsibility up and endless command chain of obsolescence. The way this dys-integrated society is structured people tend to look to preserving their little job, without interface with other sectors like blind men and an elephant. A systems approach to civilization has yet to be established, where each "level" is accountable for the integrity of their commitment to truth, beneficent reality and the sanctity of all Life. Cosmic connection is a firsthand job, you cannot borrow a secondhand God. All religion is dead, along with pretty much every other institution. The people must grow up and rise up in sanity, sovereignty and simply refuse to go along with the false power paradigm. Otherwise it is an endless road to ever increasing fascist hell.

Arrogance is the noise of human insolence born of insecurity. The arrogance of false power, protectionism and competition has resulted in a "broken culture." In a "broken, exploitative society" survival pressures make people meaner and madder by the day. Genuine HUman pleasures become scarce, and pleasures for consolation and compensation become the norm. Spiritual practice is not good enough anymore, it must be spiritual practice IN Nature — in order to counteract the myriad toxicities of the crazy dis-eased technosociety.

The body, mind and soul must be whole in order to perceive reality whole, and to Grok the wholism of the universe. Thus cosmic consciousness requires an intact HUman. The degeneration is occurring not because of any grand galactic karmic clock and the Kali Yuga, but because an unconscious species is making itself more unconscious and delinquent through its anti-life cultural habits

Only then can we stop distracting ourselves with icons, talismans, myths, potions and spells and get REAL according to cosmic design. Only then can we master karma (cause and effect). We can only see and experience ourselves and the world through our own personal and collective level of development. Both the visionary and creative levels of consciousness have been sorely ignored and misappropriated in our material-money focused industrial culture. And now with our bodies, minds and environment breaking down we are essentially stuck as a species in this truncated and aborted level of spiritual development. Unless of course we make an applied effort to live true to the sovereign cosmic being held captive within us and redeem the whole sovereign HUman within. Visionary capacity IS the growing edge most needed at this stage in our human evolution.

The five-sensory attenuated consciousness of the material Flatland conditioned human has conveniently fragmented reality into the physical, psychological and spiritual aspects, wherein the mysticism and visionary capacity are somehow "separated" from creation and our practical lives in human society. This schism lies at the heart of the Borg's blind destruction of the planet, and the Illuminati's program to eliminate the majority of the global population. If the destroyers actually awakened to a "scientific-mystical" view of life in the universe, the origin of the world, the role of man in it, and the nature of good and evil they would be healed of their madness and their homicidal passion for destruction. We ride on the back of billions of years of the evolution of life in the universe.

314

Anyone who really groks this cannot be engaged in a scorched earth campaign…thus what is needed is the greatest of all epiphanies — to really take in the miracle of Life. By misunderstanding what Life is and what it needs we sell out and settle for the lower end of consciousness, and thus we miss out on the opportunity for cultivating higher faculties of creative consciousness including analysis, strategy, focus, concentration, gnosis, imagination, precommitment, intent, visioneering, leadership, social inspiration, love and cooperation etc… False power, codependency and Thanatos arise when the Hindbrain defaults into fear mode, cutting off access to the self-reliance and empowerment of the prefrontal sovereign decision maker.

Sovereign choice means that we are drawn forth by our desires rather than pushed around by our fears. By imagining our desired destination and destiny we can then gather the inner and outer resources to bring about the success of our ventures and ultimate future. Because visionary imagination kicks in the executive parts of the brain that allow for initiative and innovation, our success can only come about through following our desires and not our fears.

When children are socialized into self-diminishment, self-hatred and blind obedience at the expense of initiative and self-compassion, as adults they become addicted to the stress of self-abuse and being socially terrorized. Social toxicity such as invalidation, shaming, intimidation, demeaning criticism, negative competition and manipulation etc... reduce prefrontal activation, thereby breaking down self-initiative and autonomy,. With sovereignty thus diminished this leaves the victim under the control of dominators, subversives and perpetrators. Negative attention is better than no attention at all to those who have been socialized into self-hatred and disempowerment by negative bonding.

Humans are such predatory animals that if you fear negative attention, you for sure are going to attract it, and probably go out of your way to generate negative attention from others and then cry victim. It was this kind of understanding I was approaching in trying to work out why a silent eugenics war is being waged against the people around the globe. How did we call this on ourselves? Was it self-hatred, ignore-ance, lack of individual and action, or inability to organize? No, it is because the people left governance to the most corrupt sector of society. Is the chemtrail holocaust occurring simply because the wicked few have the power and the technology to do so, and through default are we the people are funding our own demise?

It is a form of mental and spiritual immaturity to simply go along with the fear tactics that the corporate world uses to manipulate gullible populations. Hoodwinked suckers are addicted to self-harming GMOs, processed foods, pharmaceuticals and vaccines etc... Pretty much everything in Borg civilization is harmful to our well-being and to the planet, because the presets to the perception of reality are wrong and consequently precipitate death rather than life. We must lift the moratorium on the truth — thus allowing the growth of cogno-spiritual development beyond the current consciousness operating system of false power, pathological dominance hierarchy and entrenched authority. Truth is the ultimate elixir — the path to love, radical openness and unbroken connection.

In the wild an animal's nervous system quickly returns to normal after being attacked as they follow nature by running, shaking and self-soothing etc... Animals do not take the struggle, suffering and trauma of jungle politics personally. Whereas we humans, ruminate, remember and wallow in the stress of being held in captivity or a prey animal. The human enculturated into and trapped in an exploitative culture is essentially a prey animal held in perpetual captivity. To rise above the victim mentality of slavitude we must throw off the stress and trauma of hostility, competition and captivity, and recover our sovereignty and work towards an advanced, free humanity. We must not despair that all we seem to find is pieces to the puzzle. We must be good little detectives and document and collate all evidence. Every citizen must become a citizen journalist hot after truth and justice. As sovereigns we have to act response-ably to create the kind of world we WANT to live in.

HEALING BORG PSYCHOSIS

The End of Power Addiction and the Beginning of Civilization Next

We are caught up in a predatory regime of global conquest that originates from the command seat in the eye of the centuries old pyramid of power. We must investigate and rectify our cultural sickness in order to heal it. But we must not get caught up in that—we can notice it, and move on. Together we are making the clandestine known, and its machinations brought out in the light of day. Eventually such supreme evil will never again ensconce itself like a cancer over the face of the globe, and we will be free from the tyranny of out of control power, once and for all time.

The **piratearchy** (malpatriarchy) is not really a man's world. It is the Dark Masculine for it serves neither man nor woman, and is at war with "the people" and the planet. The corporate military economy is the product of a forestalled developmental stage gone horribly bad. This attenuated evolution has led to runaway Hindbrain dominance, void of whole brain and higher brain function. Humans came into this sorry state through fear and greed. Masters and slaves to material gain, at the expense of the security of divine connection.

For our folly, we are now condemned to impoverished lives, slaving after material objects and moving them around constantly from one place to another, as if this frenetic busywork could constitute meaning and purpose. But there is still time to awaken, redeem ourselves as a species, to make amends and regenerate the planet. The connection between ecocide, inflammation and trauma is that the PTSD brain inflammation consequence of Hindbrain false power is a self-fulfilling prophesy of cognitive regression that keeps humanity back in a state of woeful spiritual retardation. We are simply not actualizing the creature that we were born to be.

Basically the entire culture is sadomasochistic because it is operating from the Hindbrain hijacking of the prefrontal lobes—making for an immoral, unempathetic and robotic form of human. The culture itself reinforces this pattern of dominance and submission (Master/Slave) and so it is almost impossible to break out of the socio-psychopathic mindscape that is plainly insane and largely evil. The end result of "we the people" not standing up to pathological authority, is that pathological socialism, the mean green meme and covert fascism combined with dark militarism and global deep state eugenics create the breakdown of social uplift and sustainability within the 1st world countries.

If we have a master/slave relationship with ourselves our own self-abusing critic can prevent the higher cognitive faculties by which we can move forward. The sadomasochistic master/slave dynamic is a codependent bond that prevents both parties from exercising their higher HUman consciousness. Such a bond is made in fear. The collapse of consciousness into fear and contraction means our higher HUman faculties cannot be accessed. So when you have a civilization based on fear and false power the internal mechanisms of suspended growth and development lead to the corruption and breakdown of civilization…because the culture itself was diseased.

The drive for power dominance should not be called the "patriarchy" for that term assumes care of governance, whereas Hindbrain man is a predator/parasite that consumes and destroys everything he/she touches. The dominance/submission dance is merely a symptom of the retardation of evolution at the brute animal level. However with humans the power-hierarchy is sub-animal, because Homo sapiens is insane, whereas most other animals (other than domestic animals), are not insane, nor inherently sadistic or stupid. We domesticated or "farmed" humans have all but lost the inherent gifts of health, cosmic resonance, lucid observation and super-consciousness that is our species birthright.

To disengage from the trauma of the primate power paradigm, the Emancipator, The Inner Arts and Fasting are the fastest route to re-engaging with the sovereign self from the master/slave, push-pull confusion of Borg psychosis. Immersion teaching permaculture and restorative land management skills to children is a good place to start. We need to also establish a **Punitive Polluter Pays Policy** across the board in civilization and industry, and that includes the diabolical chemtrailers who are without a doubt killing the planet by day and night. Any government, army, company, community or individual that willfully poisons the air, land, ocean or biosphere is liable to pay full damages and restoration costs—without exception.

The Hindbrain "power problems" of war, usury, debt slavery, populations exceeding earth's carrying capacity, anti-life technology, chemical Ag and Med, predatory capitalism, inequality and indoctrination into The Borg— "aka machine mind," have already been solved. Thrival is a matter of "implementing" higher HUman consciousness across the board in human existence and evolving beyond the institutionalization of Borg psychosis. It is hard to find the narrow path between the wishful thinking of childish Pollyannaism, and the morbid depression of facing the train wreck of a failed civilization, and the cruelty of the underlying law of the jungle…"kill or be killed." First we must give up the predatory-parasitic attitude toward our Self and stop toxifying ourselves into unconscious oblivion.

The Hell of human existence is not going away anytime soon, but we can learn to make the best of things. To not fear the darkness, nor embrace it, but to rise above it. We are only undone by our own anger, indignation and inability to rise in the face of in-just-as. You cannot deBorg when remaining in rebellion, resistance or resonance with the Borg! Thus deBorging requires raising cell voltage, detoxification, increasing VO2, remineralizing, reNaturing, full-spectrum exercise/movement and socializing with sovereigns. The decline in metabolic energy due to decline of Omega 3 with respect to Omega 6 is one of the principle reasons the species is mentally and physically messed up.

To restore the Ethical Relationship Between Humans and the Planet we must eliminate predatory capitalism, central banks, the Federal Reserve, war profiteering, religious financial extortion (tax churches), state drug cartels using military, proxy wars, false flags, sacrificial fake mass shootings, blood sports, wild-life safaris, trophy killing, Secret Societies, outlaw geo-engineering and geo-warfare, stop oil wars, support new energy invention, eliminate the deep state and install transparency in all government agencies.

There are already multiple energy alternatives but the oil cartel men in black keep them suppressed, and the financial support is not forthcoming to support the New Energy development. The world would be a better place tomorrow, if the money would simply flow to the light side instead of the dark side. That is towards life technology, rather than death technology.

Furthermore we must reinstate common law, natural law, the Natural Step, the right of the commons, the wild commons (as wild-food heritage), permaculture land management, Schauberger water-care principles and the Native American perspective on land "ownership" as much as is possible, in moving towards a new ethic of human relationship with planet earth. The future is not explosionist, but implosionist. "Implosionist" means they use mathematics and philosophy of the feminine force of centripetal vortical action towards Zeropoint.

DeBorging is an inside job! More and more people around the world are now standing in their own power and becoming free.

THE DIVINE MASCULINE

Restoring the Divine Masculine is important at this time of confusion to set the balance of power upright on a universal moral standing. The integrated male, balanced in the hemispheres, connecting head-heart-genitals, decorporatized, disengaged from hierarchy, knows their own mind, not phased by social intimidation, able to have an open heart and mind in a sick world by standing in their own light, resistant to coercion and deceit via a meta-ethical position. To be a teacher/influencer of the divine masculine someone can either be a teacher of the subject itself, or an example of divine masculine traits or embodiment. The great women of history whom we respect are also examples of the divine masculine at play.

To study the qualities of "kingship" and the evolved (Third Tier) masculine:

David Odorisio, Joseph Campbell, David Wagner, Robert Moore, Neil Kramer, Douglas Gillette, Waller Newell, Harvey Mansfield, Jason Christoff, Paul Levy, Warren Farrell, Stefan Molyneux, Jordan Peterson, Jordan Greenhall, Mark Binet, Daniel Schmachtenberger, David Deida, Bernhard Guenther, Marco Missinato, Charles Eisenstein, Mads Palsvig, Michael Tsarion, Derrick Jensen, Garwin Redman, Max Igan.

Plus rights of passage with Aundrieux Sankofa. Books like Iron John, by Robert Bly and King, Warrior, Magician Lover: Rediscovering the Archetypes of the Mature Masculine, by Robert Moore and Douglas Gillette encouraged men to find meaningful male rites of passage. Scientists like Tesla, Walter Russell, Rudolf Steiner, Buckminster Fuller and Viktor Schauberger also exemplify the divine masculine through channeling great genius and the supreme effort it too them to convey their message.

13

OVERCOMING OMNICIDE

SURVIVING THE GLOBAL EUGENICS AGENDA

Overcoming "extermination anxiety" through a self-care routine, exercise and spiritual practices is vital to establish a Warrior's attitude in order to boost the immune system and promote detoxification and regeneration. Exercise increases brain size and function, while chronic stress and high levels of cortisol create long-lasting brain changes, reducing brain size and function. Chronic stress has a shrinking effect on the prefrontal cortex, the area of the brain responsible for memory and learning.

We are experiencing a genocide and so our psychological state can be compared to the Jews in Europe during the holocaust. However, we have not been carted off to the gas chambers...the gas chambers have been bought to us. Unless we address this mental-emotional challenge, we will not have the "strength" to be able to meta-adapt to the situation, in order to maintain our health and work to stop the ecological devastation. We are in Ecoshock from experiencing man-made collapse of the environment, human culture and exclusion from the sense of a "future."

Due to the chemtrail assault on our daily lives, Ecoshock is now the most common form of PTSD in NATO countries, thus we must deeply study the condition, and identify and learn practices and protocols that help us deal with both the biochemical onslaught AND the psychological trauma of the 6th great extinction. If we fail to get real with the consequences of what is occurring, we will not have the focus to formulate a plan nor the strength to carry it out. If you have no forward-thinking plan, then you have no predictable results. Discipline is strength.

Observe and document the planet-murderers ways, and teach others. The more they try and kill us off, the more we make ourselves stronger. It is as though we need an evil, malicious and mindless force that seeks to destroy us and dismiss our "value" in order to overcome our own self-destruction and self-negation, and thus rise up to a higher order of inherent wholeness and realization. Each "strong" person that learns how to thrive in the chemtrail holocaust...is one more citizen who is fit enough to build Civilization Next.

The absence of apology for wrongdoing is a blight on the soul of the universe. The more we flagrantly allow social crime, the more social crime occurs. It is up to the victim to be "Victim No More" and stand up for their rights as a HUman Being. Eventually when the human race reaches critical mass of becoming self-empowered, those who wish to manipulate and control us will be left behind, as they will have no-one else to control. Then and only then will the people of the world become free. The responsibility starts with each and every one of us.

FIXES FOR EXTERMINATION ANXIETY

Modern humans are already not present and in a dissociated state, and by necessity we have to be selective in ignoring the colossal wrongs, errors and evil of our contemporary civilization in order to get through our day. Thus we might call ourselves *"cultural schizophrenics."* Schizophrenic, in that we must compartmentalize our psyche, and become emotionally ingenuous in order to survive in the Hindbrain world. We cannot speak our truth, nor can we allow ourselves to fully grasp the prospect of a terrifying future born of compounded life-harming technologies that we are inflicting on ourselves and the planet.

We were on the verge of a global spiritual awakening into an enlightened civilization. However, the accruing consciousness destroying aspects of the exploitative consumer culture are holding us back. If we can get rid of the chemtrailing and the other eugenics/genocidal programs we still might make it…and make it we must for HUmanization itself is at stake. Hindbrain man is breaking spaceship earth for petty power and profit. A perfect storm is brewing, of abject piracy and greed meeting criminal lawlessness and homicidal mania. There has been no higher jinx greater than the premeditated ecocide now underway. A crime surpassing any yet conceived of by man. Chemtrailing breaks the thermodynamic laws of life in the universe, and for what?

When we destroy the immune system of the planet, we destroy our capacity to be human, and our higher human capacities are the only thing that will save us from ourselves. As we lose our minds to the chemical onslaught we are in danger of falling into a sleep so deep, we may never wake up. The enormity and unprecedented nature of this man-made disaster will require massive and comprehensive approaches to remediation, survival and thrival.

The chemtrail survival protocol is my attempt at a comprehensive survival/thrival strategy, however it is only a beginning, we need to build a complete protocol together through research and experimentation. People the world over have to get together to strategize, organize, and act. The Thrive Movement has a template for stopping chemtrailing over a certain area, but we need to bring to a close the entire evil charade and give it so much focus that the pilots will refuse to cooperate no matter how much money you throw at them.

Moral self-orientation is equivalent to the degree that we feel certain of our perception, course, direction and action in the world. Therefore the moral self is the seat of sovereignty.

INTEGRAL HEALING

Educators, policymakers and scientists have referred to ADHD (attention-deficit/hyperactivity disorder) as a national crisis and have spent billions of dollars looking into its cause. Researchers are proposing, many kids today simply aren't getting the sleep they need, leading to challenging behaviors that mimic ADHD? Could some ADHD be a type of sleep disorder? No, the sleep disorder is a symptom of ADHD which is caused by demineralization, Nature disconnection, neurosclerosis, and the chemo-industrial culture, Nature deprivation and disconnection from the earth and Unity Consciousness. Without houses, electronic devises, shoes and chemical agriculture there would be no ADHD. Earth EMF health and circadian integrity are necessary for full health, and full mental and spiritual HUman powers.

Ecoshock, Trauma, PTSD and Borg recovery gyms require a full spectrum assault (approach) on our physical, mental, emotional and spiritual shutdown and "damage." Some of the components include: rectifying mineral imbalance, Kelp and Epsom salt baths, Mud baths and Clay body packs, Thalassotherapy: therapeutic use of seawater, mud, algae, and seaweed; Spinal Shower, Grounding, Light therapy and Sungazing, Meditation, Yoga, Toning, Holotropic breathing, Infrared sauna, Steaming, improving Neurotransmitters-hormones-enzymes, Heavy metal detoxification, Hydrotherapy, GI-Liver-Brain detox, various types of Exercise including coordination-aerobic-strength-binaural-balance-martial arts-dance-circus, bodywork, Diet-juicing-sprouting-superfoods-Wheatgrass-Methylation foods, Social reconstitution with family constellation, Eye gazing, Mythological reframing, Zeitgeist-Big picture perspective, Getting on track with soul-vocation, Animal relationship building, Nature connection, reframing the Homo sapiens story, Ancestral reconnection, Cosmic reconnection, Soul recovery, Dream yoga, Sovereignty training, Entheogens and Shamanic journeys, Inner Arts Visionary immersion and Art-Crafts-Poetry-Music.

EMBRACING FEAR

A fear based society generates avarice and professional protectionism, which prevents the spiritual largess needed for systems thinking and systems vocational action. Coping with fear requires that we understand fear. Fear is an internal vibration of faint-heartedness brought about by the sense of a lack of coping, and yet it is fear which undermines our capacity to cope. Thus if you "own" your fear rather than "project" it onto entities, others or the world, then you can learn to drop the disturbing vibration of fear. Since we live in a fear driven civilization rising above the fear frequencies requires systematic attention and daily practice, but it can be done if all the bases are covered.

1. METABOLIC FEAR: Fear will not shift and leave us unless our body is detoxified, our diet raw, our soil remineralized, and the acids/plaques/poisons in our system removed. Replace all that is false, with that which is regenerated through nature.

2. FIGHT/FLIGHT FEAR: Sympathetic Hypertonicity can only be dropped by doing with the fear response what nature intended, that is to run off, exercise, breathe, punch, kick, jump, push, dance, scream and laugh off the electrical charge of fear.

3. STASIS FEAR: Paralysis, confusion, stagnation, helplessness, lostness, loneliness and desperation are symptoms of entrenched self worth fear. Thus any "movement" - physical, mental, emotional, spiritual will help to break the spell of retreat or cocooning, but you have to challenge yourself to shift.

4. UNCREATE FEAR: Fear tends to make us into reactive robots so to conquer fear we need to encourage creativity in all aspects of our lives. Most importantly we have to get creative in our mindfulness (shamanism). In dealing effectively with power vultures we have to stop being reactive, and start being creative.

5. EXISTENTIAL FEAR: Philosophy, mysticism, art and poetry are balm for the big picture fears of living in uncertain transition times. The more we move away from participation in the collapsing Borg culture and on to that of the Holy/Whole Man, the less fear and foreboding we will embody. It is then we become an example of courage and self-reliance that others can find solace in and emulate.

321

DESTRESSING PRACTICES

Chanting Thoh or Huuu! Long Huffing Outbreathing, Grounding, sungazing, yoga, meditation, dance, conscious breathing, colon cleansing, healing leaky gut, rebounding, belly massage, hanging, grounding, Inner Arts, drumming, anything with clay, infrared sauna, alternating sauna and cold shower, Liposomal Vitamin C therapy, sonic therapies, nature walks, hanging out near running water or oceans and water fasting. If you want to calm down then de-stressing practices are more meta-adaptive than smoking MJ or drinking alcohol. Alcohol is proven to cause cancer, cause brain damage, shorten lifespan, cause depression and provide negative role modelling for children. CBD oil on the neck and wrists is better than smoking if you do need an antianxiety shift, as any smoking is bad for the lungs. For existential depression and extermination anxiety you can also use kratom for a few months, NAC, wild lettuce, raw diet and lots of greens.

Mimosahuasca could provide a psychological shift to break out of fixation on limitation and the negative. Mimosahuasca is made from the root bark from Mimosa hostilis mixed with the seeds of Syrian Rue (Perganum harmala) as a source of MAO-inhibiting harmala alkaloids.

More on Ecoshock and PTSD recovery in Book 2: *"Awakening in the Chemtrail Holocaust, Liberation from Within"*

HEAL AND MIND AND RECOVER THE SOUL

The size of the chemtrail problem is so overwhelming we may be prone to thoughts like "It's hopeless. It's all over. Might as well give up and die now." There is a danger of being so focused on the games the dark side are playing that we forgo our creativity and higher culture building work. We must illuminate the dark by creating a bonfire of light, and avoid getting sucked into the abyss ourselves. A raw diet, plenty of exercise, sunshine, grounding and right livelihood will ensure that we avoid succumbing to suicidal defeatism and slip into hopelessness and defeat. Our vocational "calling" determines our journey, our livelihood and our destination. Consider the situation and condition the world is in and what is most needed, and how can you uniquely fulfill that need?

The fundamental cause of delinquency, distress and disease is separation anxiety. The domesticated human within a master/slave civilization is fundamentally violent towards themselves, others and existence. This is the result of the lack of *connection/communication/communion* due to the atomic dissonance or electromagnetic disconnection, resulting from thousands of years of anti-life human processes, practices, and sensibilities. Our bodies are composed of structure and functioning that is "out of sorts" with the unified field, out of sync with "God" and in constant distress and dis-ease...that is in perpetual separation anxiety. The Warrior Spirit is the indigenous sense of cosmic connection which provides the courage to do the right thing when facing any challenge. It may call us to put ourselves in harm's way for the greater good, and challenge us to live our truth, and to utilize our innate talents to pursue our passions. We employ the Warrior Spirit by first exploring our value system, and it is from our value system that we develop vision and intention, from which we can move forward into the challenge life presents to us with a clear purpose and good will.

REMINERALIZATION

A principal factor in this cosmic electrical disconnection is the demineralization of the soils, the earth and our bodies. The physical structure of humans is breaking down after 12,000 of agriculture and especially due to the loss of minerals in the food supply over the last 50 years. We have a lot of remineralization work to do to get up to baseline optimum mineral density and to protect ourselves from the onslaught of pollution, chemicals, EMFs and radiation. Silicon and magnesium are two of the main minerals we are deficient in. But we are also deficient in the trace minerals iodine, chromium, selenium, zinc, copper and others.

Every second of every day your body relies on ionic minerals and trace minerals to conduct and generate billions of tiny electrical impulses that drive our metabolism. Without these impulses, not a single muscle, including our heart, would be able to function. Our nerves would not fire, your brain would not work and the cells would not be able to use osmosis to balance our water pressure and absorb nutrients. To ensure you are getting the ionic minerals and electrolytes your body needs, only choose ionic mineral supplements or supplements that contain ionic minerals.

Many of the trace elements once abundant in soil have been washed into the oceans. In the oceans, they are found in the same basic proportions that are found in healthy human bodies. Fossil salt from ancient oceans in the Triassic period are the freest of impurities, that is crystallized salt deposits created such as America's Great Salt Lake, Dead Sea Minerals, La Fortuna Salina salt and Himalayan salt minerals. Black Himalayan salt, known as Kala Namak, is a special type of volcanic rock salt with a distinctive sulfurous mineral taste like hard boiled egg yolks. This sulfur and iron rich salt is a natural disinfectant, improves digestion, relieves constipation, bloating and strengthens and increases the natural hair growth. Black salt in particular will help remineralize, ease joint inflammation and ward off the chemflu and other weaponized bugs with its high sulfur content.

Mineral deficiency is behind both carbohydrate craving, blood sugar problems, diabetes and candida so take many different forms of full spectrum mineral supplements; preferably in natural form like kelp, blue-green algae, and remineralized green plants. This will ensure plentiful building materials for strong collagen. Silicon is the keystone - the architectural element to our carbon (collagen) based structure. Silicon deficiency is one of the main reasons we are losing our water holding capacity and collagen strength as we age. The stronger our collagen the more resistant the body is against microbe attack and proliferation. Hence remineralization of our bodies and our soil is essential to surviving the chemtrail holocaust.

When we eat super-ALIVE food that is grown on permaculturally remineralized soil we become more conscious and consequently we are thus more aware of the blockages to spirit or life-force within our bodies. This increase of awareness of our pain and degradation can lead to compulsive drive to reduce consciousness through eating stodgy, fatty cooked food. Thus after taking wheatgrass or eating a salad we must guard against the internal saboteur which desires for us to go back to sleep. This saboteur is as strong as our body is diseased and devitalized. Therefore, if we find ourselves constantly working against our efforts to regenerate, then we should step up our raw remineralization program and increase our spiritual/integral therapy practice.

Don't forget greensand for remineralizing your sprout and food growing soil.

FASTING FOR CHANGE

Fasting Has Been Used For Thousands Of Years For:

Disease cure and prevention — Restore human health and ward off diseases

Peak States and Flow — Prepare for fishing and hunting expeditions

Initiation — To mark a rite of passage and prepare young people for adulthood

Fitness — Increase physical strength and stamina

Ascension — Induce holotropic states directed towards wholeness

Communion — Receive guidance, wisdom, and direction from the creatrix.

Unified Consciousness — Eliminate that which blocks the Light!

Being stuck sucks, however we cannot get unstuck when we are still in the emotional funk of being stuck. The deep sadness, pain and separative contraction of those in a terminal civilization paralyzes us into inaction. Changing our habits, location, living space, entertainments, challenges and our mental-emotional-physical state is essential to experiencing ourselves and the world anew. In order to move into the abundance socio-economy we have to let go of our negative coping mechanisms and slave-mentality that keeps us addicted to the current exploitative paradigm.

That means a life overhaul routine that includes juice fasting, water fasting, detoxification routine, daily morning exercise, nootropics, super nutrition, changing over to healthy treats, self-developmental activities, daily spiritual practice, and then shamanistic journeys involving altered states and plant teachers, wardrobe overhaul, along with resetting long term and short term goals. Then through this renewal process we will figure out where we want to contribute toward the emancipation and actualization of our fellow humans.

There is a mental-emotional component to this toxic spraying that is a disorienting, destabilizing, and can make people lethargic and mentally confused, with an inability to concentrate, along with short-term memory loss. This makes focusing on the Chemtrail Syndrome Cure both more difficult and more important. Fasting is important for removing heavy metals stored throughout the body tissue.

FASTING TO BREAK THE CHAINS

Water Fasting for three days *"flips a regenerative switch"* which prompts stem cells to create brand new white blood cells, essentially regenerating the entire immune system. Combine your fasting with conscious breathing to increase immunity by 15X. Fasting for 72 hours also protected cancer patients against the toxic impact of chemotherapy. Fasting gives the 'OK' for stem cells to go ahead and begin proliferating and rebuild the entire system. Fasting cycles can generate, literally, a new immune system. When you abstain from food, the system tries to save energy, and one of the things it can do to save energy is to recycle a lot of the immune cells that are not needed, especially those that may be damaged. Prolonged fasting forces the body to use stores of glucose and fat but also breaks down a significant portion of white blood cells. Fasting for 72 hours also helps protect cancer patients against the toxic impacts of chemotherapy.

The carbohydrate addicted master/slave culture is hitting the wall - with escalating Metabolic X, insulin resistance, depression, dementia and insanity. Therefore the fail-safe way out of the mental sludge of the Borg control Matrix is a series water fasts for 3 or more days, so that the brain goes into fat burning or ketosis rather than glucose burning. As we burn up our fat stores we eliminate cell receptor resistance, insulin resistance and can undergo deep detoxification from heavy metals, pesticides, chemtrails, pharmaceuticals and all manner of consciousness impairing agents that cause so much "noise" in our system that we fail to enter into sympathetic resonance with our soul and cosmic consciousness.

When seriously attempting to detox from chemtrails we must enlist a religious zeal and moral determination normally attributed to fasting. We need the piety, sincerity and zeal of spiritual fasting in order to detox because we must stop our life harming addictions that only add to the harmful effects of EMF smog and ionizing radiation. The more heavy metals we have in our body, the more susceptible we are to damage from wireless EMF technology. These frequencies interfere the calcium channels of the cells allowing calcium to flood into the cells. Magnesium is a natural calcium blocker.

The eliminative organs cannot be further burdened by alcohol or cigarette damage while we are attempting to use them to detoxify deadly heavy metals etc… The body will not let go of its toxics nor eliminate pathogens if we engage in slow suicide by daily poisons: coffee, alcohol and whatever other acidifying, toxic, stimulants and immune destroying habits we may have. All other paths are a waste of dollars and time unless we can eliminate our internal inferior tissue, pathogens and toxic dross.

We each need to work on our own personal heavy metal detoxification and to teach our neighbors, so that we have the strength to do what it takes to stop the global chemocide. To become a beacon of light we must detoxify ourselves faster than "They" can poison us. You can take a bunch of chelators, absorbers, detoxers, immune enhances, raw diet etc... but to be really effective at removing toxins deep in our tissues we have to do interim fasting and/or longterm fasting in combination with our antichemtrail protocol lifestyle.

Does the brain have a select all and delete button too? Yes, it is behind your ears. You just flip that area up to your crown and it deletes everything, especially when done with long out-breaths.

The Fasting Path, Stephen Harrod Buhner
One Spirit Medicine, Alberto Villoldo
The Scientific Approach To Intermittent Fasting, Dr. Mike VanDerschelden

Élan Vital

Honorable therapy addresses the cause

Honorable ecology addresses the cause

Honorable spirituality addresses the cause

We must focus on the cause to live the solution!

WAKING UP TO THE ARCH PATTERNS

The dark Orks love to stack their weapons in a multi-ass-inEL attack.

We need to anticipate what will come by watching for the arch patterns: chemtrail spraying and holding back rain with high pressure systems, sending in the solar satellite or the orbital drone, lighting fires, then letting the weather go so the deluge washes away the evidence and further destroys property. Looks like community-wide focus on videotaping the firestorm attack is the way to go, to catch those lasers, which show up in the smoke. If there is no particles in the air the lasers do not show, but they are easier to see at night time.

The willful destruction of the Eugenics Regime goes into full swing during the summer with the powers that shouldn't be continuing to spray and zap Alaska/Oregon/Washington, while the West was covered with a heavy blanket of smoke from the socalled wildfires. During the "fires" Vancouver or Seattle air was the equivalent of smoking 7.4 cigarettes per day. Smoke which was laden with chemtrail fallout and radiation. Bob Nichols Veterans Today columnist points out that cities across America are receiving a million counts of radiation a week … dooming humanity to a relatively quick extinction.

Besides the incendiaries aluminum, barium and strontium, chemtrails also contain radioactive thorium. Since **thorium** and **depleted uranium** are thermally pyroclastic incendiary materials it would also increase the ferocity of wildfire…besides causing cancer, myriad diseases, mutation and act as a major ingredient in the scorched earth cocktail. Trees absorb these incendiaries and become ticking fire bombs.

USRAEL inc. has killed the north Pacific ocean with their Fukushima attack on Japan. As a consequence they are slow killing the U.S. citizens with radiation. I wonder if the masterminds in Israel planned this all along as a reprisal against American industrialists' profiting from the Jewish holocaust in WW2? It goes without saying that no individual, corporation or country should ever profit from genocide, omnicide and planetocide. The anomalous California fires are re-spreading Fukushima Radiation over the US like a deadly blanket.

Those at the top of the power pyramid are not leaders and superior human beings, but psychopaths who delight in willful destruction, genocide and the suffering of millions. The venality and greed of power addiction, like cocaine addiction rots the brain and hearts of the Powerhoes. THEY will lose control as the good guys out tech the bad guys, and the bad guys die from heart disease. Good will win out over evil. The Force of the continuity of life demands it.

If they are not cognizant of the global climate coup or the global population cull, such conferences on global climate action are worse than useless. The chemtrail program is undertaken by the Global Deep State, which is orchestrating the one world government, and I don't see them stopping anytime soon, all we citizens can do is to move beyond its present range—educate people on chemtrail survival protocols, heavy metal detox and radiation recovery etc… Point out to others the X-shaped chemtrails over the setting sun. The chemtrail pilots like to put X's over the sun at sunset, thus trying to put "The Eye in The Triangle" as a form of psychological warfare.

Authorities complicit in the UN genocide agenda are relying on this conditioned sleep, and spread their newspeak that it is an "urban myth" to those who point out the obvious chemtrails. **Newspeak** is the fictional language in the novel "1984," written by George Orwell. It is a controlled language created by the totalitarian state "Oceania," as a tool to limit freedom of thought, and concepts that pose a threat to the regime such as freedom, sovereignty, self-expression, individuality, and peace. Any form of thought that opposes the totalitarian party's reality construct is classified as "thought crime." Doublespeak is used to confuse and subdue descent among the sleeple.

Doublespeak is language that sadomasochistically obscures, disguises, distorts, or reverses the meaning of words. Doublespeak is the complete opposite of plain and simple truth, by distorting words and phrases in order to bury the truth and to make the awful truth sound more palatable. Doublespeak may take the form of euphemisms (e.g., "Downsizing" for layoffs, "Servicing the Target" for bombing, "Collateral damage" instead of multiple fatalities, "Pre-emptive strike" instead of unprovoked attack, and "Ethnic cleansing" instead of genocide.

In this fashion of "the emperor wears no clothes" the earth is being destroyed by those who refuse to admit the naked truth. *"The Emperor Wears No Clothes"* is often used in political and social contexts for any obvious truth denied by the majority despite the evidence of their eyes, especially when proclaimed by the government. When people say "The emperor wears no clothes," they point out the need for people to stop being ass kissers to political leaders and see things for what they truly are instead of denying the truth of the situation. It takes guts to speak the truth and blast through the bullshit and lies. You are not doing any favors to those who are easily assimilated by supporting them in their sleep, rather wake them up carefully, as we are living in a fascist global state.

Divide and conquer has been used as a political control strategy since land barons came into existence millennia ago. If we are made to focus on irrelevant divisive issues, we cannot get together to start focusing on the important issues, which would shift the balance back to the people where it belongs. As survival pressures build "divide and conquer" reaches fever pitch. As the mind breaks down under the weight of lies, there is usually a frenzy of symbolism, polarity and divisiveness before the catharsis of an evolutionary jump. Unbridled fascination with so-called modern technological advances has brought with it a swathe of deficits to the health and welfare of the natural environment, man, animals and all life; threatening to undermine the very fabric of planetary sustainability. It is hubris to think that we can apply our compromised, corrupted, left-brained science to the complex, integral, synergistic natural world and effect positive change. We as a species need to regrow our collective physical and spiritual senses and simply quit our all-out attack on Nature and the living planet.

The 500-1000 mile wide heat dome off the west coast has been keeping the weather from entering California for many years. Whether this heat dome be the consequence of increased ocean temperatures, El Nino or the build up of Fukushima radiation off the coast, California has been ripe for an ongoing fire apocalypse for many years due to its loss of coastal marine layer. Since there has been systematic chemical shiptrailing in the marine layer west of the heat dome for the years in which the heat dome has been established, we can assume that this weather-blocking structure is engineered to purposefully exist. As seen on NASA worldview the loss of the marine layer cloud cover has gotten worse since 2000, possibly orchestrated to stop Fukushima radiation laden precipitation from traveling into the USA from the Pacific Ocean.

If you observe the locations of the Shasta, Sonoma and Ventura California fires, it appears they are clearing out subdivisions that lie between two separate National Forest parklands, generating living corridors. This wilderness corridor creation is just one of the motives, using the wildfires to clear a path for trans-mountain oil pipelines, and consolidation of urban centers into smaller areas is another. If the geoengineers were actually proficient at weather manipulation they would make it RAIN on the fires. But no, the fires are for clearing land for their oil pipelines, bullet trains, dams, mining, wilderness corridors and their resilient cities. Redevelopment is generally prohibited after many of these fires, citing "high risk areas" designation and insurance companies that refuse to offer policies in these areas. Many times, a redevelopment plan is already in place BEFORE the fire even happened, and a contractor is ready to go.

During the **geoengineered wildfires**, please avoid breathing outside without protection and wear swimming googles when outside. The West Coast is laden with chemtrails and Fukushima radiation, which gets "recycled" when the forests burn. Is it possible that California, Alaska and Oregon are being burned with Directed Energy Weapons (DEW) in order to re-spread Fukushima radiation to increase the radiation loading on the population? chemtrailsplanet. net/. Turning our backs on the death economy requires a collective exit strategy. We know what to do, it is just a matter of believing in it and gathering the key brains, the volunteers and the community and start doing it now. Only intact nature's energy can revive our dis-eased energy and metabolism. Spirit is a river flowing back to its oceanic self, pretty much everything humans do prevents this full cycle of return. The more we turn to Nature to heal and whole us, the closer we come to Goodness, Godliness and Holiness.

Waking up is about establishing the chemistry that allows the Real you to emerge and thrive, from the imposter self that was built in response to an unreal world. We have to breed a new type of integrated, empowered, sovereign, shamanic human. Yet many in this degenerate culture are too far gone, while others are more than ready to shift over. Grand Solar Minimum will weed the flock and provide a growth exercise for those capable of meta-adaptation. Permaculturalists are the solution to sane and integral land management on a global scale.

Permaculturalists maybe self-satisfied that they are on the correct path ,which gives them a false sense of optimism. However permaculturalists are only slightly more equipped to deal with the repercussions of the chemtrail holocaust than the rest of society. Chemtrails will still cause raging infernos, destroying permaculture units, along with regular farms and houses. Radiation from Fukushima will still sicken Permaculturists and their land, nearly as much as conventional farms. Man-made weather warfare along with climate chaos from the natural cycle of the grand solar minimum will still decimate Permacultural harvests, almost as much as regular farms. We need to organize and build disaster-proof growing units, and find locations that are less likely to be hit by fire, ice and flood. Famine and the loss of seed stock for replanting is already on our door step — we must prepare.

Those in California and Colorado may know the extent of the destruction. There needs to be a conference on permaculture/survivalism/community building/climate chaos/geoenginneering, as we only have a few more years of stable culture before the food runs out, and societies break down. Moving forward is not just about getting back to the land and creating a nice little hamlet for ourselves when the entire biosphere is reaching "life support failure."

We can govern our survivability by the health of the forests.

The Kauri, the redwoods, the Amazon and boreal forests will ALL die from massive geoengineering and chemtrails, drought creation, Agenda 21 DEW wildfires, Fukushima radiation, demineralization since the end of the last ice age, death of the soil microbiome, lack of soil organic matter, reduction in the earth's magnetic field--consequent loss of ozone--and increase in UVC--plus changes in the solar spectrum due to the onset of the Grand Solar Minimum, and asphyxiation from increased methane and ozone emissions. Disease and insect infestation of forests is only a secondary effect.

The business as usual world is plainly psychotic, but by connecting the dots and making sense of the disorder, we can understand that this is a temporary sickness, and that there is a deeper reality and magnificent future waiting to be born, should we choose to accept it. Homo maniacal is ending his days on earth. We need not preoccupy ourselves with the dying of the old ways, but open ourselves to be informed and transformed by full Lifeforce and the luminous future beyond.

By reverting to a raw fruit and wild diet (moving away from commercially grown and hybrid foods) and undertaken a higher path towards returning to the spiritual state of Eden we can save ourselves from falling further into the collective mental asylum. Shamanic methods of whole-brain retrieval such as the entheogens, vision quests, trance dance, coupled with techniques such as prolonged sleep deprivation, extended fasting, extreme sports, nature connection, and shifting to a raw diet on route to a varied raw fruit diet are some methods of whole-brain recovery that we could base our life path around, to get on the right path to a sane future.

Plant trees and buildup a healthy biosphere and the crispy scorched earth is avoided — continue with this machiavellian nightmare and it is goodbye world. Everything THEY do reduces the earth's oxygen levels and we need to be well oxygenated to find our way out of this mess! Re-Evolution demands that we wake up and counteract the mechanisms of dehumanization, deforestation, ecological degradation, and irreversible biocide. Besides chopping down the trees for 5G, and the dieoff of trees from chemtrails, they are deforesting to reduce the oxygen in the atmosphere to increase hypoxia, cancer and infection. Dane Wigington said they were deliberately burning forests for solar radiation management, using the smoke as a sunshield, however this seems rather extreme. Mind you everything the climate disrupters do is extreme. How is Solar Radiation Management even possible when countries are already bankrupt?

 Geoengineering is bad for the planet in so many ways — many of which we have not yet realized — contributing to the sickening of the planet, and desecrating cultural integrity. Even without these sudden violent catastrophes, Stratospheric Aerosol Geoengineering is an extinction level phenomenon that rapidly breaks down the fabric of life on planet earth. An unholy addiction to false power is the force behind the debacle of the geoengineering program. It is a collective malaise symptomatic of the compartmentalized, fragmented, limited and machiavellian thinking that constitutes an insane drive for power over Nature, the Earth and its people.

See: "Transforming Our World: the 2030 Agenda for Sustainable Development." (2015).

MOVING BEYOND THE DEATH CULT

This fallen civilization is on its way out. What each of us do now will determine the nature of Civilization Next!

The main problem of Borg civilization, in no uncertain terms, is that our moral development and our understanding of Natural Law has not kept up with the pace of our technology. To deliberately, or unknowingly create conditions that thwart the emergence of the sovereign individual, enlightened society and the evolution of life on earth is not only evil, it is a lie against Nature, and it is deeply stupid! You cannot hold back or pervert evolution without dire consequences, for we are Nature. It shows the state of preoccupation and dissociation of the general public that they forgot or never knew what nature is, how it looks and how the physical electromagnetic world is designed by nature on certain laws and principles which make it VERY different than man made climate fuckery.

The global average atmospheric carbon dioxide in 2017 was 405.0 parts per million. Carbon dioxide is only a small faction of the % of atmosphere, and anthropomorphic carbon dioxide contribution is only 5% of the total the earth produces. The issue is that spending billions of dollars on planes, fuel and toxic aerosols that act as a heat blanket which only exacerbates the climate extremes and biosphere collapse by killing the soil bacteria, the trees and the vegetation turning the surface of the earth into a desert—baked to oblivion under extreme UV caused by the destruction of the ozone layer by the aerosol spraying. Chemtrailing is the most efficient method of killing a planet! And there is no need for it because we are already in the Grand Solar Minimum—the freeze of which will increase every year, preventing the methane bomb. After which we are scheduled for the large ice age proper.

If the geoengineers knew anything about planetary management they would have spent billions on building soil organic matter, erosion protecting ground cover, reforestation and remineralization, all of which would BUILD up the ozone layer by increasing oxygen production, thus preventing the radioactive, burnt-out planet that idiots in high places have managed to bring about. The notion of Global warming was conceived by the rich powerful polluters as an excuse to extract more money out of the public to fund the extermination program, using industrial waste dispersed in the atmosphere to depopulate the planet. They had to come up with fake science to concoct a reason why they would need to be spraying poisons and pathogens daily, over every corner of the global for decades.

Predators, Perpetrators and Pawns Must Pay! The solution to the diabolical aberration of geoengineering with chemtrails and microwaves is to stop it with international laws that force disaster capitalists and polluters to pay cleanup, remediation and recompensation to both economic damages, along with the rehabilitation of the ecosystems at large. Planet killing via spraying of toxic chemicals is obviously the most criminal endeavor for psychopathic predators short of setting off atomic bombs. All occult cabals, Wall St pirates, criminal banksters and corporations involved in planet killing technologies must be eradicated, and all those complicit in the crimes of planet killing (whether they do so consciously or in ignorance) must be charged with genocide, ecocide, and omnicide—the greatest of all crimes. We need teams of experts carefully watching Wall St for put options or hedge stocks by disaster capitalists and profiteers of the global cull and start locking these vermin up.

Since the bureaucratic leaders and protectors of society have failed the people and the planet, it is they who should pay for the clean up, restitution and regeneration programs. Since it is largely the military that are carrying out the crimes of the Global Deep State, they should be the ones to chop down every single tree they have killed with their poisons. The geoengineers and their industrial poison suppliers need to be held accountable. The solar radiation management criminals must pay! The American Elements Corporation is the largest metals and chemicals supplier in the world. How is it possible that Michael Silver, CEO of **American Elements**, is not charged with the ultimate treason of planetary omnicide, since he is culpable in profiting from the crime of spraying layer upon layer of toxic aerosol "chemtrails" in the sky above our heads on an almost daily basis for decades.

The macabre geoengineering industry must be brought to its knees, the perpetrators re-educated to see the folly of their ways, and international environmental law established to prevent such omnicide via chemtrail holocaust from ever happening again. The perpetrator's wealth needs to be applied to correcting the damage they have done, so that such compound evil never gets the chance to be let loose on Earth ever again. Let us grow up as a species and deal with our problems "intelligently" rather than killing ourselves and the rest of the planet off.

Meanwhile for the sake of all life we must do everything in our power to raise up our own energy and spiritual consciousness and come into our full inheritance as bearers of the Light. Closure' is a failure of flow. Energy must flow. When a system can no longer accept, absorb or dispel energy, it moves into 'free fall status' and becomes a runaway system that is no longer connected to its Source. We forever walk home towards the light, for we are the Light!

Nothing could be more primitive than contemporary culture as it can only lead to the breakdown and death of all life on earth. Fear-mongering is how our governments have been operating, and bereft of vision we can barely conceive of life beyond the Death Culture. And yet all of us are called by the Great Spirit should we care to listen deep enough. Without effort, determination and applied lifestyle it is hard being awake in a sleeping world. In order to save our soul and fortify ourselves against outrageous knowledge — we must train as a warrior of transformation. Others may awaken simply by witnessing the awakened in action. All come to back to "Life" in their own time.

It is overwhelming to contemplate how far Homo sapiens has fallen from sublime Nature and the embrace of cosmic consciousness. However all the wrongs point directly to the path of correction so that we can change course and arrive at a sacred, high integrity future. In our own lives and in our communities we must do everything in our power to bring about the type of society that we aspire to live in. I think it helpful to preempt and address every demon we encounter, but to do so in a "teaching mode," to help raise the zeitgeist out of the toilet. As Einstein said, we cannot *solve our problems with the same level of consciousness that created them.*

"Dismantle the current poison based control grid through non violent, non participation. Power to the people." ~ Jason Christoff

"No civilization that pollutes the air, water, soil and genetic integrity of its people, is truly advanced." ~ Andrew Faust

DYSTOPIAN SOCIAL ENGINEERING

The UN Charter of Global Democracy - In 1999 a charter to achieve "Global Governance," was developed for presentation at the Millennium Assembly. Global Democracy and is in fact International Socialism. If the UN government is presently killing every person and animal on the planet with their chemtrails. How will the one world NWO will govern? The UN-NOW is annexing the planet and trying to establish global hegemony. They can be stopped by establishing superior technology that frees the people from the control mechanisms of the global fascists. Such as getting off of hydrocarbon fuels, unplugging from the grid, extract ourselves from the banking system, creating abundance apart from the monetary system, avoiding the Borg medical industry and resist dependency on social security. If we resist dumbing down and numbing out, and raise self-reliance and sovereignty—if we come alive and freely express our authentic self we can throw off the pathology of master/slave once and for all.

A bizarre demonic force with a paradoxical sense of humor, a satanic inversion called "Wetiko," has taken over the human species. The end result of "we the people" not standing up to pathological authority, is that pathological socialism, the mean green meme and covert fascism combined with dark militarism and global deep state eugenics create the breakdown of social uplift within the 1st world countries. The straw that broke the social contract's back, was the realization that after observing the Paradise fire military attack in 2018, any trust in the established cultural model fell away. Meaning we became aware that we are living in a full-on anarchy, because "government" has come out in the light of day as the devil itself. And now with the social contract broken—we all already free in ways that we can barely begin to understand .

This is a turning point in civilization. What should each of us do now that the devil has shown us his true colors with technology we can barely describe, to destroy countless lives in the name of sustainable land redevelopment, resource utilization, bullet trains and eliminating useless eaters? I don't intend to watch the carnage of the collapse blow for blow. Rank survivalism and poverty mentality entrap us into the luciferian control matrix. Thus we must "imagine" our ideal outcome or transcendental future, establish a close relationship with the universal spirit and set about creating, not from what we fear or the existing paradigm, but via the heart's vision.

• The people need a global movement to resist Hindbrain Borg assimilation.

• A clearing house and network for sharing methods, solutions and education.

• Friendly ways of teaching children what is happening.

• Social engineering resistance training and deprogramming.

• Disaster response and preparedness.

• Collective food, seed and supplies bank.

• Stress and depression relief network.

• Unslaving, unshaming, spiritual strength building.

• Resiliency training and martial arts.

• Non-Hollywood movies and post establishment futurism.

• Soul recovery by regenerating and permaculturing the land and water.

• Training in lucid dreaming, visioneering and proactive executive traits.

14

CIVILIZATION NEXT

THE THRIVOCRACY

In order to stop this criminal program we must first learn how to thrive within the chemtrail holocaust.

The eye in the pyramid is traditionally meant as the symbol to describe the All Seeing Eye of Horus, the emissary and messenger of the Olympian gods, and son of Zeus. The Eye of Horus is an ancient Egyptian symbol of protection, royal power, and good health. And yet in today's world the eye in the pyramid is a symbol used to depict the Illuminati, those dark one's who clawed their way to the top of a corrupt pyramid of power. We must overcome our moral blindness and amnesia regarding the crimes of the Deep State by understanding the sociobiology, the history and the hermeneutics of false power. Least we forget who we are and our potential, and we don't know what we have got until it's gone!

You have to reach the level of enlightenment of the great geniuses who divine the secrets of nature to know the Hermetic structure of the arch template that creates the Universe. Through learning and divining the arch template we become enlightened. Only those who are enlightened into the arch template of the organization and mechanics of the cosmic creatrix have the right to rule or are fit to rule. A "system" is only as good as the individuals within the system, and for a system to flourish it is the responsibility all members to create a "system" in which all can thrive. Thus a thrivocracy is the only rational approach to the arch template of governmental and organizational systems.

The USA industrial-military-intelligence-security complex has a $1 Trillion annual budget. This is not money spent on "defense" when the US already has the ultimate deterrent of a nuclear arsenal. This is the people's money wasted on "offense," or military aggression and troublemaking around the globe. Imagine what a wonderful world it would be if that $1 Trillion a year was spent on global regeneration, instead of global destruction. The breakaway civilization has stolen an estimated 50 trillion dollars according to Catherine Austin Fitts, while the official number is 21 trillion dollars. She said: "You can't steal 21 Trillion Dollars without mind controlled slavery." The American public had no say in how the misplaced trillions was used, and that money never served the good of the people, for it was spent on survival structures for the criminal ĒLite and resource wars for the industralists and for the Ashkenazic global central bank total dominance control system.

The fight against the satanic oligarchy (ie: the Global Evil Empire) is the last war. This is WW3. The adversary are institutionalized, prostituted, brainsullied, co-conspirators (*Cocons*) of death and destruction. A condition arising from the separate self sense of a de-natured humanity running from scarcity by scheming to acquire personal material wealth beyond their wildest dreams. This is a one world demon that we must all respond to as faithful one world citizens.

The mechanics of Human social dynamics are similar to Newton's 3rd law of motion: "For every action, there is an equal and opposite reaction." If you push against and resist the negative you manifest more of the negative. Reacting against something with "The Negative," locks us into resonance with it, instead of transcendence of it. Nerves only respond positively to positive messages. This is referring to apriori wholeness, magnificence, attainment, success, well-being, goodness, actualization, happiness etc... That is, instead of focusing on the negative—focus on building up the positive. Indulging in negative maladaptive coping techniques only takes energy away from ascension.

Fascism only takes hold when good people float along without questioning the existing culture, instead of evolving and pushing culture forward. I am talking about the ongoing fascism of the military industrial machine, and the THEY (Tyrannical, Hegemonic, Evil, Yahoos) who have been accruing false power for thousands of years. Complaining and bringing the globalist ĒLite criminals to justice is not enough. Rather each person of conscience must wake up to new levels of creativity to change the socioeconomics of civilization itself to that which humanizes and works with nature instead of against her.

We fight to establish the freedom to be remain truly human. All citizens of the globe are responsible for either bringing about the end to the grotesque subhuman regime. Citizen slaves unite and rise up above the faceless robot hordes that want to suck the marrow out of our bones for eternity. Join the REHUMANIZING MOVEMENT! To save ourselves and the planet we must build a human world based on love, abundance and regeneration.

We must throw off the primitive, frustrated, angry simian that is rapidly losing consciousness by the day and live up to our full stature as Homo sapiens—the wise man. We are far more than we will ever know ourselves to be, had we not been intimidated, dismissed and exploited by the culture of rank competition and willful neglect. Let us not waste our energy in resistance to ignore-ance and evil, but simply expand into the full life of our authentic, ultimate and primordial "true nature."

The big fish corporations are only concerned with dominance, money and exploitative strategy, and humanity is under survival pressures from every angle because of it. Our job is to stay vigilant, avoid the life-destroying aspects of this degenerate culture and work diligently to become increasingly healthy ourselves. We can try to educate friends and/or the public, but we cannot be concerned about outcome, as the extermination regime is proceeding full force, and so there is not much we can do about species suicide on a global scale, but save our heritage seed, remineralize the soil and grow our own food. We cannot legislate that exploitative capitalism stop being exploitative, but we can boycott their businesses.

Until the vanguard of the forward moving wave gathers force, most are better off being asleep, for if they have not yet awoken they have few skills or capacity to deal with reality, and what is actually befalling our species and the planet. Best to focus on facilitating and positioning ourselves for maximum creativity and sovereign development in cooperation with those people who have taken the red pill and are already out of the Matrix.

The people stuck in the Matrix will come to the realization of global military empire, the worldwide cull, the global famine, and corruption on every level in their own time, or never — it's their karma.

Compartmentalized, dys-integrated Flatlanders enmeshed in hive mind or group-think do not have the capacity to put two and two together and see the big picture, and every day, the darkside gets ever more devious in its mind control and dumbing down tactics. The controllers' efforts to stop the evolution and enlightenment of the population are extreme! But we cannot be reactionary, instead we must turn our backs on the demonic and set about with renewed intention, enthusiasm and commitment to create the life we want, and the world we know should be.

The foundational teachers for the new civilization are both mystics, implosionists and renaissance men. Walter Russell, got the divine download of the overarching template of the metascience during 32 days of visionary trance. These amazing preceptors of Civilization Next offer Phi technologies that can be employed to counteract Borg culture's anti-life technologies: *John Ernst Worrell Keely, Nikola Tesla, Rudolf Joseph Lorenz Steiner, Georges Lakhovsky, Walter Bowman Russell, Viktor Schauberger, Richard Buckminster Fuller, Wilhelm Reich, Thomas Galen Hieronymus.*

The implosionists were all on the same track—the Phi vortical track. "Implosionist" means they use mathematics and philosophy of the feminine force of centripetal vortex action towards Zeropoint. It is it also the implosion or conjugation of consciousness and the cellular and DNA tapping of zeropoint that allows mystics direct access to nature's secrets through quantum or immanent intelligence or Nature Mysticism. When you start to tune into New Energy—that is, the energy of What IS, not what has been, then you pick up and ride a wave of creative exuberance. The day that mankind discovers that love is the greatest force in the universe, is the day he becomes sane.

"New Energy" whether it be new consciousness and creative vitality, ORMUS, zeropoint, HHO, Magnegas, Magnetic Motors, plasma vortex generators, new solar generating architecture, photosynthetic cells, fuel cells, photovoltaic glass, sewage-methane plants, or Magravs Power (Plasma capacitors and magrav coils)—all this and everything else in human enterprise is all part of the same picture of "reinventing" ourselves as a cosmically moral animal with a sane respectful attitude toward the karmic nature of Reality.

"Atomic Suicide," by Walter Russell and Lao Russell outlines the threat to our planet from mining radioactive elements, largely due to loss of oxygen and ozone layer. Nuclear material belongs where it is supposed to be, in the ground Pretty much everything "nuclear" is saturnic, that is evil, and symptomatic of the darkside of Homo sapiens.

No part of human existence can be excluded from the understanding of the cause and effect loop of Reality and how everything is part of everything else. Without an intuition for the infinite interrelatedness of existence there can be no real growth toward regeneration, sustainability and the continuum of humanity. Within anything is the seed of everything.

The most profound, eloquent article on the big picture of culture and economics you will likely ever read:

https://civilizationemerging.com/new-economics-series-part-iv/ — New Economics Series: Part IV. Overlapping Models Exploring the Nature and Evolution of Economics, **Daniel Schmachtenberger**.

CULTURAL CHANGE

The search for meaning is the great underlying driver of HUman evolution.

The inability to think outside the box and intuit expanded possibility is probably due to laziness and the reluctance to grow. Those who profit from old exploitive systems seek to perpetuate their ill-gotten income streams. This builds up a lot of negative karma from not facing reality, which drives intensifying crisis and breakdown—resulting in either death or growth. A predatory culture, trauma, enslavement and the lack of actualization of personal sovereignty narrows our worldview and perpetuates resistance to change (ie: laziness). This regressive hijacking appears to be a fatal flaw that runs automatically by default in Homo sapiens, which initiates the manifest destiny of depression, death, destruction, war and disease.

Hindbrain man is compromised and regressed by power (dopamine) addiction and is perpetually trying to shake the money tree. This is why we have the 1% spraying toxic poisons and infectious agents from airplanes to try and kill the 99%—because we are too consciousness and will not put up with power abuse, spiritual rape and criminal wars any longer. We cannot simply be the dumb crowd fighting against the evil agenda of an even dumber crowd. This has to be the smartest re-evolution ever undertaken, requiring incredible feats of maturity, intellect, self-development, insight, communication and community. The re-evoluton has to be extreme fun or it won't work. Exuberance, love and openness are magic!

Technical changes are "lateral developments," where we change what we do including establishing new skills, practices and tools. Adaptive changes are "vertical developments," that require new levels and structures of consciousness to change how we see the problem and arrive at solutions and advancements. Meta-adaptive applications are "synergistic developments," which are able to alter both the models and the adaptation process through establishing a strategic meta-model that helps to structure a meta-adaptive system.

Unconscious patterns are not a choice, they are the abdication of conscious choice. Then of course there is the people's culpability in their own demise. When opiates are used to reduce the fear, pain and anxiety this reduces the immune system. Plus our escape drugs of choice: carbohydrates, sugar, alcohol, provide the perfect medium for feeding the pathogen load in the body. Thus if we go along with the program we are doomed from the outside by the dominator culture, and doomed from the inside through our own maladaptive escape routes and soporific cultural rituals. When we source energy externally from a place of separation, we create that reality.

The existing culture we have created is a Hindbrain culture, which is self-reinforcing, entropic, unsustainable and an evolutionary dead end. It is the Hindbrain that runs on the dominance/submission circuitry of the old mammalian brain that is enlisted in the service of the master/slave paradigm, in which warmongering, ethnic cleansing and industrial ecocide are an inevitable consequence of deferred responsibility and addiction to false power. Political and religious dogma obscures the objective truth of Nature, as the regressed, fragmented sadomasochist goes to war on the planet, themselves and the universe. Both brain hemispheres, the Triune Brain and the Heart Brain (and more) are necessary for whole HUman consciousness whereby conscience, foresight, intuition, visioneering, telepathy and "spiritual" awareness are possible.

With our focus still on the **logistics of profit making** there is not enough brainstorming of new methods, new designs, organizational models, products, tools, services and commerce beyond the exploitative-capitalist model. The only thing holding us back is lack of imagination, selfish withholding, avarice, and resources going into the dying degenerate culture instead of being redirected into the regenerous culture. Only by pushing against entropy can we establish ever increasing syntropy. For starters we could start spreading Buckminster Fuller synergy philosophy everywhere.

By working on making it through the transition and provide the technologies, philosophy and social organization necessary for advanced culture, we will find our passion and our spiritual family. When we transcend Hindbrain mode we encounter a holodigm of Peace, the energy of awe, or the Mysterium Tremendum of our life, and the tacit sense of limitedness. If we are not actively working to create the world we want we stagnate and succumb to a quagmire of fear.

PHARMA MANIA

The pharmaceutical fix to problems whether they be medical, psychological, agricultural or environmental is plainly antievolutionary (evil), because it does nothing to fix the problem, while destroying lives, ecosystems and evolution in the process. What to do? It requires deprogramming from the degenerate culture — and we have been moving in the direction of the dis-ease model of existence for well over 10,000 years now. I am saying the industrial, pharmaceutical, "chemical remedial premise" is incompatible with a healthy living planet.

Nature provides ALL our corrections, alignment and balance within all domains be they medical, psychological, agricultural or environmental. The mercenary premise of capitalizing on sickness and problems is the wrong way to go about human existence. It can only create more problems down the line through ever increasing disease, disharmony and environmental collapse. The pharmaceutical premise is an attempt to "cheat" reality rather than learning from it — as such humanity descends further and further from the truth — into madness, destitution, hardship, war and planetary omnicide.

Our conditioning and schooling right from birth is now focused on manipulating the material world, rather than on understanding it and "working with" it. Thus humanity pits itself against existence and each other to the detriment of ALL life on earth for eternity. Things will change once we are enlightened, however we cannot become enlightened through the pharmaceutical fix and Borg psychosis. In this primitive state of consciousness we are bound for endless suffering and ultimate extinction — an anathema to all existence.

The forces of death and destruction have been institutionalized and are getting worse and more idiotic every day. Not sure how we can halt the avalanche of stupid. Parasitism, predation and usury must become a thing of the past in the entirety of human existence. Parasitism, predation and usury are behind the out-of-control pharmaceutical regime and exploitative socioeconomic-political civilization. The only thing that will heal the gnawing depth of need in the human spirit is spiritual evolution. The doublebind is that this life-violent culture prevents the awakening and development needed for us to get out of this mess and save ourselves and the planet. Talking about it s a good place to start.

The answer to this cultural insolvency is spiritual understanding of the natural science of the universe and enlightened human presence on earth. We already know the basics of doing this via the Essene law, rawfoodism, permaculture, Natural Step, implosion science, Walter Russellian cosmology, kundalini science and spiritual practice, Taoism, etc... Through being a living example and teaching the children we may redeem the lost Homo sapiens species.

There needs to be a fundamental change in the human organism that shifts it towards evolution, rather than devolution. We need a sea change, for if it is not 1080, Glyphosate or chemtrails it will be something else. The corporations (chemical companies) fund universities and research, poisoning the minds of students into the retarded chemological point of view. Teaching natural science via Schauberger/Steiner/Russell/Buckminster Fuller to preschoolers will save lives and souls from the huge ravenous gaping maws of the Beast! Each individual must do their part—and it will become easier the more each of us take up our true vocation towards planetary uplift.

TRANSCENDING OBLIVION SYNDROME

"All the Goyim, without exception are to be reduced to the state of human cattle by a process of integration [migration] on an international scale." Satan; Prince of The World by Admiral William G. Carr.

The nefarious effects of geoengineering are accumulative, synergistic and systemic—affecting all life on earth. If the perpetraitors would read Fertile Earth by Viktor Schauberger they might understand how they are breaking down the electromagnetic, ionic and atomic basis of all living things. The poisoning of the food supply with life killing chemicals, and the poisoning of the watersheds with 1080 in combination with the biocidal effects of geoengineering and the nuclear industry means it is a downhill slide to oblivion for Homo sapiens. And as we suicide, we appear to murdering the planet.

The chemtrailing, weather manipulation, disaster capitalism, water toxemia, resource wars, environmental collapse, predatory-fascist medicine, deliberate crop destruction, deforestation, poisoning of bushfood, and the forced migrations are all evidence of a global eugenics plan well underway. The Global Deep State (GDS) is at war with planet earth—and it is we the people who gave them the power to do so. They are euthanizing the world population and claiming all things of monetary value for themselves. The world citizens must get rid of the exploitive paradigm and the exploiters and send them all off to their own little prison island where they can exploit each other.

Their methods are obvious for anyone with the brains to put two and two together. However the majority are authority-whipped into a stupor of compliance and do not even see the chemtrails overhead on saturation spray days. Global Deep State Zionazi collaborators (ie: government workers) have been hoodwinked into carrying out various components of the eugenics program, whether it be fluoride, vaccines, chemtrailing, 1080 poison, abominable Monsanto's deathly combo of Roundup and GMOs, quake-attacks, fake wild-fires, hurricane manipulation, dam releases, deluges and catastrophic crop loss.

We all knew there would be migration due to biosphere collapse, but this current migration series in various conflict ridden areas of the globe has more to do with the Leviathan's stranglehold on the resources of those countries, and the harvesting of the gold treasury — thus preventing countries from ever being sovereign and free of the cancer of the central banking system. And we all know who has the major influence in the international banking system and the International Monetary Fund, the Turkish Ashkenazi Jews. The federal reserve is a major contributor to the IMF, and the Rothchild's are in that orbit. The Turkish Ashkenazi Mafia and their minions run the world.

Multiculturalism does not mean cultural destruction, assimilation and homogenization…and the invasion by migrant hordes from deliberated conquered and decimated foreign lands. Rothschild and Soros are deliberately using mass immigration to destroy western nations. Under Agenda 21, is planning immigration into the US with the goal is to create chaos and to lay the foundation for breaking up the United States – and the end of America as a sovereign nation. This is part of a carefully planned plot which has been in place since the early 1900's. It is called The Kalergi Plan, and the nightmare is presently ramping up in frequency and intensity.

f was devised by the predecessors of the European Union between 1923 and 1925. The Kalergi Plan declared that the Jews would take over the power, first in Europe and then in the whole world. The Japanese-Austrian politician, geopolitician, philosopher "Nikolaus Kalergi," together with his Free Mason colleagues devised a conspiracy of global conquest through destroying the spirit of nationalism by rapid mass migration, combined with "ethnic" separatist movements and inflaming political divisiveness. The Kalergi Plan proposed to destroy Europe and to exterminate the white race via the invasion of immigrants to Europe. In this way breeding a passive, less intelligent "mestizo race" or mixed-race goyim, which could be easily tamed, making it possible for an Ashkenazi ELite to rule over the world forever.

This invasion is camouflaged with words like multiculturalism, progress, mercy, humanism, fraternity, social justice, inclusiveness, equal opportunity etc. But principally it's a brutal and merciless criminal plan to destroy the European nations, and by extrapolation, other caucasian nations in the name of global conquest. As we see throughout Europe with the rape, pillage, burning cars and city street occupation…these immigrant hordes have been tasked with besieging the peacable residents of European cities…and they will continue to do so in America, or any other country they are "sent" into to do the bidding of the Kalergi Plan. "The Kalergi plan is the New World Order plan, and it's not just for Europe. White genocide is very real and is playing out exactly as Kalergi and his handlers envisioned it." https://redice.tv/search?s=The+Kalergi+Plan

It is actually Hindbrain functioning that is hindering human evolution, as the old brain structures have hijacked the neocortex. The Abrahamic Mythic religions are an expression of the Hindbrain seizure of spirituality. But it is not just spirituality that has fallen into its saturnic, demonic or regressed expression, it is science, politics, government, business, medicine, law, agriculture and all aspects of Borg society which are plainly an expression of the tenacious

Hindbrain hijacker. People normally talk of cognitive hijacking with regards to PTSD, trauma, compulsiveness and addiction—but I am talking about it in terms of arrested development of the culture-as-a-whole, that is retarded evolution. This regressive hijacking appears to be a fatal flaw that runs automatically by default in Homo sapiens, which initiates the manifest destiny of depression, death, destruction, war and disease. We cannot understand the Madness of our current civilization and our fellow humans, nor ourselves without understanding this **cerebral hijack**. If you go through a massive kundalini awakening and experience consciousness beyond the regressed/repressed and aborted state—you can clearly experience this. What it means is that we could set the world to rights really fast if we could get the creative edge to break out of the Borg psychosis and more fully wake up.

The compartmentalized, fractured psyche of industrial civilized man is skewed towards being dominated by the simply calculative, mechanical, adaptive functioning of the linear, intellectual mind. In a culture of competition, war, exploitation, poor self-esteem and false-power the higher functions of the rightbrain, wholebrain and even the executive and creative consciousness are not exercised, and are indeed "punished" and discouraged by a competitive, shaming and power hungry society. This process of spiritual dumbing down and soul castration has been occurring for over 20 thousand years, although some isolated populations by have been less affected by the cultural illness of acquisition and violence. Remnants of the "whole HUman" can still be found in pre-industralized countries and places like the forests of South America, the South Pacific, the Bushmen of the Kalahari.

The "whole HUman" also exists in those less violent populations that are less autocratic and more affiliative and matriarchal in nature, which have been saved from the brain damage and disassociation that comes from patriarchal abuse…for as industrial slaves men have not been allowed to realize their true masculinity and come into their full power, and thus weak men are self-destructive and bully others instead of protecting and mentoring the clan. By enslaving the cosmic human within a false and terminal civilization, people no longer know what it is to be HUman, and thus are held captive within a dying Borg (wetiko) kingdom, without the wholebrain functioning and cosmic soul intelligence, nor futuresight to build those bridges that will transport us from this madness. It is so that living comfortably as slaves within the belly of the beast we are wasting our lives and setting up our children for the slaughter by the heartless machine.

The Borg or wetiko is simply the 8-circuit human held in suspended animation at the lower self-centered (self-imploded) circuits due to the terror of fully taking in and integrating this terrible human world we have made for ourselves due to our social and psychological dysfunctions. Remember in Leary's Eight-Circuit Brain model "intelligence" remains latent or repressed to the degree that we are unable or unwilling to fully absorb, integrate, realize and transmit it. If we make our human world so terrorizing with our collective insanity that we cannot digest and process it, then we clearly undermine the humanization process that differentiates us from a rabid predacious beast.

Since "higher intelligence" requires the synthesis, synergy and cohesiveness of the Eight-Circuit Brain, why don't we consciously work towards exercising and realizing the genius of all Eight-Circuits. Let us embark on a new course of cosmic evolution through clear vision, to establish the healing and maturation process toward an optimized breed of human whom is no longer focused on the barbaric and life-harming level of existence, but appreciates our unbelievably rich species heritage, to preserve the future of the biosphere and its immortal evolutionary Tree of Life. I doubt there is one person alive on earth at present that truly appreciates the profound miracle of the whole HUman.

As Borg humans we have been running on barely conscious circuits, however when we awaken we begin to open up into the super conscious circuitry which Nature has graced us with. In childhood we had glimpses of these capacities, but the enslaved society and Borg culture quickly deadened these expanded levels through shaming, belittlement and vehement denial. Emotional indigestion interferes with wholebrain consciousness, future sight and executive functioning. Thus we become trapped within a sick society without the skills and strength to save ourselves, as our life energy, life-purpose and meaning slowly ebb away.

Emotional needs can only be assuaged through the right-brain soul-heart connection. We normally interpret the overly emotional as being deficient in the left brain and over active in the right brain. However, the overly emotional is a Hindbrain (reptilian and limbic) hijack of the left adaptive brain. If the right brain soul-heart connection was more dominant then the individual would not be "overly emotional" they would be at peace and in whole-brain functioning. That is, being emotion and rational as well as One with Their Maker. When we meet the occasional person who is whole-brain dominant and liberated in their right brain-heart connection, we get to experience, perhaps for the first time, soul to soul connection. It is then that cosmic consciousness (Christus, Buddha, Brahman, Allah, Manu, Tawa, Manito, Altjira) is realized and the "mystic heart" can grow. We have to love ourselves more to come alive and become healing stewards for mother earth.

The Hivemind of industrialized humanity is spiritually retarded and so their science is morally retarded — as it their politics and most everything else. Probably the best basic books for understanding this "species hijacking" is Prometheus Rising by Robert Anton Wilson, and Exo-Psychology is Timothy Leary's introduction to the Eight-Circuit Brain model. The Eight-Circuit Model of Consciousness by Antero Alli is an elaboration of a hypothesis first proposed by Timothy Leary. Also expanded on by Robert Anton Wilson that "suggested eight periods [circuits] and twenty-four stages of neurological evolution." The Triune Brain by Paul D. MacLean and The Precambrian Mind by Julian Jaynes are also great ground work.

See also all of Paul Levy's books including his most recent Dispelling Wetiko: Breaking the Curse of Evil, by Paul Levy and Catherine Austin Fitts, (2013). Quantum Revelation: A Radical Synthesis of Science and Spirituality, by Paul Levy and Jean Houston, (2018). A good place to start for Self-recovery is Breaking The Habit of Being Yourself: How to Lose Your Mind and Create a New One, by Dr. Joe Dispenza, 2013. Also the 4th way method by Gurdjieff and Ouspenskii. And David R Hawkins' book Power vs Force, and his levels of consciousness scale is a good road map to utilize for moving up the scale.

"When the mob governs, man is ruled by ignorance; when the church governs, he is ruled by superstition; and when the state governs, he is ruled by fear. Before men can live together in harmony and understanding, ignorance must be transmuted into wisdom, superstition into an illuminated faith, and fear into love." ~ Manly P. Hall.

TRANSCENDING THE SCARCITY PARADIGM

The resources on earth are bountiful and regenerative, if they are not poisoned, mutated and incorrectly used and abused by humans.

As we "divorce ourselves" from nature, the scarcity paradigm generated by the anxiety and competition of Hindbrain Dominance is compounded. By un-naturing we undermine the supernal synergy of the universal complexity, and reduce it down to products to sell and consume. This process began as our species left the tropical forests and moved away from the original highly complex food sources that fed our large brain. Our brain is presently devolving and deforming—void of the supernatural consciousness that is our species birthright. As the planet degenerates we are losing our capacity to be human-sublime.

The rape, poison, burn and fry model of the war against nature has come to an end. We have better ways of solving our deficiency, disease and imbalance problems. We can use our intelligence to work-with Nature instead of against her. As the planet is being killed we have only a few short years left to wake up and change our ways over to the regenerative, restorative health model of human existence—or humans and most other life will become toast.

Saving the true human and the planet are one and the same task as the salvation of our individual and collective lives. This means creating communities and ecovillages that use technology that works "with" nature instead of against it. As we reconstitute our genetic, cerebral and spiritual potential, we undergo a U-turn in the Fall of Humanity and return to the path of eternal grace to ever expanding glorification. A continuous, give and take process of recovery and redemption. By imagining Homo lumens we become Homo lumens.

"The ne'er-do-wells" are dumping their industrial wastes around the world for carbon credits, and to destroy the natural abundance of the land for the covert purpose of inducing worldwide famine to cull the population. We must use the unconscionable wrong of the chemtrail holocaust (solar radiation management) to rise up to soulful excellence, our true vocation and radiant health—rebuilding nature and building perma-civilization. The Whole Civilizational Structure Needs To Be Permaculturalized! Now is the time to change over to ice age farming...and create ecovillages with escaping city dwellers money.

The most important things we need to focus on during this time on the precipice of the collapse are: Water purification, EMF protection, Soil organic matter/composting, Storm-Proof Greenhouses for Food Production, Seed breeding and saving, Regenerative Health Education, Revolutionary Hazard Safe Housing Design and Materials, Community Cash and Barter Systems, The Aggregator Business Model (also termed as On Demand Delivery Model for Skills/Services/Resource exchange in communities. We also need a revamping of the music industry by musicians who are living WITH the circadian rhythms and living earth. We also need to bring back traveling sociopolitical intellectual theater that doesn't focus on the problems so much as modeling the path to Apotheosis and showing the people the way.

"The Sovereign Individual: Mastering the Transition to the Information Age." by James Dale Davidson and Lord William Rees-Mogg.

VISIONARIES

Viktor Schauberger, Callum Coats, John Worrell Keely, Dale Pond, Walter Russell, Rudolf Steiner, Buckminster Fuller, Tom Bearden, Tom Valone, John Searl, Brian Desborough, Lloyd Zirbes, Nikola Tesla [Wolfgang Wiedergut], Edwin V. Gray, Thomas Henry Moray, Nathan Stubblefield, Stan Meyers, Dennis Lee, John Hutchison, John Kanzius, John Moray, John Milewski, Hal Puthoff, Wilhelm Reich, Rudolf Steiner, Nassim Haramein, Marko Rodin, Stuart Hameroff, Eric Learner, William McDonough, ORMUS-Barry Carter, Laurence Gardner, David Radius Hudson. Douglas Rushkoff. Peter Joseph, Douglas Rushkoff, Catherine Austin Fitts, Jacque Fresco, Charles Eisenstein, Jeremy Rifkin, Chuck Blakeman, Frederic Laloux, Michael Tellinger, Paolo Lugari (Gaviotas), Paolo Soleri (Archosanti), Yasuhiko Genku Kimura, Fritjof Capra, Stuart Kauffman, Permaculture Tech: David Holmgren, Bill Mollison, Andrew Faust, Geoff Lawton.

FUTURE THOUGHT

Future thought is thinking with your headlights on, ie: integrally and holistically. Thinking about the future engages the Frontopolar cortex, which governs precommitment, intent, vision, delayed gratification, prioritization and planning functions. This then activates both the Dorsolateral cortex for will power and the Orbital cortex for morality or impulse control (discipline). Thus we see that when we are on default or autopilot mode and we do not have our headlights on, we are more reactive, embedded and vulnerable to the given stimuli from our environment and cannot be said to be "creating" our world.

If we are not creating our world then it is not really "our" life that we are living. Without engaging the higher-mind for a visionary overview - the willpower, sovereign empowerment and inner authority needed to "change and create" is not forthcoming. If the sovereign decision maker is not in charge we can expect a more hellish experience of reality than we otherwise would have. If however we can educate and develop enough creative individuals to transcend the Hindbrain culture, and allow them to succeed and survive the current homicidal mania — we may go on as a species to establish Civilization Next. Four Futures: Life After Capitalism by Peter Frase

Science Fiction and Utopian writers are a great source of future thought: Arthur C. Clarke, Aldous Huxley, George Orwell, Philip K. Dick, Robert Heinlein, Frank Herbert, Ursula Le Guin, Kurt Vonnegut, Isaac Asimov, Dan Simmons, Richard E. Friedman, Robert Anton Wilson, Lyman Tower Sargent, Kim Stanley Robinson.Utopian Horizons podcasts on iTunes.

Transcendental geniuses - the founding fathers of civilization next:
John Ernst Worrell Keely (1837–1898)
Nikola Tesla (1856 - 1943)
Rudolf Joseph Lorenz Steiner (1861 – 1925)
Georges Lakhovsky (1869 - 1942)
Walter Bowman Russell (1871 –1963)
Viktor Schauberger (1885 –1958)
Richard Buckminster Fuller (1895 –1983)
Wilhelm Reich (1897 – 1957)
Thomas Galen Hieronymus (1895 – 1988)

BUILDING CIVILIZATION NEXT

Once awakened to our cosmic HUmanity...the very best of us can be shepherds, designers and administrators of the flock. We still need leaders of heart and consciousness in order for regular dumb-numb folks to real-eyes the higher realms of their own humanity. We don't even know who/what we are until we go through a massive kundalini awakening and experience higher mind and sensory/psychic expansion. The awakened human is a vastly different animal to the farmed human cattle. We may feel exploited when we "wake" because human culture at present is exploitative. That is all that most people know how to do, except perhaps certain grandmothers, who are endlessly giving. Other than standing up to and not falling for the social ploys of winner/loser, top/bottom, higher/lower, and the bullying that accompanies exploitation, we can learn how to have a regenerous life and no longer exploit ourselves and sell ourselves short.

One of the most important things to do at present is anthropology studies recording in films and books the lifestyle, customs, technology, adaptations, and interiors (beingness) of people still living in traditional villages. Besides distributing to the world, we need a central storehouse of this material so that we can use it to plan and design the "new village" for ourselves and future generations. By following the proven path of the way "things should be" it is easier to disengage and liberate ourselves from the old world. So another thing we can do is look for people and places where they have already turned away from the profane, regressive society and embraced the new.

The stars in the heavens draw the human heart into the larger cosmic field of life, but the stars have been all but banned from city life. Human cities are a primitive design for collective human life that date back to from the period circa 3800 BC. To live in a city, the "whole human" must be broken down to mere Flatland consciousness, made paranoid and greedy in order to undergo debt slavery without revolt. True spiritual community and divine creativity must be suspended in order to keep people focused on the feeding on the commercial matrix as being the be-all-and-end-all of existence. Humans need mystery, magic, and awe, for without a greater connection to source—we are all slaves to a pathetic and obsolete God—Mammon—or materialism void of love and earth stewardship.

If you want to hijack a planet, what could be a better way of doing it than by controlling the populace without them ever knowing. Illegal wars for stealing resources, destroying infrastructure, implanting puppet leaders, creating central banks and genociding populations is the modus operandi of the malignant one world empire. Malignant power is a sickness, and a fundamental missunderstanding of the true nature of HUman existence. It is the global citizen's job to be filled with awe and excitement about working with Nature to create higher civilization and a garden planet. To this end those who are currently opting for absolute power and planet killing must be "re-educated" on that which is most valuable...Life in the Universe.

"As above, so below, as within, so without, as the universe, so the soul — to accomplish the miracle of the One Thing." ~ Hermes Trismegistus

COOPERATION AND BRAIN SIZE

There's an African proverb that says, "If you want to go fast, go alone. If you want to go far, go together."

The social brain hypothesis was proposed by British anthropologist Robin Dunbar, who argued that human intelligence evolved as a means of surviving and reproducing in large and complex social groups. According to the social brain hypothesis, the disproportionately large brain size in humans exists as a consequence of us humans forming large, complex social groups. The social brain hypothesis applies not just at the level of the species but also at the level of the individual. Cooperation and socioemotional reward chemistry may have been instrumental in driving brain evolution due to the challenge of sizing up others.

Cooperation, which is key to a prosperous society, is intrinsically linked to the idea of social comparison -- constant assessing, ranking and making decisions as to whether we want to help others or not. Due to enhanced survival, evolution favors those who prefer to help out others who are at least as "successful" as themselves. The complex task of constantly assessing other individuals and making relative judgments of who to help, has been a sufficiently difficult task to promote the expansion of the brain over many generations of human reproduction. Regardless of the social hierarchy of our birth origins, we can use this principle to further our own social advancement and creative freedom. By meditating, visualizing and emotional resonance on the word success (and other success synonyms) we can tweak our biochemistry and resonant frequency towards emancipation and sovereignty. Thereby stimulating others to "include us and cooperate with" our creative projects and increase consent, compliance and interest in our well-being and success.

Since we are dealing with systemic Hindbrain retarded unconsciousness, ie: ignore-ance. Prayer or Meditation on the apriori fact of an exalted outcome helps to bring it about, or at the very least heals ourself of the dis-ease. That is, by consciously generating a constant apriori success frequency we can overcome the dissociation, distraction, indifference and the lack of connection and attention that is ripping apart the fabric of our human world, and reducing the depth and complexity of our communal experience, such that it presents a very real threat to the continued development of the future "size" of the human brain.

The separate self-sense is divorced from the sense of unity between equals and of conscious connection or Presence. The separate self sense is an illusion—a fragile invention to safeguard the ego's need for permanence, self-importance and to defend against the fear of death itself. Mother Earth and Father Sun will feed you. Don't expect much from the human world, but learn to appreciate others with the kind of attention that you yourself hunger for. When raising children it is "indifference" or lack of connection and attention does the greatest harm. Being deprived of acknowledgement, recognition and appreciation in childhood, reduces our capacity for conscious self-love.

When we are not resonating in the frequency of love we are alienated from unity consciousness and cosmic connection, and it is this separate self-sense that is the driving force behind all conflict, violence, inequality and selfishness. If a country is run by principles, laws and goodwill it doesn't need leaders, because every citizen SHOULD be a leader…and "sovereign" ie: in touch with the divine. If there are leaders they should only be those who exhibit a genius level degree of divine grace.

Water is the life-giving fluid that is always at the heart of creation. Its presence supports life, and its absence brings death. The importance of water to life cannot be emphasized enough. Water changes in response to light, sound, EMFs, galactic cosmic rays, thought, emotion and lifeforce—recording and storing in-formation. Water itself responds to focused love. It is apparent that the earth is dying from the lack of loving attention. It is apparent then that the contemporary human has lost the capacity to radiate love and live by actions born from loving attention. We must ask ourselves why that is. To overcome our own fragmentation and dissociation we can impart both the love vibration and success frequency into our water, our food and every moment of our lives.

How to regard the chemtrails? Well, it seems they are not stopping, and I am not sure whether they will stop even during the Grand Solar Minimum, since the United Nations is behind the devils who are chemtrailing us, and the One World Empire, or New World Order, is the brainchild of the UN (Rothschild and Rockefeller). The Grand Solar Minimum has already begun and so the earth is in for some really extreme times. After which the ice age proper may arrive. These symptoms are in keeping with the effects of the reduction in the solar wind, lowering of the magnetosphere and consequent increase in galactic cosmic rays, producing more cloud cover and consequent rain. The whole solar system has moved out of alignment with the milky way, so that the sun is now rising in Virgo instead of Scorpius.

Let us not "ignore" the negative—such as chemtrails, weather/geo warfare, radiation, GMOs, industrial agriculture, resource wars, man's inhumanity to man, DEW fires, 5G, 1080 ecocide etc... Let us see them from a higher perspective as the insane manifestations of an immature and dying species—and walk away into a brand new sunrise. Create the new communities, new education, new food production, new financial systems, new science, new art and creativity and attend to our own spiritual growth without the burden of the MAD world (Mutually Assured Destruction World) on our backs or our conscience. The best we can do is grow our own food, build a winterized greenhouse, plant a medicinal herb garden, grow medicinal mushrooms, make and sell potions to our friends, eliminate any bad lifestyle habits, and to move away from the Fukushima radiation fallout zone, to non-chemtrailed locations if possible.

Complacency is not compliance, it is a failure of sovereignty, individuality and imagination. However, rather than fight the dumb predatory Beast, it is best to put our energies into creating the new world and the new culture, otherwise we are held captive to a dying regime. We must use the unconscionable wrong of the chemtrail holocaust and the MAD world to rise up to soulful excellence, our true vocation and magnificent health—restoring nature and building perma-civilization together as globally responsible world citizens. It is a potent time to start effectively making the world a better place to live and thrive. Reversing planetary degradation is now the most urgent call to action for all. Rather than commodifying and exploiting our ecological demise, we need to become a new species, with NEW FORMS of social cohesion and contribution.

"When you take away the sense of freedom where people feel that they can do anything, then people withdraw and economies collapse." ~ William Binney Ex Director, NSA

UNCULTING THE HUMAN SOUL

Commodification has destroyed community so all that is left is consumption.

The average American has been institutionalized, seduced, terrorized and so programmed from every front that they have forgotten their essential Spirit, their daemon or divine genius. (Daemon in ancient Greek belief is a divinity or supernatural being of a nature between gods and humans.)

The other day I showed a stressed woman how to turn on her parasympathetic and tone down her sympathetic by doing "The Three Kings" — (Tongue drop, Inner Smile and Gentle Throaty Breath.) She asked where I learned that from and I said I discovered it myself as I have built an extensive spiritual practice called "The Inner Arts." She was aghast and disbelieving that a "commoner" was also a "genius." Her programming in the Cult of America resigned her worldview to be a consumer of ideas and things, not a CREATOR of ideas and things.

If the world could work-with the masses in such a way that they could free themselves from the dominant meme of the "follower" of all-consuming empire, to discover their inner geni, we may help them break free from the prison of unquestioned material fascism and global conquest. The institutionalized and corporate mind is a sad half dead thing. The disempowered glom onto facets of power from the external world whether that figment be traditions, gurus, university degrees, clubs, commercial brands, political parties, or compliance to world hegemony. *Followers are the grease in the wheels of world tyranny.*

Within a context of cultural collapse the value of our contribution seems to whittle away to nothing, and it becomes harder to keep up our Dharma within an increasingly stressed and hostile environment. Dharma means cosmic law and order, achieved via inner peace through the still point within, when we surrender to Universal Will. If we first establish peace within our minds by training in spiritual paths, outer peace will come naturally. As we grow towards the light and the darkness becomes mere food for our blazing brilliance. To support an evolving future freedom and the growing impact of individual sovereignty is fundamental. Make a wish, dare to dream and have an action plan. We need to support each other in becoming **creactivists** in the manifestation of the world we want to live in.

Socio-political contraction or regression of consciousness is used by the psychopathic controllers to maintain dominion over the victim tax-payers – thus all Hindbrain (unenlightened) civilizations ultimately descend into some form of fascist holocaust (or harvest) as rising consciousness comes up against the controlling hegemonic forces. It is time for the average world citizen to become NOT so average anymore, and to dismiss being defined by the ambient derelict cult to uncover their wild, cosmic, arcadian soul. Our job for the rest of our lives is to shift the balance of power back towards the Good, the True and the Beautiful. We need to keep an eye on what THEY are doing, but to focus intently on manifesting the world we want to live in and the future our heart's desire. To come back alive and to be a force for planetary renewal, we must divest and divorce ourselves from all the proinflammatory aspects of Hindbrain culture that are stimulating a chronic stress response, destabilizing our nervous system and preventing our evolution to the sovereign HUman of Civilization Next.

Don't look at the bull, look at the gate as you are running towards it.

EXULTATION OF A WARRIOR OF LOVE

The skynet of 5g satellites, the metallizing of the atmosphere with chemtrails, the fried mutant skies, the anomalous microwave fire-wars against cities scheduled for "redevelopment," the collapse of environmental protection law—it is apparent that humanity is on a track of global genocide. The techno-kraken is out of control, or should I say "in control." They vote themselves into power and conspire worldwide to rid the planet of the majority of people so they can expand their regime and appropriate whatever land and resources they covet for themselves.

Law itself has been stolen by the lawless for their own ends, and the Babylonian money magic cabal have designed the game so that the people's taxes are funding their own demise. The trajectory of this dark game is not good, for the techno-kraken is gaining total dominance via its capacity to kill (anything and everything) without remorse or a second thought. However there are 7 billion of us against a small minority of psychopaths. If we commit to waking up and using our superhuman powers to counter their march of death we can develop the technology, systems, cultural design and global networks necessary for Civilization Next.

Self love is an inside job! If we abandon ourselves others will abandon us, and if we hate on ourselves others will hate us. If we don't love ourselves, nobody will. By raising our self-love we become a Warrior of Love who takes the high road to positively impact the world. To be a Warrior of Love means to, first of all, believe that ONLY LOVE IS REAL. Through deepening our self-love all wrongs can be made right, and we can grow up to overcome our fear-based beliefs and assumptions that undermine our journey and leave us vulnerable to the global cull and collapse of the environment.

To be a Warrior of Love means to be overwhelmed with the beauty of love and to stand up for what we believe. To be a Warrior of Love means to cultivate our jour de vive and mana so that we are forever in love with the world. The darkside doesn't stand a chance against the global movement of Love Warriors who live to love. We can systematically and mystically set about on a journey to raise our love quotient. It is up to the sovereign to be responsible for liberating themselves from their own cage. How our hurt rubs up against others shows us the work we need to do on ourselves to open more fully to love and the divine.

When we get to the point of conscious appreciation for that which we are triggered by, we are well on the road to genuine healing and freedom, rather than being trapped, repressed and suspended by the constant retriggering of debilitating pain. That which infringes on our sovereignty causes us pain—surmounting that pain is how we grow towards sovereignty. Only through learning, growing and transcending can we embrace the evolutionary edge. Sovereignty is the expression of our ability to respond skillfully to our environment using the facets of learning. Embracing the evolutionary edge is the only real healing there is, for we are not whole without being alive to change. We each need to become a higher breed of enlightened, philosophical leader who is genuinely visionary, shamanic and transpersonal.

"We, all of us, are rapidly running out of time. If the biosphere is not soon freed from the ongoing global climate engineering assault, there will very soon be nothing left to salvage of our once thriving planet." Dane Wigington

15

MORE INFORMATION

ON THE PROBLEM

An unholy addiction to false power is the force behind the debacle of the geoengineering program. It is symptomatic of the compartmentalized, fractionated, limited and machiavellian thinking that constitutes the drive for power over Nature, the Earth and its people.

WEATHER AS A FORCE MULTIPLIER: Owning the Weather in 2025: A research paper produced for the United States Air Force written in 1996 speculates about the future use of nano-technology to produce "artificial weather,"clouds of microscopic computer particles all communicating with each other to form an intelligent fog that could be used for various purposes. http://csat.au.af.mil/2025/volume3/vol3ch15.pdf

GEOENGINEERING TEACHERS: To follow the global empire's full spectrum dominance campaign see Chemtrail experts including: Deborah Tavares, Peter A. Kirby, Jim Lee, Dane Wigington, Michael Murphy, Patrick Roddie, Elana Freeland, Mike Morales, Cliff Carnicom, Ben Davidson, Sofia Smallstorm, Rosalind Peterson, Scott Stevens, Malcolm Scott, Dr. Nick Begich, Curtis Bennett, Leuren Moret, Dr. Paul LaViolette, Dr. Judy Wood, Robert M Deutsch, Retired USDA Biologist Francis Mangels, Kristen Meghan, Ted Gunderson. John Whyte of the "Consciousness Beyond Chemtrails Conference."

Peter Kirby — Geoengineering History and the perpetrators of climate crime. *CHEMTRAILS EXPOSED, A New Manhattan Project by* Peter A. Kirby.

https://weathermodificationhistory.com/

http://exopolitics.blogs.com/peaceinspace/2017/12/planetsizedlaboratory.html

Dr Harry Wexler, *Chief of the Scientific Services Division of the U.S. Weather Bureau,* revealed his concerns about geoengineering and ozone destruction in the 1962 paper *"On the Possibilities of Climate Control. "* Geoengineering methods he mentioned included increasing world temperature by several degrees by detonating up to ten H-bombs in the Arctic Ocean; lowering global temperature by launching powder to shade the equatorial orbit; warming the lower atmosphere and cooling the stratosphere by artificial injections of water vapor or other substances; and notably, destroying all stratospheric ozone above the Arctic circle or near the equator using a relatively small amount of a catalytic agent such as chlorine or bromine.

StopTheCrime.net — **Deborah Tavares** says that 5G is a eugenics sterilization program. 5G is mainly for sterilization to reduce population, and crowd suppression by frying mental functioning. 5G inflammation will speed the trajectory of all diseases, and exacerbate the Metabolic X basis of the Fall of Man.

FK21 DANISH POLITICAL PARTY, Mads Palsvig: See Very Important Youtube - "Banksters vs. Slaves & 5G Depopulation Agenda."

 https://chemtrailsplanet.net/ eg: Cooking of Humanity - amazing interview with **Barry Trower**.

https://www.YouTube.com/watch?v=qp51PiMrEq0 **Leuren Moret**, Google controlling your DNA?

www.stayonthetruth.com/what-do-we-tell-the-people-prof-curtis-bennett.php

Adjunct Professor **Curtis Bennett** - Stay On The Truth: WBN episode no. 4. This is an EXCEPTIONAL talk on wireless exposure, smart meter, 5G dangers etc... microwave cooking of all life, and electro-deterioration of building structures etc.... 5G Millimeter wave spectrum is generally considered the band of spectrum between 6 GHz and 100 GHz. Curtis Bennett says the combination of metal aerosols and microwaves will produce dys-consciousness, madness, sterilization, mutation and the breakdown of society. It will also change the physics of the environment to produce unprecedented anomalous wildfires.

Joe Imbriano says that the 5G uses the oxygen molecule signature, and that 5G will be used to create new bizarre diseases to subdue and cull the population. Listen to his interview with Jeff Rense.

1984: The New World Order—This is an excellent documentary with the heavy hitters David Icke and Michael Tsarion and others which gives the big picture of the leviathan of social control.

The USA is no longer America, it is USRAEL. No wonder the US government appears to be attacking its own citizens without mercy with geoengineering, weather warfare and the 5G genocide, and sending its troops into endless illegal wars in the Middle East for the Greater Israel Project. The U.S. Senators and U.S. Government Representatives that are Israel Dual Citizens are so numerous as to constitute a coup and take over by a foreign power. 89% of US Senators and Congress hold dual citizenship with Israel. This is also why Israel gets the most aid, and why they have the biggest lobbying groups. The Hades warmongers run the show, and they are all mentally ill.

To learn about the methods of the worldwide holocaust read Naomi Wolf's The End of America: A Letter of Warning to a Young Patriot, fascism in 10 easy steps; and watch the youtube: Culling The World's Humans.
The Anatomy of Slave Speak by Frederick Mann
The Emotional Plaque, Charles Konia, M.D.
The Mass Psychology of Fascism, by Wilhelm Reich

The Matrix Revealed; Exit From The Matrix; and Power Outside The Matrix, *by Jon Rappoport.*

A great Geoengineering Documentary to get family and friends to watch: **OVERCAST: Climate Engineering** (Chemtrail). http://overcastthemovie.com

"Manmade cloud cover from flight traffic has a bigger impact on global warning than all the CO2 emitted since the beginning of aviation." ~ German Aerospace Center, Contrails are Real Climate Killers.

ON THE SOLUTION

www.sehn.org/ppfaqs.html — **THE PRECAUTIONARY PRINCIPLE**: When an activity raises threats of harm to the environment or human health, precautionary measures should be taken even if some cause and effect relationships are not fully established scientifically.

Precautionary principle is a translation of the German Vorsorgeprinzip. Vorsorge means, literally, "Forecaring." It carries the sense of comprehensiveness, integrity, foresight and preparation not merely caution.

The principle applies to human health and the environment. The ethical assumption behind the precautionary principle is that humans are responsible to protect, preserve, and restore the global ecosystems on which all life, including our own, depends.

http://www.permaculture-media-download.com/2011/11/best-permacul-ture-homesteading-books.html

David Holmgren's "Permaculture: Principles and Pathways Beyond Sustainability".

Rollin McCraty: He's part of the Institute of HeartMath and the Global Coherence Initiative.

Left in the Dark Revised by **Tony Wright** - Metabolic origins of the Fall.

Return to the Brain of Eden: Restoring the Connection between Neurochemistry and Consciousness by Tony Wright

NATURE CONNECTION: Check out **Jon Young**'s YouTube videos. He lays the foundations for forward movement by learning/remembering from the indigenous cultures. His information is vitally important to the building of future society culture — especially the download from the Kalahari Bushmen. The are supposedly the original DNA of Homo sapiens who still embody HUman capacities of consciousness which the rest of us have lost thousands of years ago. In this sense they are our Grandparents or superiors. No other culture/genetic line can exhibit the degree of ESP and sense of Nature Connection that the Bushmen are born into. A people who live beyond Chronos TIME and MONEY, are superior in Eternal Principles. Those who live by Kairos time are superior to the war addicted master/slave culture in every way that matters in the scales of Truth and Justice. Strangely the most uncivilized ARE the most civilized. It would require in-presence-resonance to pick up what they have.

INTEGRAL SOCIETY: Herman Hesse's Nobel Prize Winning Novel, "*The Glass Bead Game*" lays the foundations for an Artistic/Conceptual Game, which integrates all fields of Human and Cosmic Knowledge through forms of Organic Universal Symbolism, expressed by its players with the Dynamic Fluidity of Music. The Glass Bead Game is, in Reality, an Age Old metaphor for what has been called, the "Divine Lila" (Play or Game of Life). This metaphor has been expressed by every great Wisdom Tradition known to man, and its players, the Magister Ludi (Masters of the Game), use as their instruments Ancient and Modern modes of Symbolic Wisdom traditionally presented through Sacred Art, Philosophy, Magick and Cosmology. http://www.glassbeadgame.com/

"The game as I conceive it," Knecht once wrote, "leaves (the player) with the feeling that he has extracted from the universe of accident and confusion a totally symmetrical and harmonious cosmos, and absorbed it into himself."
~ Hermann Hesse, The Glass Bead Game

www.psychotronics.org/ — **U.S. PSYCHOTRONICS: Bridging Science, Spirit, Mind and Technology.** The United States Psychotronics Association (USPA). We carry on the research of Royal R. Rife, Wilhem Reich, Nikola Tesla, Marcel Vogel, Georges Lakhovsy, Albert Abrams, Ruth Drown, Jacques Benveniste, T. Galen Hieronymous, and other pioneers in the psychotronics field.

Beating Cancer with Nutrition (Fourth Edition, 2005) Rev, Patrick Quillin

MEDICAL ATTENTION: The American medical world is very exploitative and not to be trusted. Someone told me that Bumrungrad International Hospital | Bangkok Thailand is like a luxury hotel and patients are treated with the utmost respect, and it is 1/8th of the price of healthcare in the USA. https://www.bumrungrad.com/

CIVILIZATION NEXT LIVING LEGIONS:

Julian Rose, Geoff Lawton, George Monbiot, Jordan Greenhall, Daniel Schmachtenberger,

To move on to create a new vision of humanitarian society read Guardian columnist **George Monbiot**'s books and listen to him on YouTube on topics of rewilding and moving beyond neoliberalism. His new book is "Out of the Wreckage: A New Politics for an Age of Crisis, 2017

CHARTER OF BRUSSELS: END ECOCIDE ON EARTH
http://eradicatingecocide.com/the-law/factsheet/

END ECOCIDE ON EARTH have prepared 17 draft amendments to the Statute of the International Criminal Court (ICC) to add to the list of the most serious international crimes: genocide, crimes against humanity, the crime of aggression and war crimes, the crime of ecocide. www.endecocide.org/

PLANETARY MOVEMENT FOR MOTHER EARTH: *"There cannot be a greater crime: to destroy Mother Earth through the military-industrial complex's planetary system of war that is currently under construction; to commit the ultimate matricide!"* Dr. Claudia Von Werlhof, Planetary Movement for Mother Earth.

In the **Symposium on Science and Spirituality** in Germany in 2013, Claudia Von Werlhof pointed out that the officially propagated thesis of CO_2 as the reason behind the growing climate chaos in the world is not true. This cover story is instead hiding the consequences of 70 years of development of a new military geo/climate warfare, applied internationally. www.pbme-online.org/

UN OFFICE ON GENOCIDE PREVENTION AND THE RESPONSIBILITY
www.un.org/en/genocideprevention/genocide.html
www.genocidescholars.org —International Association of Genocide Scholars

THEY must be sued by class action and in international environmental courts. According to Article 2 of the **1948 United Nations Convention on the Prevention**

and Punishment of the Crime of Genocide defines genocide as "any of the following acts committed with intent to destroy, in whole or in part, a national, ethnic, racial or religious group, as such: killing members of the group; causing serious bodily or mental harm to members of the group; deliberately inflicting on the group conditions of life, calculated to bring about its physical destruction in whole or in part; imposing measures intended to prevent births within the group; [and] forcibly transferring children of the group to another group."
www.law.cornell.edu/wex/genocide

NEW CIVILIZATION

www.integralvisioning.org/ —Visionary Integral
http://via-visioninaction.org/—Yasuhiko Genku Kimura
http://bioneers.org/ —Visionary, practical earth restoration
http://gen.ecovillage.org/ — Global Eco Village Network
www.newciv.org/ — The New Civilization Network
www.permacultureinternational.org/ —Bill Mollison, Permaculture
www.permaculture.org.au/index.php —Geoff Lawton
www.holmgren.com.au/ —David Holmgren Permaculture Founder
http://bfi.org/ —Buckminster Fuller Institute
www.chelseagreen.com —Sustainable Living Publisher
www.acresusa.com —Eco Agriculture
www.pfaf.org/index.html —Plants For A Future
www.tradewindsfruit.com/ —Seeds of exotic plants to grow
www.eco-logicbooks.com/index.cfm?fa=home —Books for sustainability
www.wwoof.co.nz/ —Weekend Work On Organic Farms
www.howtosavetheworld.co.nz/ —Biodynamic revolution in India
www.globalresonance.net/ —The Global Resonance Network

PLANET X -NEMESIS DARK STAR

The sun appears to being cannibalized by a visiting dark star system, **Our Binary Twin** and is also being fed a lot more asteroid and comet material than usual. The Grand Solar Minimum may be a phenomena related to this cannibalization causing massive coronal holes and messing up the normal circulation and conveyance patterns in the corona. The catastrophic symptoms we are seeing around the planet are a sign of the visitation of our bianary twin star. The red (iron) rain in Russia in Jul 5, 2018 is a sure sign of the Nemesis brown dwarf star system is in our vicinity. Seventy per cent of all stars in our Galaxy are red dwarfs. Most stars are born as binary twins. Nemesis is a hypothetical red dwarf or brown dwarf, originally postulated by Richard Muller in 1984. This hypothesis proposes that the Sun may have an undetected companion star in a highly elliptical orbit that periodically disturbs our solar system at intervals leading to mass extinctions.

1/19/17: I was dreaming profusely last night. I was cleaning and ordering hotel laundry closets when it wasn't my job to do so, then I went outside and there were these cute baby skunks that didn't particularly look like skunks, but they were really friendly so I picked one up. Someone warned me they were skunks and very dangerous so I let the little beastie go, but it didn't spray me. Then after I let the skunk go I looked up and saw Nemesis, the dark star, in the sky. It was about 20 times the size of the moon, a faded red-pink with lighter cream colored markings on it. I think the dream was suggesting to drop all lesser fears (skunks), for there is something far greater to fear — something of great beauty, "Nemesis," and I was not afraid.

That woke up my consciousness level and a word popped into my head that was the antithesis to "end-times" superstition, but in the morning I had forgotten what that word was. It started with "A" so perhaps it was ATTENTION. Could be attention, awakened, accountability, adequacy, ascension — all "doing" words. It was a strange occurrence to have a word forcibly present itself, only to have forgotten it on waking. In the morning I went for a walk and subsequently remembered what the "A" word was. It was "**Acceptance**."

This was quite the shock to me when it forced its way onto my mindfield, and my brain wanted to rejected it. But I knew it was the answer to existential superstition. Existential superstition is the angst that comes from never good enough, not quite right, bad, not condoned, not up to snuff etc. If we are coming from a 'cup half empty" sense of deprivation and deficiency, then everything we see, hear or do is flavored with a sense of insufficiency. Only by viscerally stopping and embracing the skunk without fear, and observing the nemesi with wonder instead of fear, can we let go of our paranoic, superstitious reaction to the world.

Acceptance as the answer to existential superstition is unacceptable to the orphaned soul who wants to make a more linear active approach to fulfilling deprivation needs, and yet the more yin, relaxed and step-back solution of "acceptance" is the only thing that will preserve energy and consciousness for one's own evolution. The child of the patriarchy — the presovereign, orphaned self wants to reject "Acceptance" as being too passive a response to intolerable danger or deprivation. And yet acceptance, in that it preserves energy, consciousness and presence for "higher transcendent" action and effective direction, is after all the most proactive stance.

The Luciferian NWO may be out to get us, but if we "accept" that deeply in our bones, then our immune system and neuroendocrine system can fully engage in healing even as danger looms overhead. The effort to order other people's lives is symbolic of the need for affirmation (a poor substitute for acceptance) and worthiness. Existential superstition undermines our sense of self-value, rigidifies our identity to that which panders to others and is many times removed from the deeply lived life of the sovereign.

"Acceptance" is a method of finding peace within astronomical circumstances beyond our control. Acceptance may be the first door into finding the inner peace (stillness) to arrive at right action, but then we have to ACT — or why the heck are we here? Certainly not to serve as food for the death machine. The non-superstitious existence is the self-contained life, a being sufficient unto itself, and answerable to no man, beast or specter, but guided by themselves and their singular connection to the cosmos. *"Nature" is the ultimate Guru.*

SURVIVING THE PLANET X TRIBULATION: A Faith-Based Leadership Guide, by Marshall Masters.

"Preparedness begins with a sharp focus on the ability of survivors to communicate with like-minded others without the constraints of suppression." Marshall Masters, http://yowusa.com/

See the National Geographic Documentary, **Nemesis: The Sun's Evil Twin.**

OTHER PLANET X AND SKY PHENOMENA EXPERTS ARE:

Terral Croft on the BlackStar; Gill Broussard and his the Planet X (7X) hypothesis; Steve Olsen-WSO; Dave Dobbs and SuspectSky. Terral's videos are great for the geometry of the electromagnetics of earth's proximity to the Dark Star, explains earthquake, volcano up-tick, magma movement effects.

PREPAREDNESS: To prepare for the Great Tribulation - if it occurs, the ultimate preparedness book is "When Disaster Strikes, A Comprehensive Guide for Emergency Planning and Crisis Survival," by Matthew Stein.

ESCAPE OPTIONS:
We all need multiple options for the upcoming upheavals. These links provide some inspiring ideas

www.escapeartist.com/

https://www.sovereignman.com/

https://theexpatfiles.podbean.com/

THRIVAL ASSURANCE

Rather than survival insurance we might start preparing for thrival assurance. Adapt 2030 and the Oppenheimer Ranch Project YouTube channels provide information on the upcoming Grand Solar Minimum, which we are now in.

COMMODIFIABLE SURVIVAL ITEMS: Silver and gold coins, seeds, dry goods, survival gear, batteries, generators and fuel, tools; passive-nature-technology such as ceramic water filters, solar distillers, solar dehydrators, solar lighting, passive solar water heating units; log cabin/hempcrete and earthship building skills; medical supplies, Pioneer skills and How To books, wool clothing for Grand Solar Minimum, Non-radiated Kelp, clean compost, hydroponic units; water cars and new energy devices.

THRIVAL COMMUNITY: Building community either virtual or real is the most important imperative to thrival in the coming era. Establishing an alternative economic and exchange system prior to collapse is ideal. Lessons could be learned from Michael Tellinger (The Ubuntu Movement), Charles Eisenstein (The Gift Economy), and The Damanhur and Gaviotas communities.

The Millennium Quest —A **Damanhurian** book.

Utopian Dreams, **Tobias Jones** —Book on some of the world's ecovillages

David Holmgren, *PERMACULTURE: Principles and Pathways Beyond Sustainability*

Frederic Laloux, Reinventing Organizations

Larken Rose youtubes for envisioning a post-governmental world.

James Scott, The Art of Not Being Governed

https://nexusmagazine.com/— Alternative news and information magazine.

CHARLES EISENSTEIN: One of the most forward thinking! *The Ascent of Humanity*, describing the history and future of civilization, the gathering collapse. www.ascentofhumanity.com

http://thrivemovement.com —**THRIVE** Network community and change templates. Foster and Kimberly Gamble.

GLOBAL COHERENCE INITIATIVE—The Solari Report gives you **Catherine Austin Fitts** unique perspective on what's really happening with world issues affecting your assets and your life.

www.rushkoff.com — **Douglas Rushkoff** - Technology, Media, and Popular Culture

www.tpuc.org/node/535 — *"The principal reason why money has not thus far been eradicated and replaced by pure cooperation is due to the blinkered collective mind of the masses, their lack of imagination, incapacity to comprehend, myopia, and obstinate misguided beliefs."* Dan Hughes

https://resonance.is/— Resonance Science Foundation, Nassim Haramein

www.electricuniverse.info/ and https://electroverse.net/ Wallace Thornhill and David Talbott. Electric Universe Theory

www.bfi.org/ —"You either Make Money or Make Sense, they're mutually exclusive." So said the great Richard Buckminster **"Bucky" Fuller**

www.zeitgeistmovie.com —**Peter Joseph**. The second film, *Zeitgeist: Addendum*, attempts to locate the root causes pervasive social corruption, and offers a solution based understanding of what we actually are and how we can align with nature, of which we are a part. www.blogtalkradio.com/peter-joseph

www.thevenusproject.com/ —**Jacque Fresco** of the **Venus Project** envisions a future of a resource-based economy rather than an outmoded monetary-based economy. In Venus Florida

www.ascentofhumanity.com/ — **C**harles Eisenstein advocates the change to a gift economy. "Again, I do not advocate the abdication of our human gifts of hand and mind. Only the motivation, and therefore the direction and application, of technology will change."

www.foet.org/ —**Jeremy Rifkin**, The Distributed Energy Economy. See on YouTube: *RSA Animate - The Empathic Civilization*

www.vironika.org —The book, *The Love Mindset: An Unconventional Guide to Healing and Happiness* by Vironika Tugaleva is a good place to start.

HELIOSPHERE MAGNETOTAIL EXPLOSIONS

On 12/14/18 a US presidential panel made a public announcement that there was an the eminent threat to the power grid due to an EMP from a solar eruption or terrorist attack. The public were warned to prepare for the grid going down for up to 6 months. On the evening of 12/27/18 there was a massive explosion that lit up the sky bright blue over NYNY and a consequent power outage. A so called Minor G1-class geomagnetic storm from a large **coronal hole** produced auroras in the northern latitudes in response to the solar wind. Next month that same coronal hole was earth facing again when there was another light-explosion/power outage event on the early morning of 1/20/19 in Crossville, Tennessee. Watching videos of these events I realized the earth is experiencing Matter:Antimatter explosions in our heliosphere magnetotail due to cosmic rays from the massive coronal holes associated with Grand Solar Minimum.

Metallizing the atmosphere with nanometals (as in chemtrail Stratospheric Aerosol Geoengineering) is a surefire way to convey more solar energy back down to earth during a Matter:Antimatter heliotail explosion or a CME equal to the force of a billion megaton nuclear bombs. In an electric universe increasing the conductivity of the atmosphere leaves civilization vulnerable to mega-disasters and destructive environmental impacts. This fact will be the Achilles' heel to the Hindbrain global fascist cabal which has been undertaking geoengineering to ionize the atmosphere in order to increase EMF conductivity for surveillance, military and weather manipulation.

There is even the possibility of the collapse civilization by increasing the conductivity of the atmosphere in the advent of solar flares, coronal hole wind-stream magnetogasms, supernovas, solar novas and lightning from asteroid and comet (NEO) flybys. Even the lightning effects from storms are amplified via metal aerosols, and ionization by radar and HAARP technology. Besides leading catastrophic ozone depletion, large Solar flares, Grand Solar Minimum coronal hole wind streams, Solar Nova, nearby supernovae and galactic gamma-ray bursts are all candidates for a EMP explosion that could wipe out half the earth's electrical grid causing the death of billions via famine, cold or civil unrest.

Heliosphere magnetotail explosions travel back along the field lines and BLAST the polar vortex down towards the equator, creating dangerously cold conditions, at the same time as a potential power outage. We must be aware that an EMP event caused by the sun can occur at night from these Matter:Antimatter spacegasms, and we can anticipate them by watching the coronal holes on spaceweather.com in combination with the heliosphere patterns on SWMF-RCM. *See*: https://iswa.gsfc.nasa.gov/IswaSystemWebApp/

They chop the antimated SWMF map for up to 30 minutes when there is a heliotail plasma explosion that lights the night sky and causes power outages on earth, thus the government is hiding the fact that massive space weather connected to solar minimum is affecting the grid. Smart meters on gas and electric systems make the contemporary electrical utilities extremely dangerous under solar coronal hole/heliotail plasma explosion conditions. The government is culpable for this energy grid vulnerability, both in allowing smart meters and not telling the public about the danger of heliotail plasma explosions so people can opt out of smart meters, and install protective electrical and backup systems.

Full article on the heliosphere magnetotail explosions at:
www.academia.edu/38222458/HELIOTAIL_PLASMA_EXPLOSIONS.pdf

The animated maps to follow are the **SWMF 2011+ RCM Magnetosphere - BATSRUS - Y-CUT Magnetic Field Lines**. Pin this and the **SWMF 2011+ RCM Magnetopause Position** in your Bookmark. When there is a night time magnetosphere sky explosion and grid failure get the correct UT time stamp and go save the video from the SWMF — and you may save the explosion prior to them cutting it out. Twitter and Instagram are useful to get the correct time.

***For more on creating Civilization Next see Book 2 in the Chemtrail Meta-adaptation Series: *"Awakening in the Chemtrail Holocaust: Liberation from Within."* This part 2 in the series covers psycho-spiritual and cultural meta-adaptive methods, and information on the electromagnetic effects to the biosphere from aerosol/microwave geoengineering. Book 2 gives environmental remediation methods, and gardening in the chemtrail holocaust and much more.

Love!
No Fear
We will be victorious
For we are legion and we are glorious!

www.ingramcontent.com/pod-product-compliance
Lightning Source LLC
Chambersburg PA
CBHW070841300326
41935CB00039B/1335